CONTENTS

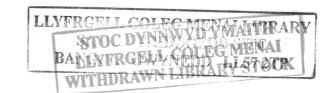

D1332447

ACKNOWLEDGEMENTS

City & Guilds would like to thank the following:

For their invaluable hairdressing expertise

Shelley Dalton

Eugene Davis

Sam Grice

Denise Johnson

Maurice Lister

Diane Mitchell

For the cover photoshoot

Photographer – Squiz Hamilton

Creative Hair Artist – Eugene Davis

Stylist – Deborah La Touche

Makeup Artist – Sian Duke

Models – Dennis Okwere AMCK Models and Ruby Payge Johns – Agency Model

Studio – FTWS 'the WORK space'

Thank you also to Selina Davis, Shelley Dalton, Diane Mitchell and Hannah Cooper.

For their help with the photoshoots

Thanks to creative hair artists Eugene Davis, Hector Obeng and Shelley Dalton, photographer Andrew Buckle, makeup artists Laura Hunt and Jessy Berry, models Katty Jennah and Karla Jones, and Selina Davis/FTWS 'the WORK space'.

Thanks also to Maurice Lister; Adam Sloan and the Men's Hairdressing Federation; Billy Moore at Central Training Group; Melissa Birch, India Flaherty, Sarah Hawtin, Melanie Mitchell and Alison Pick at Cheynes Training; Chris Connors at Coco's; Maria Howard and Kate Meek at Enfield Training Services; Lorraine Pamenter, Donna McClelland, Liz Dickinson, Avril Hall, Sandra Griffin and Danielle Skeats at Epping Forest College; Pav Sagoo and Tracey O'Connor at Havering College; Jo Newland, Tracey Shakeshaft and Terri-Ann Neighbour at Hertford Regional College; Mandy Cresswell, Chanel Turner Rowley, Leslie Smith and Tracey Hesson at Walsall College.

PICTURE CREDITS

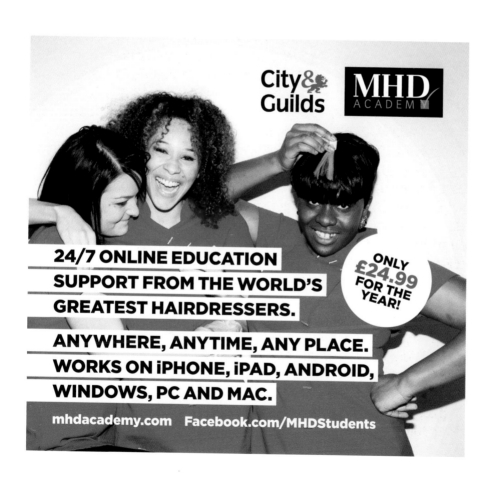

ABOUT THE AUTHOR

My mum is a hairdresser and I grew up wanting to be a hairdresser too. I started working in a salon the day after I left school, over 20 years ago, and completed the youth training scheme (YTS). I then travelled to London, struggling on £65 a week and paying £48 for fares – but when you want something badly enough, you are prepared to work hard for it and I now have a career to be proud of.

I started teaching and assessing 18 years ago, where my love of hairdressing and training has gone from strength to strength. I have taught both full-time and part-time students, NVQ Levels 1, 2 and 3 and VRQ Levels 1, 2 and 3. In my current role as a Senior Manager and Group Head of Curriculum, I train new assessors, manage the hairdressing training team, carry out teaching observations and develop the curriculum across all the centres at Central Training Group.

Sharing my skills and knowledge with new learners throughout my teaching career has been a highlight. Watching someone master the art of hairdressing or achieve summative assessments is what training is all about, and I love it.

Keryl Titmus

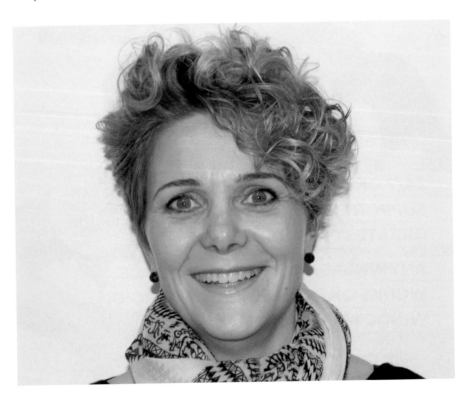

ABOUT THE CONTRIBUTOR

With 30 years' experience in the hairdressing industry, Shelley Dalton has a reputation as a technical and business expert. With outstanding knowledge in all aspects of hairdressing and the hairdressing industry, Shelley's experiences range from creative and technical salon work, salon ownership, technical consultancy, product development, business development, account executive, project management, recruitment consultancy, mentoring and business consultancy and she is also a qualified assessor. In 2014 Shelley fulfilled one of her dreams and along with her friends launched The Curl Care Project – this project helps carers, social workers, foster parents and anyone within the care system to understand the needs of people with excessively curly hair - her list of talents are not only endless but all proven.

Investment in ongoing development and understanding of all hair types is what sets Shelley Dalton apart from other education providers. Shelley has worked with and educated some of the world's leading hairdressers. Her education delivery is insightful, innovative and profound.

Shelley Dalton, author of chapter AH2

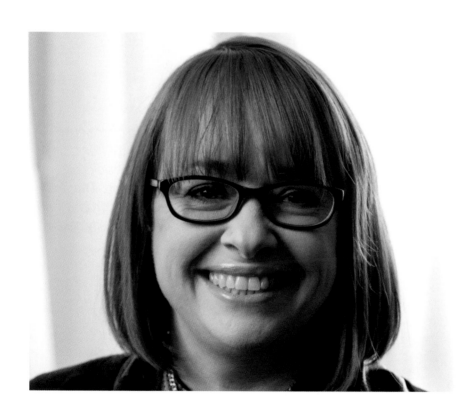

FOREWORD

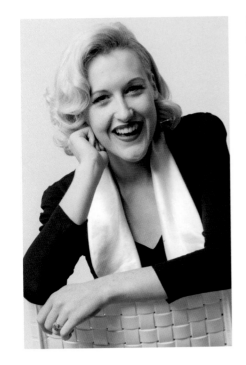

I think the greatest thing about hairdressing is it can be whatever you want it to be. Even though, when you first start out, you may think there is only one career path, once you get going suddenly you start to see all the possibilities around you. I have friends that use hairdressing as the perfect job while raising a family, and I've got friends that work in spectacular day spas in Barbados. I've got friends that own their own salons, friends that teach in academies, friends that work on cruise ships and friends in fashion. My own career path meant that I spent a long time doing competition work to build a name for myself and now I work in Central London and do hair shows all over the world!

Now lets get one thing straight: your Level 2 diploma is a starting point. It's your initial introduction to all aspects of hairdressing - and it's fantastic. But after you have qualified, it is up to you take yourself to the next level and that means constant education. You need to be going on a hairdressing course every year. Whatever career path you want to take, you need to be the best you can be.

In hairdressing you will always work hard for your money, it's a physically and mentally tiring job. But believe me, if you work a little bit 'smarter not harder', by reinvesting in your education, you will become a great hairdresser and all that hard work will pay off tenfold.

Trust me.

Sophia Hilton

Sophia Hilton is an international educator, teaching in over seven countries worldwide. Now one of L'Oréal's most sought-after UK educators and the artistic co-ordinator of Brooks and Brooks Hairdressing, she is positively obsessed with hairdressing. The face of the Hairdressing Council, winner of the L'Oréal Colour Trophy and the British Hairdressing Awards, at the age of 27 she's really taken the UK by storm.

HOW TO USE THIS TEXTBOOK

You will find that your City & Guilds Level 2 Diploma in Hairdressing and Barbering textbook is laid out in a similar way to your City & Guilds Level 2 Diploma in Hairdressing and Level 2 Diploma in Barbering logbooks to aid your navigation and understanding of both. The chapters on values and behaviours and health and safety are the exception. Each unit in your logbooks makes reference to values and behaviours, and health and safety. This textbook has two separate chapters dedicated to these areas, so you can refer to the chapters directly for in-depth information.

The units in your logbooks and in this textbook are divided into hairdressing units, barbering units and combined hairdressing and barbering units.

The 'CH' in the unit number means 'classification of hair' types; this covers hair classifications from straight to very curly hair. Units that start with 'CH' are hairdressing units, units that start with 'CB' are barbering units and those starting with 'CHB' are combined hairdressing and barbering units. For example, CHB11 is combined hairdressing and barbering – this is the 'Shampooing, condition and treat the hair and scalp' unit, and CH4 is hairdressing – this is the 'Colour and lighten hair' unit and CB2 is barbering – this is 'Cut men's hair using basic techniques'.

Each chapter in your textbook covers everything you will need to understand in order to complete your written or online tests and practical assessments. Each chapter starts first the theory and then covers the practical skills for the hairdressing skill described. The assessments in CHB and CH units can be carried out on male or female clients, but for the CB units, all assessments must be carried out on male clients.

Throughout this textbook you will see the following features:

HANDY HINTS are particularly useful tips that can assist you in your revision or help you remember something important.

> **HANDY HINT**
>
> You must ensure that you remove hair cuttings during and at the end of the service. Wet and dry hair can be slippery and cause accidents. Sweep up the hair and place it in the salon's designated hair bin.

KEY WORDS in bold in the text are explained in the margin to aid your understanding.

> **Protruding**
>
> Sticking out.

WHY DON'T YOU ... boxes suggest ideas to help you practise and learn.

> **WHY DON'T YOU ...**
> Ask a colleague to pretend to be your client. Ask them to visualise a style and then ask the relevant questions to identify the image and look they require.

ACTIVITIES help to test your understanding and learn from your colleagues' experiences.

> **Activity**
>
> Discuss with a colleague how you think a client would feel if you used combs, scissors or clippers with the previous client's hair still on them!

VALUES & BEHAVIOURS boxes link to the sections in the values and behaviours chapter for you to recap learning.

> **VALUES & BEHAVIOURS**
> Refer to the values and behaviours chapter for more information on maintaining effective, hygienic and safe working methods.

HEALTH & SAFETY boxes link to sections in the health and safety chapter for you to recap learning.

> **HEALTH & SAFETY**
> Refer to the health and safety chapter for more information on the health and safety Acts you need to follow when cutting hair.

The green IMPROVE YOUR MATHS badge identifies items that combine improving your understanding of hairdressing with practising or improving your maths skills.

The purple IMPROVE YOUR ENGLISH badge identifies items that combine improving your understanding of hairdressing with practising or improving your English skills.

At the end of each chapter are some 'Test your knowledge' questions. These are mostly multiple-choice questions, designed to prepare you for your written or online tests and to identify any areas where you might need further training or revision.

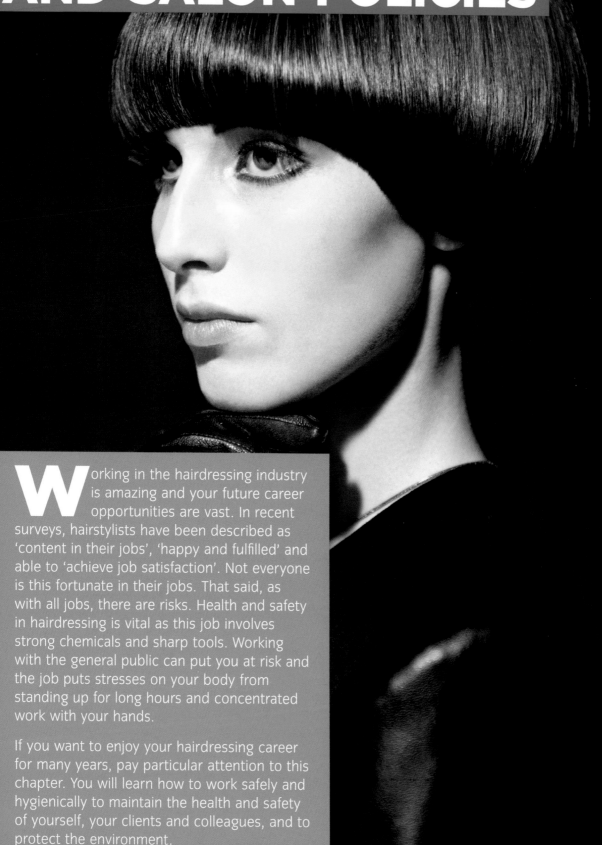

HEALTH AND SAFETY AND SALON POLICIES

Working in the hairdressing industry is amazing and your future career opportunities are vast. In recent surveys, hairstylists have been described as 'content in their jobs', 'happy and fulfilled' and able to 'achieve job satisfaction'. Not everyone is this fortunate in their jobs. That said, as with all jobs, there are risks. Health and safety in hairdressing is vital as this job involves strong chemicals and sharp tools. Working with the general public can put you at risk and the job puts stresses on your body from standing up for long hours and concentrated work with your hands.

If you want to enjoy your hairdressing career for many years, pay particular attention to this chapter. You will learn how to work safely and hygienically to maintain the health and safety of yourself, your clients and colleagues, and to protect the environment.

Health and safety

As with everything else in life, there are ways of doing things, right and wrong. So to ensure we do things correctly we have to follow some rules. In your salon, your employer makes the rules and these form your **salon policy**.

If the government passes a law (**Act**) and calls it, say, 'The Health and Safety at Work Act', we have to know what its rules are. These rules are called **regulations**. As you can imagine, there are lots of rules (regulations) to cover such a large subject as health and safety.

The health and safety legislation covering your job role consists of:

- The Health and Safety at Work Act (HASAWA)
- The Reporting of Injuries, Diseases and Dangerous Occurrences Regulations (RIDDOR)
- The Health and Safety (First Aid) Regulations
- The Regulatory Reform (Fire Safety) Order
- The Manual Handling Operations Regulations
- The Control of Substances Hazardous to Health (COSHH) Regulations
- The Electricity at Work Regulations
- The Environmental Protection Act
- The Management of Health and Safety at Work Regulations
- The Health and Safety (Information for Employees) Regulations.

The Health and Safety at Work Act (HASAWA)

The Health and Safety at Work Act covers the responsibilities that you and your employer have.

Your employer's responsibility is to staff, clients and visitors.

Your responsibility is to yourself, your colleagues and your clients.

The Health and Safety at Work Act is the overarching Act that covers all health and safety legislation.

This Act covers everyone – employees, employers, self-employed people and visitors including clients and representatives. This Act outlines everyone's responsibilities, including your own and is about your health and your safety in your place of work.

Your employer's responsibilities under the Health and Safety at Work Act are to:

Salon policy

Your salon's rules.

Act

A government law.

Regulations

The rules of the Act.

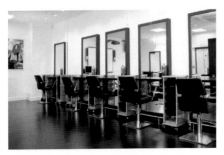

Clean and tidy workstations

HANDY HINT

Along with your salon policy and government laws you will also need to follow other rules or regulations. These are the instructions provided by the manufacturers of your equipment and products, and your local by-laws. Local by-laws are your local council regulations, rather than government regulations.

THE CITY & GUILDS TEXTBOOK

- maintain the workplace
- give staff appropriate training and supervision
- keep access and exit points clear and free from hazards at all times
- provide a suitable working environment and facilities that comply with the Act.

Your responsibilities under this Act are to:

- maintain the health and safety of yourself and others who may be affected by your actions
- co-operate and communicate with your employer about health and safety issues, so that your employer can keep within the law.

Who is the person responsible for reporting health and safety matters? YOU are!

If you see a health and safety problem, you must deal with it or report it. Everyone is responsible for putting it right.

Training staff to use electrical items

Activity

With a colleague, discuss some examples of health and safety matters that you would need to refer to someone else and identify who you would refer them to (for example, a leaking pipe in the salon.)

The Reporting of Injuries, Diseases and Dangerous Occurrences Regulations (RIDDOR)

The Reporting of Injuries, Diseases and Dangerous Occurrences Regulations include reporting the following to the HSE (Health and Safety Executive):

- a fracture, other than to fingers and toes
- amputation of digits or limbs (fingers/toes or arms/legs, etc)
- death to workers and non-workers if they arise from work-related accidents
- crush injuries that lead to internal organ damage
- unconsciousness caused by a head injury or asphyxia (crushing of the wind pipe)
- injuries that requires admittance to hospital for more than 24 hours or resuscitation.

The following diseases (made worse by work) are also reportable under RIDDOR:

- occupational dermatitis
- carpal tunnel syndrome
- occupational asthma.

All of the situations listed above need to be reported to the HSE – this can be done online. To confirm what needs to be reported, visit www.hse.gov.uk/riddor/do-i-need-to-report.htm.

Your employer's responsibility under these regulations is to:

- report and record any of the above occurrences.

Your responsibilities under these regulations are to:

- report any work-related diseases to the person responsible for health and safety
- prevent any work-related disease by wearing **personal protective equipment (PPE)** such as gloves, etc.
- report any accidents or injuries that you sustain
- prevent any accidents or injuries by maintaining a safe and tidy working environment.

All accidents must be written in the accident book with clear details recorded. The salon's accident book must be kept in a safe place and every member of staff must know where this is.

Ensure you record the date and time of the incident, the name and address of the person involved and of any witnesses. Record the treatment given or that none was required. This must be completed in case of any legal consequences from the injury.

Since personal details are recorded, these pages must be removed in order to follow the Data Protection Act and keep personal details confidential. Forward the page from the accident book to the person responsible for health and safety.

Activity

Research other occupational diseases that need to be reported.

Personal protective equipment (PPE)

Your personal protective equipment, not your client's!

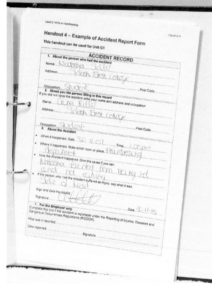

A page from an accident book

Activity

A 'walk-in' client asked for a full-head colour service which was carried out that day. The following problems occurred:

- A few days later you are signed off work with occupational dermatitis because you applied the client's colour without wearing gloves.
- The client suffered from an allergic reaction.

1 Which legal Acts have been not been adhered to?

2 What are the causes of these problems?

3 What are the potential consequences to you, the client and the salon?

4 What is the correct procedure that should have been followed?

The Health and Safety (First Aid) Regulations

These regulations were updated in 2013. They apply to all workplaces in the UK, including those with fewer than five employees and self-employed staff. Their aim is to protect everyone in the workplace by ensuring risk assessments are carried out to prevent accidents and injuries at work.

Your employer's responsibilities under these regulations are to:

- take immediate action if employees are injured or taken ill at work
- consider providing a first-aider
- nominate an appointed person to be responsible for the first aid arrangements
- provide a well-stocked first-aid container.

According to the HSE website http://www.hse.gov.uk/firstaid/changes-first-aid-regulations.htm, there is no mandatory list of items to be included in a first-aid container. It recommends (as a guide only):

- a leaflet giving general guidance on first aid (for example, HSE's leaflet *Basic Advice on First Aid at Work*)
- 20 individually wrapped sterile plasters (assorted sizes) appropriate to the type of work (hypoallergenic plasters can be provided if necessary)
- two sterile eye pads
- two individually wrapped triangular bandages, preferably sterile
- six safety pins

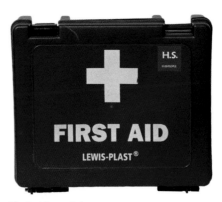

First-aid container

- two large sterile individually wrapped unmedicated wound dressings
- six medium-sized individually wrapped unmedicated wound dressings
- at least two pairs of disposable gloves.

The appointed person should check the contents of the first-aid container frequently and ensure it is restocked soon after use. They should ensure the safe disposal of items once they reach their expiry date.

Your responsibilities under these regulations are to:

- avoid taking any unnecessary risks that might put you or others in danger
- report any first-aid shortages to your appointed person.

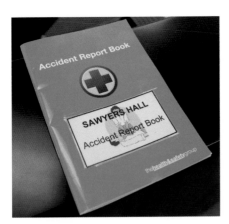

Accident book

The Regulatory Reform (Fire Safety) Order

The Regulatory Reform (Fire Safety) Order came into force in 2005 and was set in place to ensure that appropriate steps were taken to protect human life. The order consolidates previous fire safety legislation and aligns fire safety legislation and health and safety law.

Every building, structure or open space to which the public (such as clients and employees) have access is covered by the order. The order puts the onus onto a 'responsible person', the person accountable for the business or property; this could be the owner, occupier, employer or landlord.

The responsible person must ensure they:

- protect any persons on the premises or those who may be affected by a fire at the premises
- provide adequate safety measures to minimise risk
- carry out a risk assessment – checking the possible dangers and risks – consider who may be at risk, reduce the risks, make sure there is protection available (fire-fighting equipment), create an emergency plan (fire evacuation procedure), and keep the risk assessment up to date.

The Fire and Rescue Service is responsible for extinguishing fires, promoting and providing information and advice and carrying out audits and inspection visits to premises. Failure to comply with audit and inspection recommendations could result in:

- low risk – receiving an informal notification
- serious risk – receiving an enforcement notice, which could lead to prosecution, resulting in a fine or even imprisonment.

Your responsibilities are:

- to know where the fire-fighting equipment is located in the salon
- to know which extinguishers should be used on different types of fires
- to know your evacuation procedure and identify your meeting point.

Activity

Draw a simple plan of your salon. Label the fire extinguishers, exits and meeting point. Add the name of your salon's responsible person.

Fire-fighting equipment

The most widely used extinguishers in salons contain water or carbon dioxide (CO_2). Currently most extinguishers are red and can be identified by their coloured label. The types of extinguisher found in the hairdressing industry are listed in the table below, which explains where they should be located, how they should be used, how they work and the dangers of using them incorrectly.

Type of extinguisher	Identified by	Used for	Location	How to use	How it works	Dangers
Water extinguisher	Red label and a thin hose	Class A fires involving wood, paper, hair and textiles	Salon Staff areas Corridors	Point the jet at the base of the flames and move across the burning area until the flames are out.	Water has a great cooling effect on the fuel's surface; with the spray nozzle covering a wide surface area using the water pressure, it cools the fire down and extinguishes the flame and heat source.	Do not use on electrical fires as electrical shock may occur and the fire may spread.
Foam extinguisher	Cream label and a thin hose	Class B fires involving flammable liquids except cooking oils	Salon Staff areas Corridors	Aim the jet around the side edge of the fire – do not aim the jet directly into the liquid. Allow the foam to build up across the liquid.	As the extinguisher is mainly water-based with a foaming agent, the foam floats on top of the burning item and breaks the contact between the flames and the fuel's surface.	Do not use on electrical fires, as electrical shock may occur and the fire may spread.

Type of extinguisher	Identified by	Used for	Location	How to use	How it works	Dangers
CO$_2$ extinguisher	Black label and wide nozzle	Class C fires involving electrics and flammable gases	Salon Office area	Direct the nozzle at the base of the fire and move the nozzle over the flames.	CO$_2$ does not burn and it replaces the oxygen in the air. Fire needs oxygen to burn; CO$_2$ suffocates the fire by the removal of the oxygen.	Not good at cooling fires. The extinguisher horn gets very cold and can cause 'freeze' burns and blisters, so it must not be touched when in use.
Dry powder extinguisher	Blue label and a thin hose	Class C fires involving electrics and flammable liquids	Salon	Aim the jet at the base of the flames and sweep over the flames.	Dry powder helps to reduce the chemical reactions needed for the fire to continue.	Not good at penetrating into appliances, so electrical fires may re-ignite. Not very good at cooling fire down.
Fire blanket	Blanket	Class F fires involving cooking fats. Also to be used to wrap around people if their clothes are on fire	Staff kitchen area	Wrap the person on fire in the fire blanket or cover the item on fire.	Suffocating the flames by removal of oxygen whilst the person is wrapped or item is covered.	Needs to be left to cool, to prevent re-ignition when the person is unwrapped or item uncovered and exposed to oxygen.

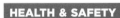

HEALTH & SAFETY

If water or foam extinguishers were used on an electrical fire, the fire could spread and electric shocks could occur.

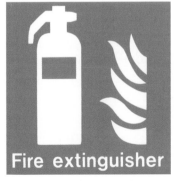

Fire extinguisher

An extinguisher sign indicates where to find an extinguisher

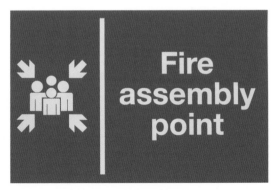

Fire assembly point

A fire assembly point sign indicates where people should assemble in case of fire

THE CITY & GUILDS TEXTBOOK

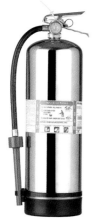

If the style and appearance of your salon is important, your employer may choose to purchase stainless steel or polished alloy extinguishers. The labels are colour-coded in the same way but the extinguishers are not red in colour like the majority of extinguishers.

Polished stainless steel fire extinguisher

The Manual Handling Operations Regulations

You are sometimes required to move equipment and stock around the salon. This is called manual handling. There are correct ways to lift to avoid injury.

According to the HSE more than a third of all injuries resulting in over three days' absence from work are caused by manual handling. Recent surveys have found that over 12.3 million working days are lost each year due to work-related **musculoskeletal disorders** that have been caused or made worse by poor manual handling.

Your employer's responsibility under these regulations is to:

■ carry out risk assessments on all employees for manual lifting.

Your responsibility under these regulations is to:

■ always ask yourself 'Can I lift this?' If the answer is no, then don't! Ask for help.

If you are able to lift it, remember to bend your knees and keep your back straight. Lift the weight with your knees not your back and keep the item you are lifting close to your body.

Musculoskeletal disorders

Muscle and bone disorders.

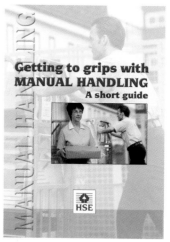

The HSE guide to manual handling

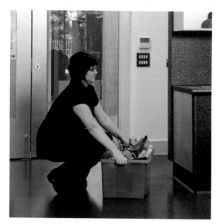

STEP 1 Check the area in front is clear and hazard-free. Bend your knees.

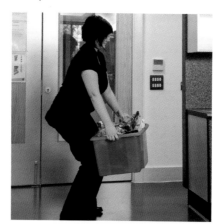

STEP 2 Keep your back straight.

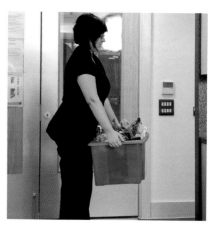

STEP 3 Lift the weight with your legs.

The Control of Substances Hazardous to Health (COSHH) Regulations

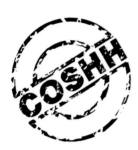

Chemicals and hazardous substances can enter the body through ingestion, absorption and inhalation so they present a high risk to salon staff. According to the HSE website, every year thousands of workers are made ill by hazardous substances; contracting lung diseases such as asthma or cancer, or skin diseases such as dermatitis. These diseases cost many millions of pounds each year; for the industry to replace trained workers, for society in disability allowances and for individuals who may be unable to work and lose their jobs.

Hazardous substances must be:

■ stored correctly, ideally on a low shelf and in a cool, dark, dry, secure, fireproof cabinet

■ handled correctly, ensuring that PPE (personal protective equipment) is worn when mixing chemicals

■ used correctly, ensuring that you and your client are protected from chemicals

■ disposed of correctly in an environmentally friendly and safe manner.

We refer to this as SHUD:

    S – Store

    H – Handle

    U – Use

    D – Dispose

When following SHUD you must do so following the manufacturers' instructions (MFIs), the local by-laws and your salon policy.

The MFIs will instruct you on how to store, handle, use and dispose of the chemicals or substances; the local by-laws will tell you how to dispose of the chemicals/substances, to suit the environment and follow the local authority's guidelines on waste and refuse. Your salon policy will explain where to store and mix the chemicals and where to dispose of them in the workplace.

Your employer's responsibilities under these regulations are to:

■ ensure COSHH information sheets are available for substances and chemicals in the workplace

■ supply PPE

■ ensure waste disposal is suitable for the environment and follows the local by-laws.

Your responsibilities under these regulations are to:

- follow SHUD
- read and follow MFIs, follow local by-laws and your salon policy
- know where to find the COSHH information sheets.

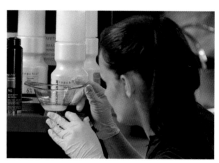

Chemicals being safely mixed

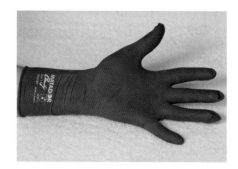

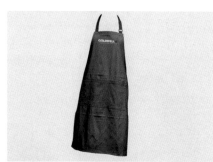

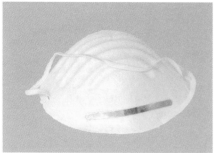

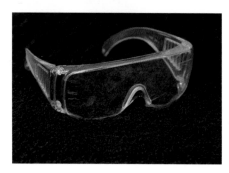

Wear your PPE

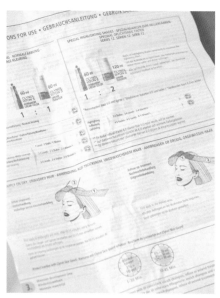

Always follow MFIs

Activity

Substances include all powders, liquids, creams or lotions in your salon – everything from washing powder to peroxide. Take a look around your salon, laundry room, staff areas and bathrooms, and identify all substances that need to be controlled under COSHH. How many can you list?

The Electricity at Work Regulations

Use electrical appliances with caution. Electrical equipment must be handled correctly, checked and tested. Plug sockets must be safe and faulty electrical equipment must be labelled, removed and reported to the relevant person. After use, equipment must be correctly stored.

Your employer's responsibilities under these regulations are to:

- ensure that a qualified electrician completes a portable appliance test (PAT) on electrical items in the salon each year
- keep a record of these tests.

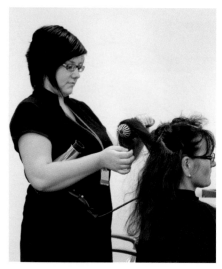

Incorrect handling of a hairdryer

Your responsibilities under these regulations are to:

- not use electrical appliances until you have been trained
- use appliances correctly and switch them off after use
- check each item is in working order before using – check wires, switches and plugs
- report, label and remove any faulty items.

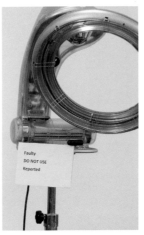
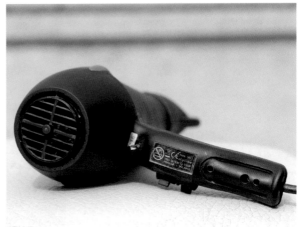

Faulty dryer and climazone – report, label and remove from the salon floor

The Environmental Protection Act

The Environmental Protection Act fundamentally protects our environment. It is a huge Act consisting of the control of emissions into the environment and waste management. Of course this Act affects every business – from large factories emitting masses of fumes and excessive waste to small hairdressing salons with marginal waste and minimal emissions.

Activity

You can estimate your own carbon footprint using the online calculator and entering details about your home, your travel and your appliances. The calculator estimates how many tonnes of carbon dioxide you produce each year.

http://carboncalculator.direct.gov.uk

For more information on reducing your carbon footprint visit http://www.energysavingtrust.org.uk/Take-action/Reduce-your-carbon-footprint

Whatever the size of the business, each owner/employer has a duty of care to protect the environment and dispose of waste on land in an appropriate manner. In fact every individual has a duty of care, as this Act covers dog fouling, litter – including fast food waste,

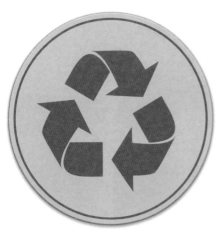

Reduce, reuse and recycle

cigarette butts and chewing gum – and fly-tipping and graffiti to name but a few. Not following the Environmental Protection Act can cost you £300 as a fixed penalty and may result in criminal prosecution.

The Management of Health and Safety at Work Regulations

The Management of Health and Safety at Work Regulations require employers to carry out risk assessments, make arrangements to implement necessary measures, appoint competent people and arrange for appropriate information and training.

Risk assessments

A risk assessment of the workplace and its contents is important to protect employees and visitors in the salon, and it is required by law. The salon owner is responsible for the salon's risk assessments. Although you may not play a huge part in the risk assessment process, you need to be aware of it. If you, your colleagues or clients are pregnant, have limited mobility, are asthmatic or have ailments that may put you at risk in the workplace, your employer must be informed. Your salon manager is not expected to eliminate all risks, but they must ensure they protect you where possible. It is your responsibility to make your employer aware of any health issues you may have that could put you at risk, so that they can assess the situation.

What is risk assessment?

A hazard is something with the potential to cause harm. A risk is the likelihood of the hazard's potential being realised. Trailing wires and hair cuttings on the floor are both hazards. If the trailing wire is neat and tidy against the wall it poses a lesser risk than if it is trailing across a workstation where someone may trip over it. Hair cuttings on the floor pose a potential risk to the stylist and the client if not swept up immediately, but there is a lesser risk to the client while they are sitting in the chair.

A risk assessment is a checklist of what could cause harm to you and others. It helps to identify whether enough precautions have been taken to prevent harm or risks in the workplace.

Advice from the HSE on risk assessment is to follow these five simple steps:

STEP 1 – Identify the hazards.
STEP 2 – Decide who might be harmed and how.
STEP 3 – Evaluate the risks and decide on precautions.

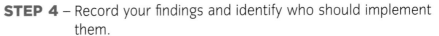

STEP 4 – Record your findings and identify who should implement them.

STEP 5 – Review your assessment and update it if necessary.

Activity

Walk around your salon thinking about the following points and then complete the chart below.

Identify potential risks.

Decide who might be harmed and why.

Decide what preventative precautions could be put in place.

Decide who is responsible for carrying out the precautions.

Refer to http://www.hse.gov.uk/risk/casestudies/pdf/hairdressers.pdf for more information on risk assessment in a hairdressing salon.

Potential risks	Who is at risk?	Preventative precautions	Who is responsible?

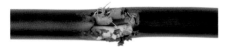

Damaged wires are a hazard – someone could receive an electric shock

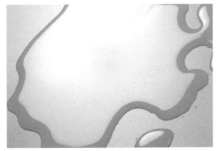

Water on the floor is a hazard – someone could slip over

The Health and Safety (Information For Employees) Regulations

The Health and Safety (Information for Employees) Regulations require employers to display a poster telling employees what they need to know about health and safety. Your employer is responsible for health and safety, but you must help by taking responsibility as well.

The following information is displayed on the health and safety poster and your employer should write the names of your health and safety representative.

All workers have a right to work in places where risks to their health and safety are properly controlled. Health and safety is about stopping you getting hurt at work or ill through work.

In line with these regulations, your employer must do the following:

- Decide what could harm you in your job and the precautions to stop it. This is part of risk assessment.

- Explain how risks will be controlled and tell you who is responsible for this.

- Consult and work with you and your health and safety representatives in protecting everyone from harm in the workplace.
- Provide you (free of charge) with the health and safety training you need to do your job.
- Provide you (free of charge) with any equipment and protective clothing you need, and ensure it is properly looked after.
- Provide toilets, washing facilities and drinking water.
- Provide adequate first aid facilities.
- Report major injuries and fatalities at work to the Health and Safety Executive (HSE) Incident Centre. Report other injuries, diseases and dangerous incidents online at www.hse.gov.uk.
- Have insurance that covers you in case you get hurt at or ill through work. Display a hard copy or electronic copy of the current insurance certificate where you can easily read it.
- Work with any other employers or contractors sharing the workplace or providing employees (such as agency workers), so that everyone's health and safety is protected.

In line with these regulations, you must do the following:

- Follow the training you have received when using any work items your employer has given you.
- Take reasonable care of your own and other people's health and safety.
- Co-operate with your employer on health and safety.
- Tell someone (your employer, supervisor or health and safety representative) if you think the work or inadequate precautions are putting anyone's health and safety at serious risk.

The above information is taken from www.hse.gov.uk/pubns/law.pdf. Visit the HSE website for more information about your rights and how to ensure you are protected by health and safety whilst at work: www.hse.gov.uk.

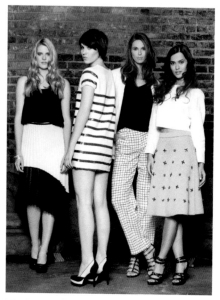

Work together for health and safety

Environmental and sustainable working practices

Consumers and businesses dispose of more than 1.2 million tonnes of waste per year – that's the equivalent of 150,000 double decker buses! Sadly most of this waste goes to landfill. More and more salons are becoming 'green' salons in attempts to be environmentally friendly. This includes using less energy, managing and reducing salon waste, preventing pollution and using eco-friendly furniture and

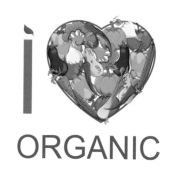

I ♥ ORGANIC

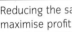
Organic
Produced without the use of artificial chemicals.

products where possible. Using eco-friendly (natural and **organic**) products minimises the negative impact on human health and the environment (such as pollution).

Reducing waste and managing waste

Reducing and managing waste relates to more than just physical stock (such as tubes of tint, bottles of shampoo and towels) – it includes resources such as team members and time, as well as energy.

Reducing waste can save money, which is great for business and potentially your salary!

Managing waste is about looking at what you use, how much of it you use, and using it correctly. It also includes how you remove the salon's waste.

You need to look at your waste and identify what can be reduced, re-used or recycled.

HANDY HINT
Reducing the salon's waste will help to maximise profit and help the environment.

Reducing

To reduce the salon's waste we need to monitor where the wastage occurs and identify the causes.

In the salon you can try to reduce waste such as:

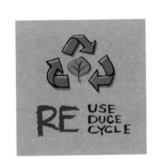

- water
- stock and products
- energy
- paper
- money
- time.

Activity

From your salon retail stand, choose one retail product and count how many are in stock. Ask your manager how many have been sold in the last two months. Do you think your salon stocks the right amount of product, too little or too much?

THE CITY & GUILDS TEXTBOOK

Activity

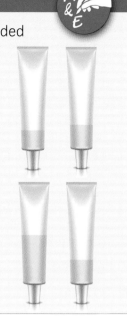

If a stylist mixed up 5% more tint than they needed for each colour client, over 20 clients a whole tube of tint has been wasted (5% x 20 = 100% – a full tube).

1 If in one week, six salon stylists all wasted 5% of tint, and carried out a total of 50 colour services – how many tubes of tint have been wasted?

2 If these six stylists mixed up ½ a tube of tint when a ¼ of a tube would have been sufficient, how much product has been wasted on the 50 colour services?

3 If one tube of tint costs £6.70 +VAT, how much money has been wasted?

Re-using

Over the years we have developed a 'throw-away' lifestyle and where possible we should re-use items.

When shopping for salon provisions, re-use carrier bags or use 'bags for life'. Shampoo and conditioner bottles can be refilled; packaging materials can be re-used for storing items; old towels can be used as cleaning cloths and scrap paper can be used for messages and notes for the team. Your manager may also consider buying 'pre-loved' or second-hand furniture, creating a retro or vintage image whilst protecting the environment too.

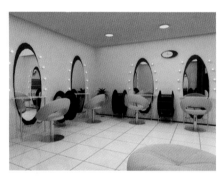

A retro-look salon using vintage furniture

Recycling

People in the UK throw away enough rubbish to fill the Wembley Stadium every day. Buying recycled and greener goods means there is less rubbish for landfill and fewer valuable natural resources getting wasted.

For many of us at home, recycling is a way of life and now businesses have to lead the way in the war against climate change.

So many items are recyclable and your local council can provide you with information on how, where, when and what to recycle. Always follow your local by-laws when disposing of rubbish or recycling.

Activity

Research and investigate where you can recycle electrical items and batteries in your area. What does your local council do to encourage you to protect the environment and recycle?

HANDY HINT

Organise your salon bins into recycling containers and separate your waste. Your salon could increase their salon profits by selling aluminium cans and waste foil through a cash recycling scheme.

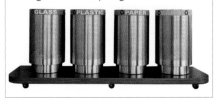

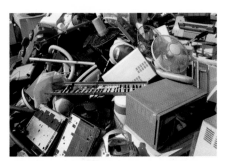

Every year an estimated 2 million tonnes of electrical items are discarded by householders and companies in the UK

Recycling electrical items

Electrical waste is the fastest growing waste in the UK and it increases by 5% every year. Seventy-five per cent of electrical waste ends up in landfill and the lead and other toxins contained in electrical goods cause soil and water contamination. This affects our natural habitat, wildlife and our health. In July 2007 the new 'like for like' Waste Electrical and Electronic Equipment (WEEE) Directive was set up. This means that if you buy a new item, you can hand over the old item and have it recycled for free. For more information on the WEEE regulations, see www.hse.gov.uk.

Salons can recycle most of their electrical goods such as:

- straighteners
- hairdryers
- clippers
- kettles
- washing machines
- computers
- phones.

Buying recycled and greener goods

You can purchase recyclable and greener everyday salon goods such as paper, stationery, toilet paper, paper towels, rubbish bags, and eco-friendly soaps and cleaning supplies.

Other recyclable items

Even the salon light bulbs can be recycled. Low-energy bulbs contain mercury and should not go into waste bins but be taken to a recycling centre. Fluorescent tubes can be recycled too.

- Batteries should not be disposed of with general waste but recycled correctly and safely.
- Printer toner cartridges can be recycled with the manufacturer.
- Tin cans, paper, cardboard, glass and aerosol cans are all recyclable.
- Some plastics can be recycled depending on their recycle symbol – symbols 1 to 3 are recyclable but 4 to 7 are not due to the mixture of compounds.

plastic symbols explained

The chart below will help you identify different types of plastics to make recycling a little easier!

Symbol	Polymer type	Examples	Recyclable?
1 PETE	**PET** Polyethylene Terephthalate	Fizzy drinks Mineral water bottles Squashes Cooking oils	✔ Recycling points are located throughout the UK
2 HDPE	**HDPE** High Density Polyethylene	Milk bottles Juice bottles Washing up liquid Bath & shower bottles	✔ Recycling points are located throughout the UK
3 V	**PVC** Polyvinyl Chloride	Usually in bottle form however not that common these days	✔ Some Recycling points in the UK
4 LDPE	**LDPE** Low Density Polyethylene	Many types of packaging are made from these materials, for example, plastic formed around meats and vegetables.	Due to the mixture of compounds these plastic types are hard to recycle and not generally recycled in the UK
5 PP	**PP** Polypropylene		
6 PS	**PS** Polystyrene		
7 OTHER	**OTHER** All other resins and multi-materials		

For information about where to recycle different types of materials please check out the bank locator on recycle-more.co.uk.

www.recycle-more.co.uk   please recycle me after use

Benefit your local community – donate hair cuttings to your local allotment group

Food and hair

We all know that food waste is great for composting but did you know that hair is too? Disposing of hair in a compost bin with food waste helps make healthy, rich soil. Some eco-friendly salons are even using human hair to insulate the salon and help maintain heat in the winter months – saving energy on heating too.

Safe disposal

Hairdressing salons and barbers should dispose of waste in the following manner: waste materials must be packaged and stored correctly preventing **pollutants** escaping into the environment. If disposing of large amounts or **toxic** chemicals then you must produce a waste transfer note for the company collecting the waste, providing an accurate description of how to handle and dispose of the materials or chemicals safety and appropriately.

Pollutants

Toxins or impurities.

Toxic

Poisonous.

HANDY HINT

For more information go to www.recycle-more.co.uk.

General salon waste must be placed in sacks and kept on the premises until the agreed collection day. The public footpaths must be kept clear at all times and the salon area left clean and tidy. The salon should recycle where possible and flatten down or bundle any cardboard boxes ready for collection. No sharp or dangerous objects should be placed in the refuse sacks and chemicals must be disposed of appropriately.

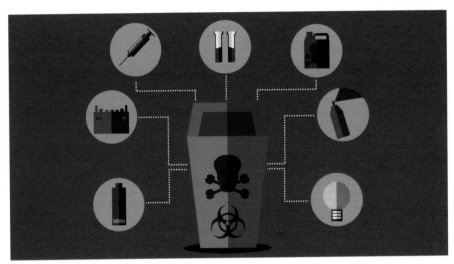

Toxic and hazardous waste

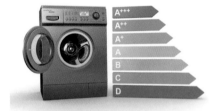

Appliance energy ratings

HANDY HINT

EU directives are forms of legislation that set out objectives for all parties in the European Union (EU) to follow. These directives are often used to enforce free trade, free movement and competition across the EU. They also establish common social policies that can affect employment issues and law, the Working Time Regulations and the Equal Pay Act 1970.

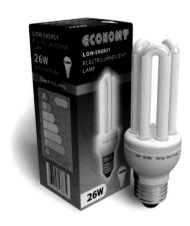

Low-energy lightbulb

Reducing energy usage

Activity

In pairs or small groups try to list five to eight ways in which you could save energy usage in a salon.

To reduce energy usage, salons should:

- turn lights off when not required
- use energy-saving/high-energy-efficiency light bulbs
- have sensors fitted for lights in rooms that are not used so often – toilets, storage cupboards, treatment rooms, etc
- turn off and unplug appliances – eg straightening irons
- use a 'quick wash' cycle on washing machines
- use airers to dry towels instead of tumble dryers
- use 'A' rated appliances (boilers, fridges, heaters, etc) – A+++ is the highest rated for EU directive labelling meaning the most energy efficient
- use solar panels for production of electricity and hot water
- use high-efficiency heating systems
- use low-wattage/high-efficiency hairdryers and electrical tools
- thermally insulate building structures.

Reducing water usage and other resources

Water usage

To save water in the salon, the most obvious thought is to turn off the taps when massaging during the shampoo service. Although this is important, we can also save water by using low flow showerheads and ultra low flush systems on the toilets. When washing up or cleaning tools, do not turn the water flow up high or waste water – instead use a washing-up bowl and fill it with the right amount of water.

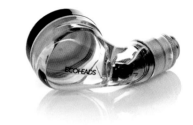

Eco head – showerhead

Activity

At your shampoo area, fill a bucket with warm water and log how many gallons of water you use in one minute. Ideally the flow should be 2.5 gallons per minute. Share your findings with your manager. To avoid wasting water, use the water in the bucket to wash up the clients' tea and coffee cups. If the water is cold, perhaps you could water the plants with it?

Do not leave taps running

Other resources

To reduce the wastage of other resources in the following ways:

Stock and products:

- Mix colours correctly.
- Measure products accurately.
- Judge the hair service correctly mixing up the right amount of product for the hair length and density and using the correct amount of shampoo, conditioner and styling products, etc.
- Understand and follow the manufacturers' instructions.
- Rotate stock so that it does not go out of date.
- Don't overorder stock.

Paper:

- You could ask clients to book appointments in their diaries or on their smartphones, rather than issuing appointment cards.
- Set the salon's printer to print on both sides of the paper as default.
- Use email or the internet to place stock orders.
- Contact the mail preference services to have the salon address removed from mailing lists to prevent junk mail – www.mpsonline. org.uk.

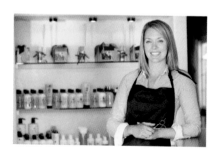

Take stock

Money:

- When calculating your client's bill, make sure you charge for the products you have used.

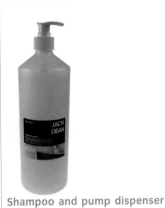

Shampoo and pump dispenser

Activity

Find out from your salon whether they charge clients more money for colouring services if they have abundant hair, or if the hair is very long.

If your salon does charge more, work out how much more money the salon would make if you had five clients with long hair book in for a colour compared with five clients with short hair.

Time:

- Organise staff rotas to ensure all staff are busy.
- Book appointments correctly so they are timed efficiently for each stylist's working day.

Possible causes of wastage

Generally wastage is caused by poor usage and can easily be prevented. Poor stock control, poor procedures, bad practice, poorly trained staff, accidental wastage and even dishonest staff may be the causes of some salon wastage.

Activity

Walk around your salon and watch the team working. List any activity you can see that could be wasting money, products, time, energy or water. Identify what you think are the main reasons for the wastage. If you have any really good ideas that would save your salon wasting time and money, then you could write an email to your employer with your recommendations. Remember to write your email professionally and to check your spelling before you send it.

Pollution

Contamination of the environment.

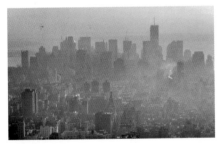

Smog is a form of pollution

Preventing pollution

Individual businesses do not generate that much **pollution** on their own but collectively small- and medium-sized salons and individuals working in people's home produce substantial waste pollution. The use of chemicals such as hair colours, lighteners, perm lotions and relaxers, and aerosol products such as hairspray, contributes to pollution.

Using hairdressing chemicals can cause poor indoor air quality – which can affect people's health. On a daily basis we are exposed to:

- ammonia – a chemical used in hair colour
- phenylenediamine (PPD) – also used in hair colours and the ingredient that can cause allergic reactions to hair colour
- hydrogen peroxide – mixed with hair colours to activate them
- sodium hydroxide – used in hair relaxers.

Installing air filtration systems will help to protect clients and staff from poor air quality.

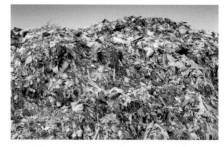
Landfill

Liquid waste, particularly chemicals, can be toxic and is banned from landfill, as it can pollute the environment. Chemical waste can kill wildlife and in extreme cases enter our drinking water. Toxic chemicals cannot be poured down the sink, but small amounts of hairdressing chemicals – such as leftover tints and peroxide – can be diluted with water and rinsed down the drain.

Aerosols have a very long shelf life; so only dispose of them when they are empty. Aerosols can be recycled as they are made from 60% tinplated steel and 40% aluminium – both of these metals are recyclable. Do not pierce, crush or flatten aerosols before recycling.

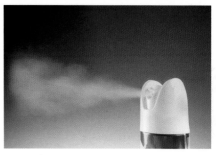
Aerosol spray

Using disposable items

Disposable towels

Using disposable towels may sound costly, but in fact they are more convenient, absorbent, eco-friendly and hygienic than traditional towels. You can save up to 25% on laundry bills and reduce energy use too. They are made from renewable sources and they're recyclable and 100% biodegradable within three months. The packaging is often compostable too, as the companies selling these products are environmentally friendly.

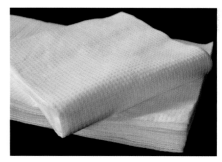
Easydry disposable towels

Using recycled paper towels in hand washing areas is hygienic and can be better for the environment than some hand dryers. Jet stream dryers are efficient to use but can be noisy and may not suit the environment.

Disposable cups

The main raw material used to make paper cups is wood, which is a renewable resource. However, collecting the wood still impacts on the environment – trees are cut down, fuel is used to collect the wood, etc. A polystyrene cup is made from oil – collecting and transporting the oil can also affect the environment.

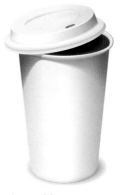
Disposable cup

A paper cup is more expensive to produce than a polystyrene cup and more chemicals are used during the manufacturing. Paper cups cannot normally be recycled because the glue used to hold them together cannot be broken down during the recycling process. But a polystyrene cup is recyclable and reusable.

Ideally salons should use mugs or cups and saucers when providing clients with refreshments.

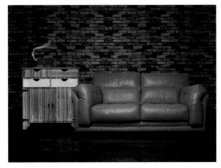

Reclaimed furniture

Using recycled, eco-friendly furniture

All salons want their decor to reflect their salon culture and image, and to look clean and tidy, but this can still be achieved using eco-friendly furniture, fixtures and fittings. You can purchase eco-friendly salon items like furniture and flooring, basins and taps, and white goods – washing machines and fridges – from recyclable or sustainable sources. Unwanted salon furniture can be donated to the homeless or non-profit organisations.

Activity

Research online how to 'get rid of stuff for free'. How many sites can you find where you can either recycle or donate items? How many of these are charities that could help your local community?

Using low chemical paint

Volatile organic compounds (VOCs) are gases given off by paints and other chemicals that contain solvents. They have an unpleasant odour and the fumes can be carcinogenic. Carcinogenic products and chemicals can cause health problems, such as irritation, lung and respiratory problems, asthma and cancer. Some paints can give off gas for many months after painting.

Eco-friendly salons are opting for VOC-free paint made from natural materials and environmentally managed sources.

Using organic and hypoallergenic hair products

Organic and hypoallergenic hair products can include shampoo and conditioners, styling and finishing products such as serums, volumiser, styling gels, protecting oils, hairspray, etc. They are made with up to 98% naturally derived ingredients that are ethically sourced. Ingredients may include essential oils, Moroccan argan oil, plant-based products and most have UV sunscreen protection too. They leave the hair feeling fresh, manageable and healthy, providing shine, body and firm control. Organic hairdressing products are less likely to cause allergies or irritate the client's skin and scalp. However, you must always ask if your client has any allergies, as you may not be familiar with the ingredients; a client suffering with a nut allergy may not be able to have Moroccan argan oil products on their hair, for instance.

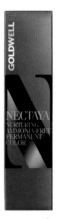

Moroccan argan oil product

Activity

Look at the ingredients in a retail product from your salon range and identify any ingredients and products that some clients may be allergic to.

Using ultra low ammonia hair colourants

The salon consumers – our clients – are requesting eco-friendly and chemical-free products for their hair. This includes colouring products too, but of course they still want vibrant colours and white hair coverage.

Several manufacturers offer ammonia-free hair colour products, where over 90% of the ingredients are of natural origin and still cover resistant white hair and achieve up to three levels of lift. These products are kind to the hair, as well as the planet.

Salons are also less likely to use products that have been tested on animals or those with animal-derived ingredients. This may be due to consumer demand or salons' choices.

Goldwell Nectaya colour product

Using environmentally friendly product packaging

When salons decide to go green and help protect the environment, they should request that their manufacturers and wholesalers use environmentally friendly packaging. They could ask if the Styrofoam peanuts that protect products during transit can be returned, re-used or recycled. The cardboard boxes should be made from recycled paper and after delivery they would ideally be flat packed and recycled.

For example, Aveda believes it 'can change the world, by changing how the world does business'. It:

- uses 100% post-consumer recyclable packaging
- reduces the size, weight and processes of packaging

HANDY HINT

Visit Aveda's website for further information: http://www.aveda.co.uk.

WHY DON'T YOU…
When selling retail to clients you could offer a reward scheme for clients using their own bags and maybe even offer a refill option for the shampoos and conditioners.

- offers packaging that can be recycled
- uses environmentally sound materials
- uses renewable energy to manufacturer and fill its packaging
- uses 100% wind power to manufacturer its products.

Fairtrade

Fairtrade guarantees that products carrying the FAIRTRADE Mark have been made with fairer trading conditions and opportunities for producers in developing countries.

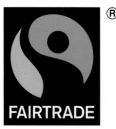

FAIRTRADE Mark

Choosing responsible domestic products

Almost everything you buy has been made; each item is manufactured, processed, packaged and then driven somewhere to be delivered. This process affects the environment and the people who are involved in its production. Even when you clean the salon, the products you use could harm the environment and a simple gesture like offering your client a tea or coffee could probably be improved by using **Fairtrade** tea and coffee.

When cleaning in the salon, use eco-friendly laundry detergent, washing up liquid and multi-surface cleaners. Check cleaning supply bottles and containers are biodegradable and in bathroom areas use recycled paper toilet roll and eco-friendly hand wash.

WHY DON'T YOU…
Take a look at the website of Emma Hellier's eco-friendly salon for inspiration: http://www.emmahellier.com/eco.

Activity

Create a mood board and design your eco-friendly salon. You must use:

- re-usable, recycled or eco-friendly furniture and flooring
- VOC-free paint
- eco-friendly and hypoallergenic hair care products and retail
- ultra low ammonia hair colours
- low-energy equipment.

Encouraging carbon-reducing journeys to work

Travelling by car to work with only one person in the vehicle increases our carbon footprint. To help reduce your carbon footprint, consider whether you could walk to work, cycle there, use public transport or car share.

HANDY HINT
Maybe your salon could provide a cycle rack and encourage clients to cycle to the salon for their appointments and offer them a reward for being eco-friendly.

Answers in the back of the book.

1 Statement one

The employer's responsibility, under the Health and Safety at Work Act, is to ensure all staff, clients and visitors are safe.

Statement two

It is the employee's responsibility to make sure their actions do not out others at risk.

Which one of the following is correct for the above statements?

a True   True
b True   False
c False   True
d False   False

2 Which one of the following is **not** reportable under RIDDOR?

a A fractured skull
b A fractured finger
c Occupational asthma
d Occupational dermatitis

3 Which one of the following is a stylist's responsibility under the Regulatory Reform (Fire Safety Order)?

a To know which extinguisher to use on different types of fire
b To be able to use all types of extinguishers
c To carry out a fire risk assessment
d To perform inspection visits

4 Which two of the following identify what is contained in a CO_2 fire extinguisher and which type of fire it is best used on?

1 Carbon dioxide
2 Carbon monoxide
3 Paper or wood
4 Electrical items
a 1 and 2
b 2 and 3
c 3 and 4
d 4 and 1

5 The acronym SHUD stands for

a Store, handle, use and dispose
b Stain, hands, use and dispose
c Safe, health, union and directive
d Stain, hands, union and directive

6 Which is the most important item of PPE to use when carrying out wet work?

a Apron
b Gloves
c Mask
d Goggles

7 Statement one

The Environmental Protection Act requires employers to dispose of waste responsibly.

Statement two

Information on health and safety laws can be found on www.healthandsafety.co.uk.

Which one of the following is correct for the above statements?

a True   True
b True   False
c False   True
d False   False

8 Statement one

It is better to recycle than to re-use waste.

Statement two

Using second-hand furniture in a salon can give it a vintage look and also help to save the environment.

Which one of the following is correct for the above statements?

a True   True
b True   False
c False   True
d False   False

9 Which of the following categories of waste is the fastest growing in the UK?

   a Chemical substances

   b Electrical items

   c Furniture

   d Plastics

10 Which one of the following is the most eco-friendly salon?

   a One that offers Fairtrade tea

   b One that uses oil-based products

   c One that uses renewable energy

   d One that has recycled flooring

VALUES AND BEHAVIOURS

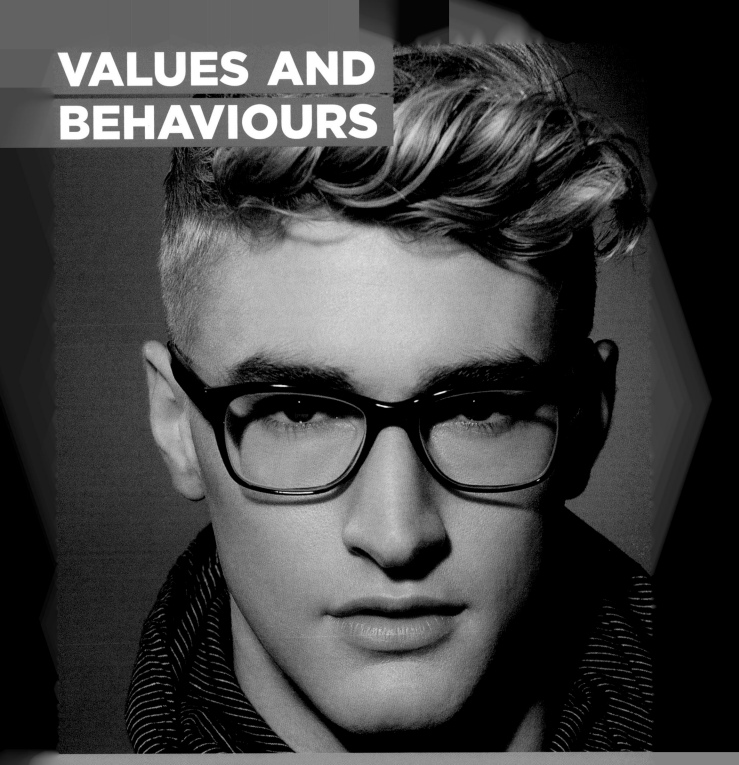

You have chosen a career in hairdressing and/or barbering, so every day you'll be in contact with other team members and salon clients, working in a 'people'-orientated industry. Good working values and behaviours can accelerate your career and boost your client base, providing you with a loyal clientele and a long future in an amazing, exciting and ever-changing industry.

The values and behaviours covered in this chapter link to each and every unit in your qualification. They clarify the key values that underpin the delivery of services in the hair and beauty sector, and the behaviours to ensure that clients receive a positive impression of both you and the salon. Look out for the following icon which highlights the key 'values and behaviours' points in each chapter.

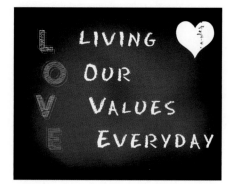

Values

Values are our working ethics, the moral code we work to, and our principles and beliefs. Every person is unique and his or her personal views will vary, but when working in the hairdressing and barbering sector we need to standardise our ideals, and follow and promote the expected industry values set out in this chapter.

Willingness to learn

When working in the hairdressing and barbering industry you must be prepared to work hard! Standing all day, working with the general public and learning new skills requires a strong disposition. You'll need motivation and enthusiasm for this kind of work, and a keenness and eagerness to learn new skills.

You'll need to be ready and prepared for every eventuality, such as:

- clients arriving without appointments
- clients and stylist running behind appointment times
- changes to appointments and services booked
- absent team members
- the ever-changing fashions and skills required to maintain your career.

Being a willing participator in the salon and focusing on the high standards required from your salon will help you to improve your performance and develop your career.

> **HANDY HINT**
>
> You will carry out services on a variety of people: some will have very different values from you, and some will have different backgrounds, upbringing, cultures, religion and beliefs and may behave unexpectedly. You will need to learn to adapt to these differences and respect other people's values, beliefs and points of view, even if you do not share them.

Completing services in a commercially viable time

Working to a commercially viable time when carrying out services in the salon is of great importance. Clients are allocated a time when they book their hair appointment and they expect that appointment to run to time. There are times when appointments will run late: this may be because clients are late for appointments or occasionally services overrun, but you will be expected to complete most of your salon services in the timeframes allocated to ensure the salon operates as smoothly as possible.

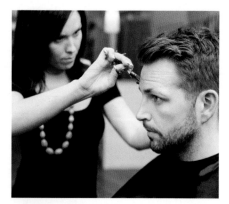

Complete the service in a viable time

> **WHY DON'T YOU...**
> Refer to chapter CHB12 and complete the activity on service times.

> **Activity**
>
> If you failed to work to commercially viable times or clients were regularly later to appointments, the salon would run behind schedule. If you have eight clients booked in your appointment column today and run 12 minutes late with every client, how late will you be leaving?

Organisational and industry standards of appearance

Within the hairdressing and barbering industry, personal appearance and the salon's dress code can vary immensely. Some salons have a uniform or a colour code, such as all black. Some salons encourage the team to express their individuality and personality through their own choice of clothing and they feel that this style may attract clients with similar tastes and personalities. Always ensure you prepare your work clothes in advance.

Your appearance

Along with the receptionist, every member of the salon team should look presentable and represent the industry and their salon. Ensure you allow enough time before work to prepare yourself for your working day.

The following diagram shows areas of appearance that are important:

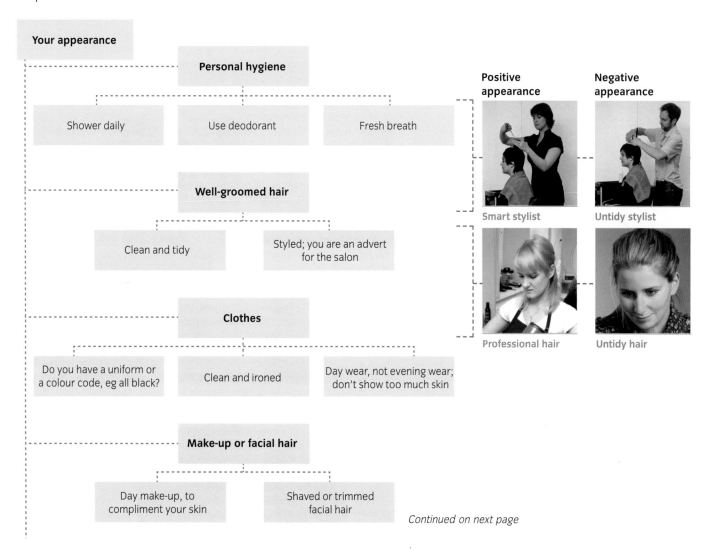

Your appearance

Personal hygiene
- Shower daily
- Use deodorant
- Fresh breath

Well-groomed hair
- Clean and tidy
- Styled; you are an advert for the salon

Clothes
- Do you have a uniform or a colour code, eg all black?
- Clean and ironed
- Day wear, not evening wear; don't show too much skin

Make-up or facial hair
- Day make-up, to compliment your skin
- Shaved or trimmed facial hair

Positive appearance
Smart stylist

Negative appearance
Untidy stylist

Professional hair

Untidy hair

Continued on next page

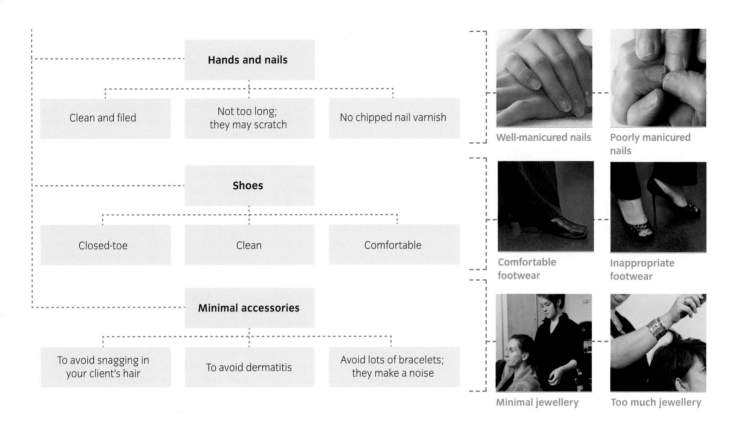

Hands and nails

Clean and filed | Not too long; they may scratch | No chipped nail varnish

Well-manicured nails | Poorly manicured nails

Shoes

Closed-toe | Clean | Comfortable

Comfortable footwear | Inappropriate footwear

Minimal accessories

To avoid snagging in your client's hair | To avoid dermatitis | Avoid lots of bracelets; they make a noise

Minimal jewellery | Too much jewellery

Activity

Which of these photos give positive impressions of the salon and which give negative impressions?

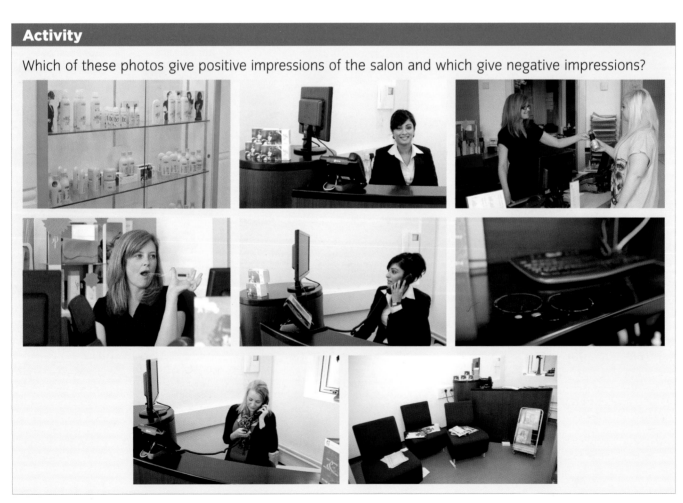

Personal hygiene and protection requirements

Start your day after a good night's rest, ensuring you brush your teeth, shower or wash before work, and use a deodorant. Wear clean, ironed clothes that are well presented. If you are a smoker, or enjoy coffee or spicy foods, always ensure you have mints or similar handy to freshen your breath. Your hair should always represent the industry you are in and look clean and tidy. Ladies may choose to wear a little make-up to help them look well groomed, and nails must be clean and not chipped if painted. For men, facial hair should be neatly trimmed.

Dress in layers that can be taken off so you don't get too hot. Becoming too hot can lead to body odour and cause offence or discomfort to others. This is especially important as hairstyling involves working very closely to your clients and often leaning over them.

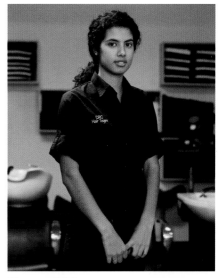
Clean and tidy

Maintaining personal hygiene

Staff should ensure that their own personal hygiene is maintained; this is how:

- shower before work
- wear clean clothes
- wear deodorant
- brush your teeth every morning
- ensure your hair is clean and tidy
- keep breath fresh throughout the day
- do not attend work with infectious conditions.

For safety reasons, wear shoes that cover your toes and are comfortable to stand in for long periods of time. Never wear open-toed shoes, as hair cuttings can penetrate the skin on your feet, and you may injure yourself if you drop any sharp objects such as scissors. Avoid wearing baggy jumpers that may get caught in equipment. Avoid wearing excessive jewellery. Long necklaces may get caught in equipment and rings could catch in your client's hair, as well as encourage occupational dermatitis. Wearing several bracelets creates a noise which may affect your client's enjoyment of the treatment, for example when massaging during a shampooing and conditioning service.

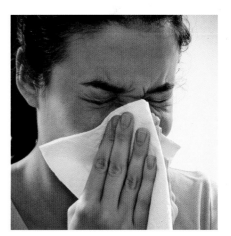
Infectious? Stay away!

Activity

Identify infectious conditions that may keep you away from work.

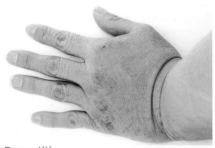

Dermatitis

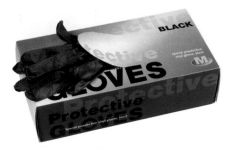

Wear non-latex disposable gloves

Protecting your hands and clothes

It is important to protect your hands to avoid occupational dermatitis. Dermatitis can occur when your skin comes into contact with substances that can irritate the skin and cause allergies. Each person's skin will react differently to substances and dermatitis can occur at any time of your career. Hairdressers are more likely to develop occupational dermatitis than any other profession. Dermatitis is not contagious to others but it can spread around your own skin. Although most commonly found on the hands, it can appear on the face, lips, arms and cause irritation to the eyes. The good news is that it can be avoided. Follow these five simple steps to healthy hands:

1 Wear non-latex disposable gloves for shampooing, conditioning, removing colours and neutralising, etc.
2 Dry your hands thoroughly after wetting.
3 Moisturise your hands regularly.
4 Use new gloves for every client.
5 Check your hands regularly for signs of contact dermatitis.

Dermatitis can be recognised as:

- dry hands
- itchy hands
- redness of the hands
- cracking of the skin
- bleeding and swelling
- blistering.

PPE (personal protective equipment) for the stylist and the assistant includes:

- gloves to protect your hands from chemicals and staining
- an apron to protect your clothes from chemical damage.

If you suffer from asthma or allergies:

- wear a mask when mixing chemicals, particularly when using bleach powders, to prevent inhalation
- wear eye protection when handling chemicals, to prevent chemicals from entering the eyes.

Flexible working attitudes

Where possible, have an adaptable approach to your daily work and always expect the unexpected! Be willing to change your working pattern to suit the needs of the business; and try to be flexible during your working day to meet the client demands, without affecting other client services. Be respectful to all staff, visitors and clients and understand that everyone has differences: this includes values and beliefs, religion and culture, and personal views.

You need to be able to adapt to different situations, such as working under pressure or dealing with a regular client.

Would you treat a regular client differently if the salon were busy or quiet? How would you react if you were short of staff in the salon, or had to deal with a power failure?

> **HANDY HINT**
>
> Treat everyone equally, ensuring that you do not make any unsuitable comments regarding age, gender, disability, sexual orientation, race, religion, marital status and so on.

> **HANDY HINT**
>
> Refer to chapter CHB12 for more information on assisting others and working effectively as part of a team.

How to adapt to different situations

A routine service	A busy salon	A quiet salon	Staff shortages	Power failure
You should already have built a good rapport with your regular clients, but this doesn't mean you don't need to try. Treat all clients like it's their first visit and impress them every time.	Make sure you give every client the attention they deserve, no matter how busy you are. Apologise if you're running a little late with the service and explain that the salon is busy. Reassure your client that you have plenty of time for their service. Don't panic and don't rush the service.	If you're not busy, don't assume your client isn't. Don't slow down the service. Use any extra time you have to discuss and promote products and services to the client and give extra aftercare advice.	If you have staff absences to cope with, always explain the situation to your clients. If they understand the situation they are more likely to sympathise and not get upset if services run late. If a stylist is absent, check whether anyone else can look after the client. If an assistant is absent, then the stylists all need to help each other. Remain calm, work methodically and do not rush your services.	Your salon should have a **contingency plan** for emergencies such as a power failure. **Contingency plan** Back-up or secondary plan. Try to contact all clients in advance to warn them of the power failure and offer an alternative appointment time. Ask if they would prefer a wet cut, if you can't dry the hair. If the power fails in the middle of a service your manager will tell you what the salon procedure is. Remain calm, reassure your client that the outcome will not be affected. Remain professional. Remember – you can cope!

Activity

Consider your strengths and areas to develop. List the tasks and roles where you are adaptable and flexible and note the ones you need to develop further.

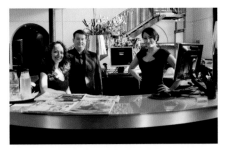

Teamwork makes a great salon

Team working and assisting others

A salon operates effectively when everyone works as one team, and with one common goal – the client experience being the main focus. Team work and assisting each other is explored in more detail in chapter CHB12.

Activity

In a team meeting, allow 15 minutes for staff to create a mission statement that creates focus and that everyone buys into. Each person should write down the end of the sentence, 'My vision of a team that works is …'

(Materials needed: pens, paper, and any team requests.)

The entire team now creates one statement or vision that represents the total of these vision statements. The desired outcome of this activity is that the team finds commonality of purpose and is more willing to cooperate.

At the end of this activity, make sure that all spellings are correct and the grammar and punctuation are accurate too.

Maintaining customer care

Client care is paramount in establishing effective relationships, so ensure you always treat clients well.

This is how to treat your clients:

- respect them
- look after their belongings
- protect their clothes
- show an interest
- listen to them
- offer advice
- question them about their hair.

Diversity of clients

If your client has mobility problems, ask if you can assist them walking to the workstation or shampoo area.

If your client arrives wearing a head scarf or burka, ask them if this is for religious purposes. If so, ask how you can carry out their hair services whilst respecting their religion. Can you ensure there aren't any males around if a Muslim lady has her hair on show?

If you have a client who is transgender, you may be unsure of how your client would like to be referred to – male or female. It is ok to ask your client how they would like to be referred, and this will prevent you from offending them.

Speaking with your client

The first impressions of the salon will start at reception so ensure that the reception area is neat and tidy. A selection of up-to-date magazines for clients to read while they wait for their appointment may keep them happy if the service is running late. Always communicate with clients, advise them if the stylist is running a little late and offer them a drink to make them feel at ease.

Salon staff should always:

- speak politely
- introduce themselves
- welcome and greet the client by their name
- generally refer to the client by name
- offer refreshments
- give advice about products and services available in the salon.

Salon staff should not:

- chew gum
- leave the reception unattended
- let the phone ring more than three times
- make a client wait to be attended to
- take personal calls
- use jargon or technical terms.

When questioning and talking with clients you are using your communication skills! Remember that how you communicate can make a positive or negative impression on your client of you and your salon.

HANDY HINT

Show all your clients and co-workers respect at all times and no matter what the circumstances.

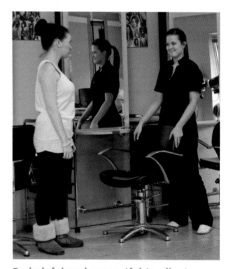

Be helpful and respectful to clients

Activity

Which of the following comments are good and which are poor? From the poor sentences you identify, how would you rephrase them to make them better?

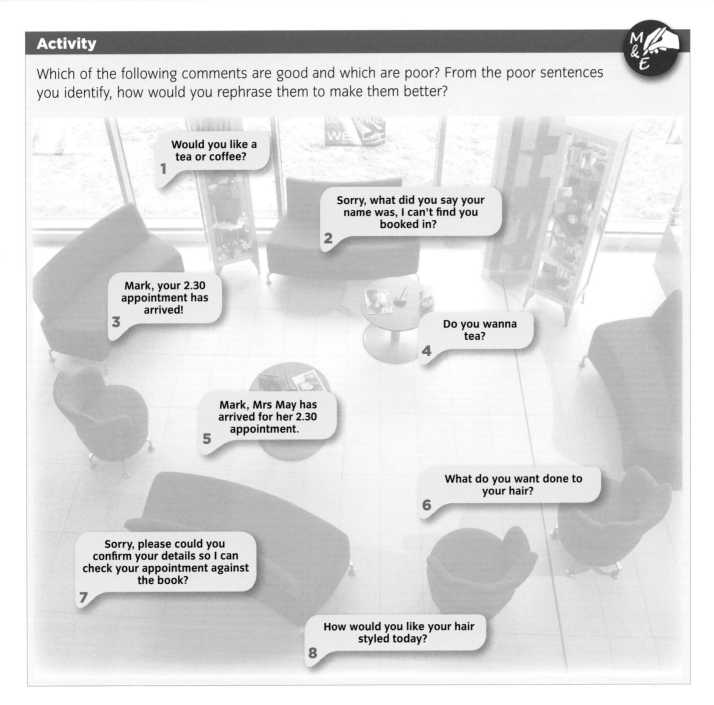

Protecting your client

When your client arrives, sit them comfortably at your workstation and after consultation, protect them suitably for the service required.

Always use:

- a fresh clean towel
- a fresh clean gown
- a plastic/disposable shoulder cape or another fresh clean towel if you are using chemicals or working with long wet hair – this may vary depending on your salon requirements)
- a cutting collar for cutting services.

A client must wear a gown during a chemical service otherwise you may cause damage to their clothes. This could easily lead to a loss of clients or **revenue** if an unsatisfied client charges the salon for damages or takes their business elsewhere.

Revenue

Income or money received from clients for services provided by the salon.

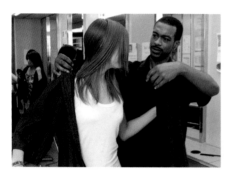

Gowning a client

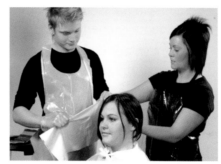

A gowned client with stylist during a colour service

Positive attitudes

You spend many hours at work, so working relationships are important. Be helpful and friendly to your co-workers; smile, avoid sarcasm, control your reactions, be appreciative, and be happy with other people's success. Offer encouragement and give compliments to others, such as: 'congratulations on your promotion', 'your client's hair looked lovely', 'you look nice' and so on.

Statistics show that people working in the hairdressing are some of the happiest people at work. Enjoy your job and have fun whilst working, look your best, remain optimistic and upbeat and get back up, even after a fall. Set yourself goals and go after them, and don't complain if things don't go your way – just try again next time.

HANDY HINT

If someone has upset you, discuss it with them face to face. Always be constructive, communicate clearly and in a friendly manner, and don't talk about them behind their back.

HANDY HINT

Remember that everyone is different and value everyone's opinion even if you do not agree with them. Treat people fairly and professionally.

Personal and professional ethics

Your personal ethics and your salon's professional ethics are often very similar, because they are about right and wrong. Although professional ethics are more formal than our personal ethics they both generally involve treating people correctly, being honest and fair.

Personal ethics

Personal ethics are very subjective and individual. Our beliefs are formed by our everyday life experiences and our background, and can vary from person to person. Personal views, those of family and friends, our communities or our culture or religion may form our personal opions and views on what is morally right or wrong. Our personal beliefs are reflected in how we interact, respect and treat people, how honest and fair we are and even how loyal we are to our employers.

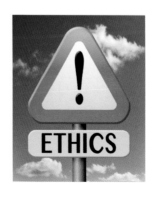

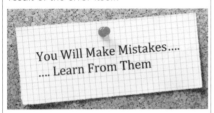

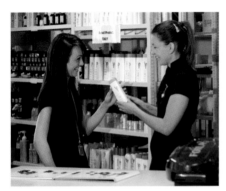

Help your colleagues

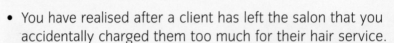

Activity

Discuss with a colleague what you would do if you encountered the following scenarios:

- You have realised after a client has left the salon that you accidentally charged them too much for their hair service.
- You have accidentally got permanent colour on the collar of your client's shirt.
- A colleague has confided in you that they have taken some hairdressing products from the retail stand for personal use.
- A colleague has taken a client's phone number from their record card for personal use.

When you and your colleague have discussed how you would deal with the above scenarios, use your skills to present your answers to other colleagues. Clearly explain why and how you came to your conclusions.

Professional ethics

Professional ethics are more about company rules and regulations, what we must adhere to when working with clients and co-workers. It is our salon code of conduct and may include client confidentiality, respecting the diversity of clients and co-workers, reporting concerns that may affect the salon business and following legal requirements. It should also include how the company and others treat you.

Self-management

Being a self-manager is important in work; it helps you organise yourself, take ownership of your own responsibilities, and take the initiative with change. Self-management is about taking charge of your own future, working towards goals, taking and managing risks, dealing with pressure and managing your emotions. It's your contribution to your work – being organised, responding positively to change, planning and managing your time effectively. If you can't self-manage, you may struggle to progress through life and advance with your career. Failing to manage yourself could lead to unhappiness and potentially unemployment.

Take the initiative, set yourself clear goals and targets to work towards, self-appraise and reflect on your own strengths and weaknesses and monitor your own progress. Ask for feedback from peers and your employer and take on board their criticism.

Self-management skills

A good self-manager:

- manages and adapts to change, takes risks and seeks advice
- has a flexible and adaptable approach to work and learning
- manages emotion, anger, conflict and stress
- thinks outside the box – problem-solving
- works towards goals, showing initiative, commitment and perseverance
- deals with competing pressures and builds self-confidence.

> **HANDY HINT**
>
> Making wise choices about your career progression and demonstrating a 'can-do' approach at work will help you to develop.

Activity

Write a career progression plan about where you want to be in six months' time, one year and where you would like to be in five years' time. Add achievable personal 'SMARTER' targets to work towards.

SMARTER targets:

- **S**pecific – what exactly do you need to do/achieve?
- **M**easurable – how will you know you have achieved the target?
- **A**greed – do both you and your manager agree on and understand what the target is that has been set?
- **R**ealistic – are you realistically likely to be able to achieve the target and is it relevant to your role and ability?
- **T**ime-bound – when do you need to achieve the target by?
- **E**valuated – what is the date that has been set to evaluate progress so far?
- **R**eviewed – what is the date that has been set to review the outcomes?

At the end of the activity, check your spellings, punctuation and grammar. Make sure it reads well and, if need be, ask someone else to check it for you too.

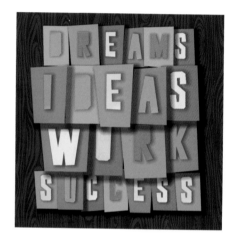

> **HANDY HINT**
>
> For more on SMARTER targets, see chapter CHB12.

Creativity skills

If you think of a great idea, but don't do anything with it, you are imaginative not creative. Creativity is about thinking of something and then acting on it. This may be artistic thinking and producing a beautiful hair-up style, or it may be developing a concept.

Being creative, using your imagination and producing ideas and having the commitment to drive these forward are skills that employers are calling out for. It can take courage to express your

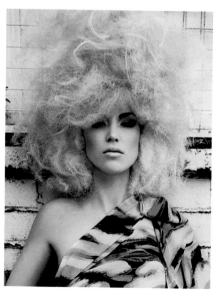

Be creative

ideas though – fear of ridicule or lack of interest can sometimes prevent us from speaking out loud and expressing our ideas. So be brave and rather than think 'I can't', think 'why not?'

When thinking creatively you need to generate and explore your ideas and those of others. Sometimes you need to work alone but at times you need to know when to work together. You'll need to explore ideas, experiment and practise, learn from mistakes and make adaptations to the original concept, ask questions and maybe observe others at work. Try keeping an ideas book, noting your visions and writing down what inspires you, as this may prevent great ideas being forgotten about.

Verbal and non-verbal communication skills

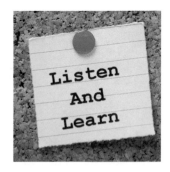

In the salon you will communicate with your clients face to face, via the telephone and, in some cases, electronically – via email or the internet. Your salon may offer a text messaging service to remind clients of their appointment or to promote special offers. When you are using verbal and non-verbal communication skills you are using your English skills. These skills are highly valued by employers and expected by most of your clients.

Verbal communication

Always speak at a speed your client can understand, be polite, well mannered and express yourself clearly. If your client is showing signs of uncertainty you can ask more relevant questions to clarify the situation and put them at ease. You will need to adapt your tone of voice and the vocabulary you use to suit your client's needs.

Tone of voice

Your voice needs to be pitched high enough to project over the noises in the salon, such as hairdryers and music, and spoken clearly but with a soft, friendly tone. Smile when you speak as it softens how you sound and look. When emphasising a point or asking a question, raise your voice a little at the end of the sentence. Always remain courteous and never talk to colleagues across your clients. If you need some help from your salon assistant, ask politely and respectfully. Never display any animosity that may be present in the team or engage in idle chat with a colleague when you should be focused on your client.

Face to face

You will need to use verbal and non-verbal communication and show you are listening. Always smile and look friendly, ensuring you display open body language that promotes a good impression, and maintain

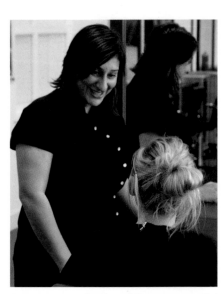

Great communication skills are essential

eye contact with your client to aid trust. You should never interrupt a client when they are speaking.

Telephone

When you answer the telephone, smile, as it shows in your voice; speak clearly and say good morning/afternoon to the caller. Always state your name, to let the caller know who they are speaking to.

Vocabulary

It is essential that your client understands what you are saying, so use words they will understand when discussing their hair. In general, avoid using slang and never use bad language in the salon. Also avoid technical words or jargon. Ensure you speak in a way which **exhibits** a professional image.

Exhibits

Shows.

Activity

From the following list, which is the best way to answer the phone and why?

- Hello, Cut Above. Can I help you?
- Good afternoon, Cut Above hair salon. Sarah speaking. How may I help you?
- Good morning, Sarah speaking. How can I help?
- Hello, Sarah at Cut Above speaking. Can I help you?

Activity

In groups, discuss examples of poor telephone manners and think about your own experiences.

Non-verbal communication

When communicating with your clients it is very important that you listen. Always give your clients enough time to express their wishes, and smile and nod to acknowledge you understand. Maintain eye contact and show an interest in what is being said.

Body language

When you communicate you do so verbally and non-verbally. Body language is a method of non-verbal communication and can be positive as well as negative. It can give away secrets about whether you are telling the truth, listening to your client and interested in what your client is saying:

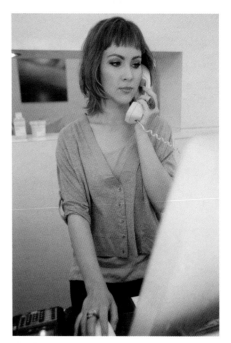

Think about your telephone manners

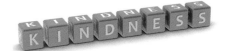

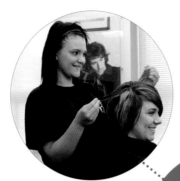

Smiling indicates you are
happy and approachable

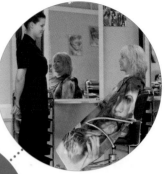

Eye contact indicates
you are listening

**POSITIVE BODY
LANGUAGE**

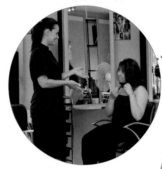

Open palms indicate
openness
and honesty

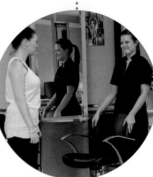

Good open body posture
indicates you are
alert and ready for work

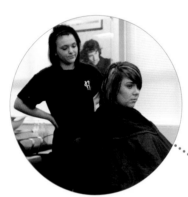

Keeping a little distance shows respect
for personal space

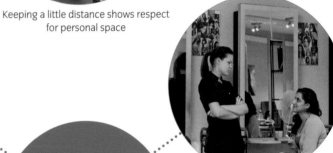

Poor posture looks unprofessional
and indicates tiredness

**NEGATIVE BODY
LANGUAGE**

Crossed arms, closed-in body
posture indicates defensive
behaviour and a closed mind

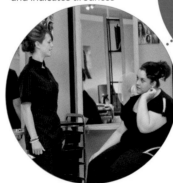

Scratching behind the ear or rubbing the
back of the neck indicates that the
listener is uncertain

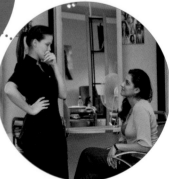

Talking with your hand in front of your
mouth indicates to your client that you are
not being honest or truthful

Email and texts

If your salon asks you to contact a client via text message or email, you should avoid using text abbreviations. Always write words in full and check the spelling. Text messaging and emails are still quite new methods of communicating with clients and some text messages can be impersonal and brief. Remember, your client can't see your smiling face or hear the friendly tone in your voice when reading an email or texts, so re-read the message to ensure it is friendly and professional, and not too abrupt or direct.

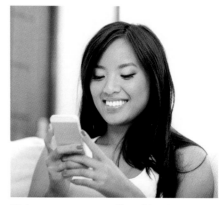

Make sure your email and text messages are professional in tone

Activity

A client emails the salon asking for a hair appointment next Tuesday at 3pm and you respond with the following email.

> Hi Jan
>
> No worries, we can def fit u in on Tues. Who does your hair? Gems free, will she do? Wot you want doing? Can U let me no? See you l8r.
>
> John.

Discuss with a colleague what is wrong with this email, list all the problems and spelling errors.

Re-write the replying email professionally.

Activity

Use the internet to search for salon websites.

Discuss with your colleagues whether you think these salon websites would be useful to clients.

Identify salon websites you like and explain why.

Identify salon websites that you would improve and explain your reasons.

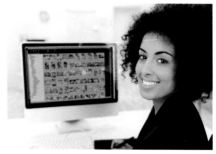

Research on the internet

Effective, hygienic and safe working methods

It is essential that salon cleanliness is maintained throughout the day. This will ensure that a professional image is projected to your clients. Always use a clean towel and gown for each client and ensure that the salon floors are kept free of hair cuttings. At the start of a service you must ensure that tools and equipment are ready for use, and when you have finished, tidy wires and put items away, and return styling products to the product area. After every service you must ensure that equipment is cleaned and sterilised, ready for the next client and to prevent cross-contamination.

Sterilising tools and equipment

Tools and equipment must be sterilised in an appropriate manner. Salon sterilisers consist of disinfectants, an autoclave and an ultraviolet (UV) light.

A common liquid disinfectant is Barbicide, but some salons may use sprays and wipes or even a bleach solution. Items suitable for a liquid disinfectant are placed in the solution for about 20 minutes; some chemicals will sterilise and destroy 'all' micro-organisms, whilst others will disinfect or sanitise by destroying 'most' micro-organisms.

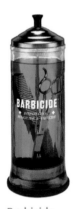

Barbicide

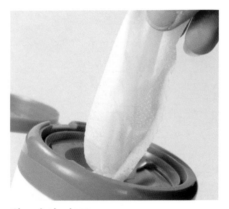

Chemical wipes

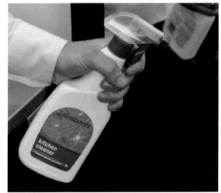

Chemical sprays

Autoclaves are the most effective method of sterilising. They use heat to steam clean and sterilise equipment, which usually takes about 20 minutes.

Sanitising using UV lights takes longer as the equipment needs to be placed in the cabinet for about 20–30 minutes and then turned over for a further 20–30 minutes. This method is effective only if used with cleaned sterile equipment and the equipment is turned properly.

Always wash brushes and combs with warm soapy water before sterilising them. A hair-covered brush will not be effectively sterilised after the UV light process and will look unprofessional and unclean. Also remove excess hair from scissors, clippers and razors prior to sterilising.

HANDY HINT

As a rule when cleaning, disinfecting and sterilising equipment and tools, clean with detergent and water, sterilise in an autoclave and disinfect with a chemical liquid or a UV light.

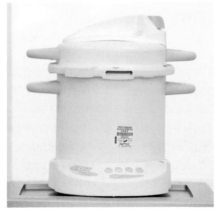

Autoclave

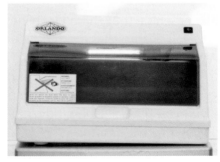

UV light cabinet

Sterilisers and their uses

Type of tools and equipment	Liquid disinfectant	Autoclave	UV light
Towels and gowns	Yes – in a washing machine at temperatures of 60–95°C	No	No
Combs, clips, plastic brushes and clipper attachments	Yes – Barbicide, sprays and wipes	Yes, although not all plastic equipment can withstand the heat of the autoclave	Yes
Wooden handled brushes	No	No	Yes
Scissors and razors	Yes	Yes, this method is the most suitable	Yes
Clippers	Yes – sprays and wipes only	No	Yes
Work surfaces	Yes – sprays and wipes	No	No

Head lice procedure

You should follow your salon's procedure if you suspect a client may have head lice. An example of this may be:

1 Always visually check the scalp before any service.

2 If you identify or suspect head lice, do not panic or draw any unwanted attention to your client.

3 Ask a senior member of staff to confirm your diagnosis.

4 Discuss the situation with your client somewhere quiet and discreet. Put them at ease and do not cause them any embarrassment.

5 Explain that you cannot treat the problem in the salon or offer any salon services until they have dealt with the infestation.

6 Rebook your client for a few days' time and offer advice on dealing with the infestation.

7 Sterilise all towels and gowns used for the consultation by boil washing them.

8 Clean all equipment used and sterilise for about an hour to ensure it is effective.

9 If you have already started work on the client's hair before you notice the infestation, complete this part of the service and stop the procedure when you are at a suitable point.

10 Inform your manager.

Head louse under the microscope

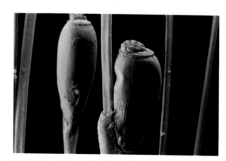

Nits (eggs) under the microscope

Comfort for you and the client

Both stylists and their assistants work long days and spend many hours standing, particularly when working on chemical treatments. It is very important you stand correctly to minimise fatigue and reduce the risk of injury caused by a bad posture. Poor posture can cause

WHY DON'T YOU…
Look up the other (Latinate) name for head lice.

back problems and long-term illness, so always stand with your feet slightly apart to maintain your balance and ensure your body weight is evenly distributed. Avoid overstretching or bending unnecessarily.

Client comfort is very important, especially as some services can take several hours to complete. To maintain your client's comfort, ensure their back is straight and supported against the back of the chair at all times throughout the service to prevent neck or back injury. This will also help you to maintain an even balance and meet the needs of the service.

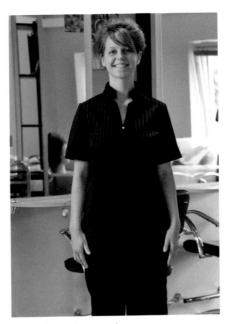
Correct way to stand

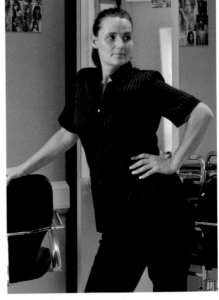
Incorrect way to stand

Always ensure that you position your equipment and trolley within easy reach for your comfort and to prevent fatigue. This will also enable you to work efficiently and save time, maintaining a professional image at all times.

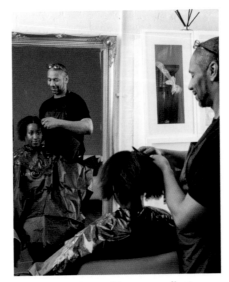
Correct way to position your client

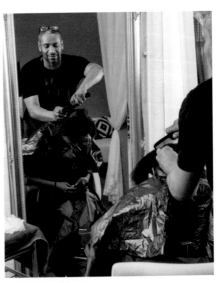
Incorrect way to position your client

THE CITY & GUILDS TEXTBOOK

Safe use of electrical equipment

Before using electrical items, ensure you check them visually for any cracks in the main body or plug. Check that the wires are tangle- and kink-free and not frayed or split. If you identify any problems or faults with the electrical equipment, make sure the equipment is safe to touch, isolate it from the electricity supply (switch off at the socket), remove it (if possible) from the salon, label it as faulty and report it to a senior member of staff.

For more information, refer to the Electricity at Work Regulations.

Adhering to instructions

To ensure the smooth running of the salon and to follow health and safety, it is of vital importance that you follow your workplace policies and those of the suppliers and manufacturers.

Workplace policies and instructions

Workplace policies are a collection of individual rules on several kinds of subjects and may include various policies on:

- how and where to mix up colours
- how and where you should do the salon laundry
- how you should meet, greet and treat clients
- how to behave in the salon
- how you must maintain the salon's hygiene
- how to dispose of the salon's waste.

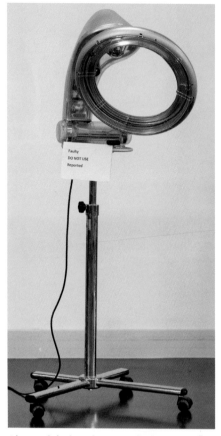

Always label and report faulty equipment

Activity

List as many of your workplace policies as you can.

Suppliers' and manufacturers' instructions

Your salon's representative or supplier may provide you with products, tools, equipment, salon fixtures and fittings as well as general salon supplies such as foil or salon towels. When you are using the tools and equipment it is important that you read any manufacturer instructions (MFIs) and follow the advice given by your supplier. Also follow the MFIs for advice on storing, handling, using and disposing (SHUD) of products.

Following instructions properly ensures that you use equipment correctly, which not only prolongs the life of the item, but also ensures the safety of yourself and others. Following the MFIs for products, such as colouring products, should ensure that the correct result is achieved and prevent any damage to the client's hair or skin.

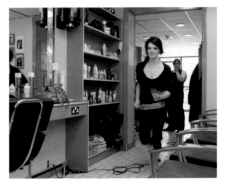

Never run in the salon

HANDY HINT

Read the 'Expected standards of behaviour' section of chapter CHB12 for more information.

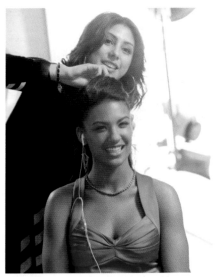

Be friendly and respectful

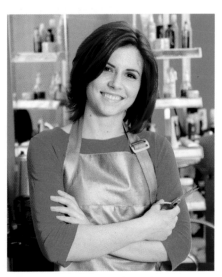

You are representing the salon

Behaviours

Behaviours are the way we conduct ourselves and perform in the workplace; they are the way we look after people and demonstrate our manners, they are the deeds we do, and how we carry out our activities on a day-to-day basis. The industry's expected behaviours are covered in this section of the chapter.

Meeting your salon's standards of behaviour

Your personal presentation and behaviour must protect the health and safety of both you and others. It must also meet with legal requirements and follow your workplace policy.

Your personal image reflects on your salon's professional image. Always ensure you are healthy for work and follow good standards of personal hygiene. Seek guidance from your manager before going to work if you have a potentially infectious condition, for example a cold, flu, eye infection or stomach bug.

Your behaviour should reflect the standard expected of you in the salon and reduce the risk of harm to yourself and others. You are representing your salon, and the image you give of yourself has an impact on the whole business. Always act professionally, speak politely to visitors and clients, and promote equality and diversity for all.

Greeting the client respectfully and in a friendly manner

When greeting clients always ensure you are friendly, courteous and respectful. Check whether the client has booked the appointment by their first name or surname and, if unsure, you should refer to them using their title and surname, until your client advises otherwise. Always be helpful and assist them with their coat: make them feel welcome and valued. Clients are visiting the salon for treatments, so the experience should be a treat.

Activity

At some point all of us have entered a shop and been poorly greeted by an uninterested staff member. Discuss with your colleagues how that made you feel, what was wrong with the service and whether you have since returned to that shop.

Communicating with clients

Salons are in a very fortunate position! More and more people are shopping online and customer service in many industries is therefore deteriorating. Your potential clients cannot get their hair cut and styled via the internet, so you have the potential for a long-lasting client base if you serve them well so that they want to return to you and not your competitor. All it takes is great customer service and a great hairdressing result.

> **HANDY HINT**
>
> Avoid discussing topics that involve politics, religion and faith, as some people have very strong views and opinions, and these topics could lead to a heated debate.

Establish effective rapport with clients

It is perfectly natural if you don't get on with everyone you meet! Personal beliefs and individual interests make people unique, but when it comes to working in the salon, you must work harmoniously with your colleagues and clients, and maintain a professional working relationship at all times.

As soon as a client walks through the door, you must make them feel valued and special. Conversations with your clients should be targeted around them, their interests and activities and, of course, their hair. Always try to engage your client in a neutral, friendly conversation, avoiding views on politics, religion and controversial subjects. Always show respect towards your client's views but minimise expressing your own opinions.

The small talk and personal details discussed with your client individualise the treatment you offer. Remembering small details of conversations from previous visits goes a long way to building a good **rapport** with your client.

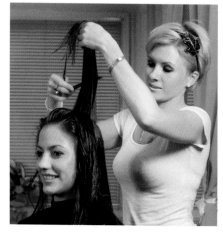

Establish a good rapport with clients

> **Rapport**
>
> A personal link or understanding between people.

Identifying and confirming the client's expectations

It is your responsibility to identify and confirm your client's requirements and expectations, and to decide if they're achievable. One of the great features of hairdressing is that not only is every head of hair different, so are your clients! Your clients will have a vision of what they are expecting the result to be; you need to take into consideration their hair type, features and lifestyle to decide the best way to achieve their vision.

Your clients are expecting advice on how to achieve the vision and maintain it. You need to consider the following:

- hair – the density, texture and hair type (abundant, coarse and curly, for instance)
- features – prominent ears, sharp jaw lines, etc.
- lifestyle – busy mothers, full-time workers or sporty.

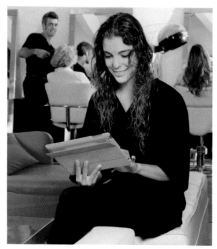

Images from the internet can shape the client's vision

Being courteous and helpful

It is important that you are always polite and courteous to your clients. Ask after their well-being, make them the focus of your conversation and be as helpful as possible. You must always provide them with aftercare advice, explain how to maintain their current style and colour, and make any recommendations for future services.

You should show them colour charts/swatches when discussing colours, images from magazines or the internet when discussing styles, and demonstrate the products and tools you used when styling their hair. Always offer a future appointment to your client and advise on costs of the services and how long the service will take.

Activity

What advice would you offer the following clients?

1 Mark (a keen motorcyclist) has fine straight hair and has just had a textured short haircut. He would like hair products that will not make the inside of his crash helmet oily. What products would you recommend?

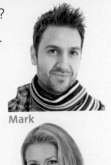
Mark

2 Jola (an office worker) has dry hair from swimming and colour services. She would like to improve the condition of her hair. What service would you recommend and why?

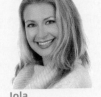
Jola

Keeping the client informed

Throughout the service you must always keep your client informed of what you are doing and why. You should confirm the service before you begin, explain what products you are using and why, clarify the amount of length you are taking off before you cut the hair, and talk your client through any colour or chemical service you are carrying out. This will ensure your client is put at ease during the service, reassure them if they have any concerns and it will give them an opportunity to ask any questions.

Responding to different client behaviours

On a day-to-day basis you will encounter a variety of clients, all with different needs. It is important that you are able to respond positively to every question and comment your clients may have. It is said that behaviour breeds behaviour: if you encounter an angry client who is talking to you in a raised voice, you must not match their behaviour and raise yours. Always remain calm, non-defensive and polite.

Types of client and how to deal with potential problems

Type of client	Potential problem	How to deal with it
Confident and bubbly	Asking for services in a way that indicates they know more than they do. Might not be open to listening to your ideas.	■ Express your advice clearly with detailed explanations of why you recommend certain services. ■ Use open questions to clarify their requirements.
Shy and nervous	May not explain their requirements clearly.	■ Make your recommendations suitable for the client needs. ■ Use open questions to clarify their requirements.
Early arrival	The salon may not be able to carry out the service before the allocated appointment.	■ Check whether the stylist can accommodate an early client. ■ See if another stylist is available. ■ Explain the outcome to the client and offer refreshments if the client chooses to wait.
Late arrival	There might not be time to carry out the service and the client may need to rebook.	■ Ask the stylist if they can accommodate the late client. ■ Check whether another stylist can accommodate the client. ■ Offer an alternative service that suits the time allocations. ■ Offer to rebook the client.
Angry	The client may raise their voice and upset you. They may cause a scene in the salon and other clients may overhear.	■ Remain calm and polite. ■ Don't get defensive but stay objective. ■ Don't raise your voice. ■ Move the client to a discreet area if possible. ■ Refer the complaint to your manager and explain clearly to the client what you are doing and why.
Confused	There is potential for the service requirements not to be met if the client is confused.	■ Look at your client's body language and use open and closed questions to identify which areas need further discussion or advice.
Limited mobility or mobility impaired	Access to all salon areas may be difficult. A client may be offended if you treat them unfairly.	■ Always follow the Disability Discrimination Act (see https://www.gov.uk/rights-disabled-person/overview) and treat clients fairly. ■ Don't patronise disabled clients. ■ Don't assume someone needs help but ask if they require any.
Hearing impaired	Clients may struggle to understand or hear you clearly over the background noise. Potential for misunderstandings.	■ Ensure you speak face to face to aid lip-reading. ■ Use visual aids to clarify understanding. ■ Reduce background noise where possible. ■ Speak clearly but don't shout.

Type of client	Potential problem	How to deal with it
Vision impaired	The client may not see potential hazards in the salon.	■ Offer guidance to the client when moving around the salon. ■ Make them aware of any steps or hazards ahead and move obstacles where possible. ■ Speak clearly to guide them to your voice and where you are.
Non-fluent English speakers	Misunderstandings	■ Speak clearly, using non-technical terms. ■ Keep the language style simple. ■ Use images, visual aids or write down what you are suggesting.

Activity

How would you deal with a client who asks why their appointment is running late?

Activity

Describe the signs of an angry client and those of a confused client.

Activity

Some religions and faiths prevent women from having their head or hair uncovered in front of men. With a colleague, research faiths and religions, and identify any that may affect hairdressing services. Why is it useful for you to have a basic understanding of faiths and religions?

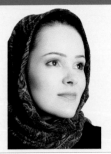

HANDY HINT

Remember to treat all clients equally and respect the diversity of the clients in your salon.

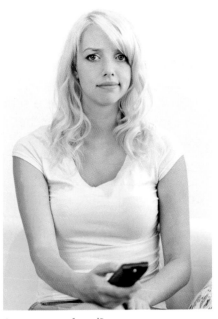

Angry or confused?

Promptly assisting the client

You will need to respond to your clients' needs in a variety of situations, such as at reception when booking appointments, during a consultation and throughout the service. Clients will also seek advice on aftercare and recommendations on retail products for maintaining the style between visits. Always ensure you work within the limits of your own authority and refer to a senior staff member or your manager for guidance when needed.

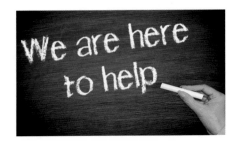

We are here to help

Communicating appropriately

You must be able to communicate with many different types of client: children, young adults, middle-aged and older clients. Each type of client needs to be addressed differently.

The table below shows how you might adapt your style of conversation and behaviour with each type of client, but remember that everyone is different so you should always be ready to change your approach.

How to adapt your conversation and behaviour appropriately

Children	Young adults	Middle-aged clients	Older clients
Talk to the child to put them at ease. You should keep your tone light and friendly; most young children do not like having their hair cut. Try to make the experience fun and behave in an informal manner. Avoid technical terms and grown-up words. Explain what you are doing every step of the way.	A more informal approach could work well with young adults to relax them, and the friendly atmosphere you create will encourage them to return. Explain what you are doing and why, and offer ideas on how to style their look in various ways to maximise their style.	Middle-aged clients expect a good customer service and are more likely to remain loyal to the salon. They may be confident in expressing their wishes and articulating exactly what they want. Ensure you listen carefully and advise alternative options if their requests are not the most suitable.	Older people may be used to old-fashioned values and customer service. Always remain respectful and a little more formal. If an older client has mobility or hearing problems, be sensitive and helpful at all times. Older clients tend to be happiest returning to a regular stylist and building a solid relationship. Some personal chat about their families often goes down well.

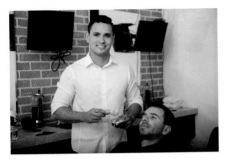

Understand your client's expectations before you start

Checking the client's expectations

You must check that your client fully understands what you are advising for their hair and that you have understood your client's requirements.

Use open and closed questions to check each other's understanding. Open questions start with 'what', 'why', 'how' and 'when' and give you the detail required. Closed questions are answered with a 'yes' or 'no' and can help to confirm what is being requested.

Always read your client's body language and look for signs of uncertainty. If your client is rubbing their neck or behind their ears, it is a sign that they are unsure and further advice/discussion is required.

Promptly and positively responding to questions and comments

It is important that you respond to your client's questions and comments promptly, positively and professionally to ensure your customer service is of a high standard.

Your client may have questions about the service being carried out, future services or products; ensure you answer these questions honestly and in a positive manner.

It is always easy to respond to positive feedback from a client but some comments may not be positive. A client may be unhappy for several reasons such as:

- the time he or she had to wait for their appointment
- the time the service took
- the end result of a hair cut or colour
- the cost of the service
- the behaviour of the stylist or other staff.

When you have to deal with negative comments you must respond in a professional manner at all times. Try to resolve the issue promptly, apologise where necessary and make any necessary arrangements to rectify the issue as soon as you can. Any comments that become complaints should be reported to your manager.

Allowing the client time to respond

Before you commence with any service, ensure your client has been given the time to consider their responses and clarify their needs. Always allow additional time if your client is still unsure and offer further information if required. You must never talk over your client and should use jargon-free language when discussing services and products to help your client understand what is being suggested to them. Listen to your client and nod or repeat what is being said so they are clear you have understood.

If your client is thinking of having a new service in the future or has expressed an interest in purchasing some products, allow them time during the service to consider the benefits. Towards the end of the service, revisit the conversation, show them the products used and repeat the benefits to the client.

Let the client respond

Quickly locating information

You must always ensure that the salon systems for information are easily accessible to you. Clients require effective responses to their questions and you must be able to locate this information quickly.

If your client requires information regarding appointment times and availability, ensure the reception is tidy and the appointment book and appointment cards are available.

A price list for services and retail products should be available to clients.

Deal with any clients' complaints politely and swiftly. If your manager needs to contact the client, ensure you have all the relevant contact details and have taken notes about the nature of the complaint.

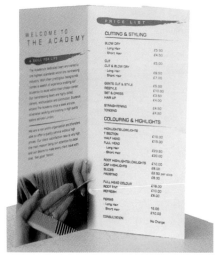

Have appointment cards and price lists to hand

> **HANDY HINT**
>
> Always give appropriate and accurate information to your clients.

Providing information about services and products

It is important that you are aware of all the services and products your salon offers. One client may see another client receiving a service or buying a product and enquire what it is. It is part of your job role and as well as being the client's expectation that you can provide them with relevant information and advice.

You should keep a price list to hand, as this lists the services your salon offers and the prices charged. You should also attend any salon training regarding new products and services to ensure you are well informed and can advise your clients effectively.

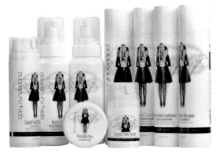

Products for clients to use at home

Activity

1 Identify two or three products that you have not used for a while; read the manufacturers' instructions on how to use each product and research the features and benefits to the client for using these products.

2 Identify any services that you have limited knowledge of, and ask your salon managers or peers to explain them to you.

Recognising complicated information and checking understanding

Check your client understands what has been decided by using open and closed questions to clarify what has been discussed and agreed. If the information is complicated, ensure you use non-technical language that is jargon-free.

Information that your clients require needs to be communicated quickly and effectively. Complicated information should be checked for a clear understanding and the reasons why client expectations can't be met must be explained.

HANDY HINT

Open questions require the client to give a more in-depth answer and may start with 'why' or 'how'. Closed questions help to confirm and define details as they are answered with one-word responses like 'yes' or 'no'.

Activity

You have used the explanation below to describe a process to your client and she looks confused. Reword the explanation into client-friendly words that she will understand.

'OK, Sheila. As you have seborrhoea, I am going to shampoo your hair using a gentle rotary massage technique to avoid activating the sebaceous glands.'

Explaining why client expectations cannot be met

Sadly, some clients attend the salon expecting a treatment to be carried out, but a consultation and relevant tests prove that the required service cannot be carried out. For example, a client may want a permanent colour service but the results of an elasticity test show that the hair is too weak. It is essential that you explain to your client why a service can't be carried out and you should suggest alternatives. Speak clearly, be polite and give the appropriate detail. Remain professional and objective as to why the client's expectations can't be met.

Explain why any services cannot be carried out

Activity

List some examples of services that clients might expect but which can't be carried out due to the results of tests or the consultation. How would you explain this to your client?

Answers in the back of the book.

1 What does the term 'values' mean?

   a Morals and ethics

   b Ethnicity and religion

   c Culture and age groups

   d Possessions and money

2 Which one of the following is the best way to deal with a client with different values?

   a Avoid talking to them so that they don't get upset

   b Ask detailed questions to try to understand them

   c Debate with them and try to change their minds

   d Respect them and adapt to their needs

3 Why is it important to have commercially viable timescales for working?

   a To make sure the salon operates smoothly

   b To make sure the salon closes on time

   c To make sure all clients are satisfied

   d To make sure no clients turn up late

4 Why is it important to wear minimal jewellery when working in a salon?

   a It can be uncomfortable to wear for long periods

   b It can tangle in the hair and cause dermatitis

   c It looks unprofessional

   d It causes allergies

5 **Statement one**

   It is recommended that layers of clothing are worn at work to regulate heat and minimise body odour.

   Statement two

   Shoes should be comfortable and have open toes to keep feet cool.

   Which one of the following is correct for the above statements?

   a True   True

   b True   False

   c False   True

   d False   False

6 Which one of the following is the best way for a stylist to avoid contact dermatitis?

   a Keeping nails short and neat

   b Rinsing hands after each client

   c Wearing gloves for wet work

   d Applying hand cream every night

7 Why is it important to have a flexible working attitude?

   a To secure a pay rise

   b To keep the salon busy

   c To work under pressure

   d To meet changing demands

8 Which one of the following is the best action to take when a stylist is running late?

   a Explain the situation to the client that is waiting

   b Tell the next client to come back when it is not so busy

   c Put a gown on the next client to encourage them to stay

   d Expect that the client can see what is happening and will understand

9 Which two of the following best describe the term 'self-manager'?

  1 Being the first in the salon every day

  2 Taking ownership of responsibilities

  3 Being flexible

  4 Working quickly

  a 1 and 2

  b 2 and 3

  c 3 and 4

  d 4 and 1

10 Which one of the following describes creativity?

  a Working well with others and using their ideas

  b Having good ideas and acting upon them

  c Being imaginative

  d Asking questions

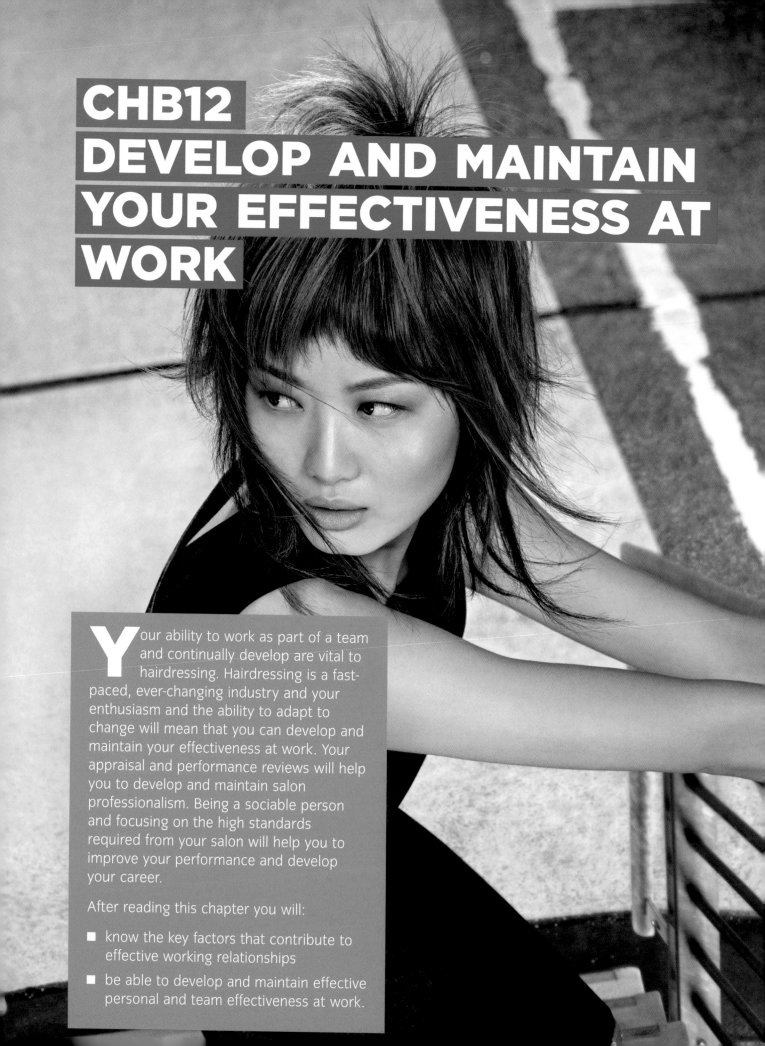

CHB12
DEVELOP AND MAINTAIN YOUR EFFECTIVENESS AT WORK

Your ability to work as part of a team and continually develop are vital to hairdressing. Hairdressing is a fast-paced, ever-changing industry and your enthusiasm and the ability to adapt to change will mean that you can develop and maintain your effectiveness at work. Your appraisal and performance reviews will help you to develop and maintain salon professionalism. Being a sociable person and focusing on the high standards required from your salon will help you to improve your performance and develop your career.

After reading this chapter you will:

- know the key factors that contribute to effective working relationships

- be able to develop and maintain effective personal and team effectiveness at work.

Key factors contributing to effective working relationships

Salon and legal requirements

Your job role and responsibilities

Everyone has a role to play in the salon. It is important that everyone works together to achieve the salon's objectives and enable the salon to work effectively. You'll need to know the job roles of your colleagues in order to understand how your own role works alongside theirs.

The flow chart below is an example of how staff might be structured in a salon:

HANDY HINT

To help you identify how your job role relates to others, ask your manager what the responsibilities of each person in the team are. For larger salons or corporate businesses, this information may also be given in the company handbook or available via Human Resources (HR).

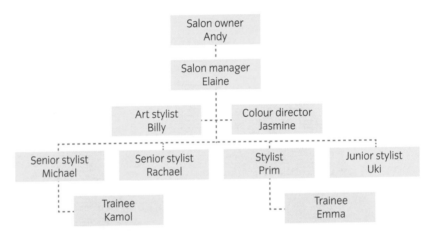

Activity

Complete a salon organisation chart for your salon and its staff and explain how your role relates to those of the other team members.

To improve your personal performance at work you need to be clear on your job role objectives. These should be clearly stated in your contract of employment, to enable you to help achieve the salon's performance objectives.

Employment contract

An employment contract would ideally be issued to you when you start working at the salon. A contract is a legally binding document that sets out working guidelines. This information may also be given to employees in a written statement, in a job offer letter or in an employee handbook.

Salon staff

If you were issued with a contract of employment it is likely that it would include:

- your name and job title
- an outline of your roles and responsibilities
- who you report to
- your start date at the salon
- your address and contact details
- your days of work
- your hours of work
- your holiday allowance
- the sick pay agreement
- the maternity/paternity agreement
- the appraisal and review procedures
- the period of notice agreement
- disciplinary, appeals and **grievance** procedures
- the pension scheme
- your pay, how often you are paid (weekly or monthly) and how you are paid (cash, cheque or bank transfer).

Grievance

Cause for complaint.

Your contract may also include any special arrangements agreed for you by the salon – this could be time off for training, medical appointments or agreements for other employment alongside your salon job.

Your job description

Along with your contract of employment, your job description will give you information about your specific job role, your responsibilities and the standards expected of you. It is likely to be updated more often than your contract and should be reviewed at each appraisal or whenever your job role changes. The job description document outlines your roles and responsibilities, to help you achieve the company objectives.

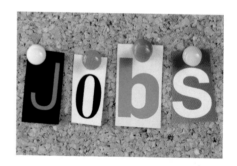

It is likely to include:

- your name
- who you directly report to
- the main overview of the salon's objectives
- your roles and responsibilities
- general roles and responsibilities that affect every employee, such as working in accordance with the salon's health and safety policy, equal opportunities policy and maintaining the confidentiality of the salon's information

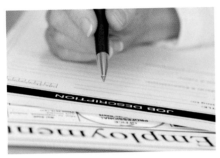

Employment contract

HANDY HINT

You should ensure that you receive and keep a copy of your contract of employment and your job description.

VALUES & BEHAVIOURS

Refer to the values and behaviours chapter for more information on the following values:

- willingness to learn
- flexible working attitudes
- the ability to self-manage
- personal and professional ethics
- positive attitudes.

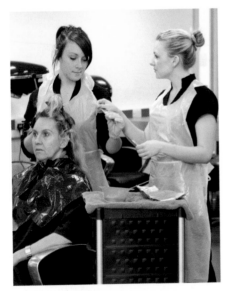

Working together

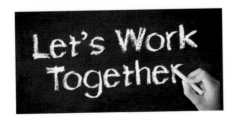

- who you may deal with on a day-to-day basis
- any people you are responsible for.

Both your contract and your job description should be signed by you and your manager and are legally binding documents. At your appraisal or review you and your manager should check whether your job description is still current or whether it needs updating. Your roles and responsibilities may change as you develop and take on extra responsibilities.

Other people's areas of responsibility

There will be elements of other people's job roles and their responsibilities that you will need to know about. Your manager or supervisor should inform you of the whole team's roles as an overview, so you know how everyone's roles interlink. There may be team members that are responsible for your training and progression too.

Activity

Identify two staff members at your workplace and explain their job roles and how they link to yours.

Assisting others

Always ensure that you work within the limits of your authority. You may assist your colleagues on a one-to-one basis, helping one staff member for long periods of time, or supporting the whole team as a group. Working outside your limitations could cause accidents or result in dissatisfied clients and have further insurance implications. It may result in you facing disciplinary action, as you have not followed your salon's policies or your job description.

Identifying your own strengths and weaknesses

It is as important to identify your strengths as it is to be aware of your weaknesses or areas to develop.

There are several ways in which you can identify your strengths and weaknesses:

- listening to those around you
- peer review and feedback
- client feedback
- manager feedback (appraisals reviews, etc.)
- self-reflection
- online test.

Your strengths are often things you are naturally good at, things you enjoy or are confident doing, or something you have a skill in. When you have identified your strengths it is important to continue to develop these skills and to maintain them as strengths.

Weaknesses can be things you struggle to do, that don't motivate or inspire you or where your skills need to be developed. We go through life learning from our mistakes, and acknowledging mistakes is an important part of life and learning. Don't be too hard on yourself or self-critical but do seek to improve and embrace change.

Activity

List four personal and professional strengths and weaknesses.

Consider how you are going to maintain your strengths and develop your weaker areas. Who could help you to develop? Consider your communication, English and maths skills too, and identify whether these are strengths or areas to develop too.

Expected standards of behaviour

You must ensure that you maintain a professional image at work: avoid bad language and shouting, don't eat or drink in the salon or in front of clients, and never gossip about colleagues, other clients or the business.

You may find that you and your clients or colleagues have very different opinions; you should avoid expressing yours. Let the client voice their opinion; if it has the potential to offend you, move the conversation forward and to a different topic.

You should avoid discussing your personal problems with clients and leave all personal issues at home. The client might use you as a 'counsellor' and tell you all their woes but they are paying for your service and you should therefore not discuss your problems with them.

Appeals and grievance procedures

If you find yourself in a disciplinary position, have a grievance or need to complain or appeal about a decision or situation, you should refer to your company handbook and/or your salon procedures.

Disciplinary procedures

The reason for the disciplinary action and the required procedure should be clearly explained to you. It is essential that salon staff follow a set procedure for any disciplinary action and that all meetings and discussions are documented. Employees can take their case to a tribunal or court, so documented evidence will be required.

HANDY HINT

Failing to work within your job responsibilities could:

- cause disruptions to the general running of the salon
- cause accidents or injuries
- result in disciplinary action.

HANDY HINT

Always help and support your colleagues willingly but be sure to work within your capabilities.

VALUES & BEHAVIOURS

Refer to the values and behaviours chapter for more information on team work and maintaining customer care.

HANDY HINT

Clients are always clients, so even if you become friends, always remain professional. Make sure that all correspondence is professional too. The use of good English spoken and written skills is very important in the workplace.

VALUES & BEHAVIOURS

Avoid discussing politics, religion and controversial subjects, as some people have very strong opinions and these subjects could lead to a heated debate. If conversations become too personal, threatening or problematic, try to move the conversation to neutral topics or seek guidance from your manager.

VALUES & BEHAVIOURS

Refer to the values and behaviours chapter for more information on behaviours expected in the salon environment.

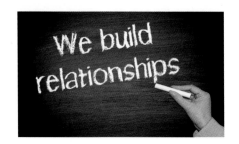

The written procedure should include:

- the nature of the disciplinary offence
- what the disciplinary and dismissal procedures are, and who is involved in dealing with it
- the appeals procedure and who to contact if you are unhappy with the outcome.

Depending on the nature of the disciplinary offence, the outcomes can vary from a verbal warning to a written warning, a final written warning and, ultimately, dismissal. Your salon should offer you support and further training to help avoid the outcome being dismissal.

Grievance procedures

Your salon's policy on grievance procedures should outline who you should refer your grievance concerns to and how to make a grievance application. If you have any concerns or relationship issues with other staff members, you should document all conversations and situations as they occur. This will enable you to have a clear, accurate record that you can present in your grievance application.

Appeals procedure

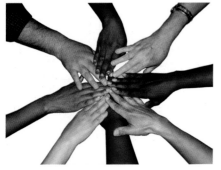

Teamwork

If an outcome of a disciplinary meeting leads to verbal or written warnings or your dismissal, you have a right to appeal against the salon's decision. You will need to submit your appeal request in writing to the manager or owner and follow the salon's procedures for appealing.

If you are appealing against a decision or outcome and submit a written appeal, make sure the spelling, punctuation and grammar are correct and that it is professionally written or typed.

Target-setting and personal performance

Continuing professional development

To help you progress in your job role, you may need further training or further professional development. Continuing professional development (CPD) is very important in the hairdressing industry as client requirements change as often as the fashions and trends do, so you need to keep up with the times.

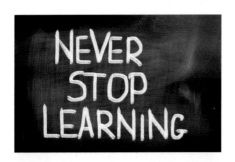

Reasons for continuing professional development:

- to achieve job satisfaction
- to keep up to date with client requirements
- to be aware of product updates and legislation

- to develop your skills
- to provide assistance to others
- to help you gain promotion
- to gain the potential to earn more money
- for career development.

National Occupational Standards

To help you know and identify your personal development targets, you could refer to the National Occupational Standards (NOS), written by the Hair and Beauty Industry Authority (Habia). They state what is required for the industry; they set the NVQ training standards and can provide you with a clear structure and pathway which allow for natural progression. You can access information on the National Occupational Standards via the internet at www.habia.org.

Awareness of current needs

Your awareness of the industry needs and your own current needs are your responsibility too. You cannot expect your manager to hold your hand throughout your career development; some actions are required by you. You should want to update your skills and be prepared to stay late to attend some training evenings or product update sessions. The new skills you learn help you to earn more money and progress in your career.

To maintain industry awareness:

- attend seminars and workshop activities
- update skills through CPD
- read trade and fashion magazines
- carry out internet and literature-based research
- attend fashion and trade shows
- subscribe to e-learning for example, www.myhairdressers.com.

Who can help you identify your development and training needs?

Always ask the relevant people to help you with opportunities to learn. You can obtain help from your manager, the salon trainer and your colleagues. Help does not have to come just from your senior staff members – it could be from a **peer**. If you or your colleagues are good at something, show each other, learn from each other and share good practice.

WHY DON'T YOU...
Think of some activities you would like to complete for CPD.

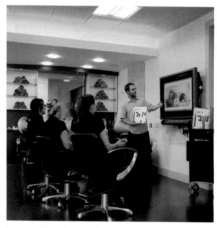
Professional development seminar

Peer

One of the same rank or position.

HANDY HINT

If there is no opportunity for training, you must discuss this with the relevant person. Your career progression depends on learning new skills.

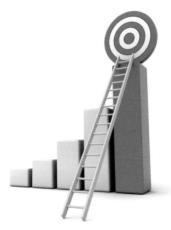

Reach your targets

Your personal development and productivity targets and timescales

Setting your own personal targets and agreeing developmental targets with your manager are important for you to advance and grow in your job role. A review of your progress is vital if you want to develop and progress. You need to know what your peers and more importantly your manager think of your performance.

Appraisals and reviews

All companies and salons will have different appraisal processes but as a guide you should expect a yearly appraisal with more frequent reviews.

When you are a new employee at the salon, your progress may be reviewed monthly for the first few months to check how you are getting on and identify any training needs. Once you are settled into your role, you may have an appraisal yearly. It is important to remember that appraisals are a two-way communication. Your manager will review your progress but you should also assess the salon's support and training given.

An appraisal should never be feared: it should be seen as a positive experience. You should be given a couple of weeks' notice of the appraisal time and date. During this time you should have a chance to review the appraisal pack and complete your areas or write notes that you wish to discuss at the meeting. Once you return your appraisal pack to your manager, a few days should be allowed for them to read it and prepare for the meeting.

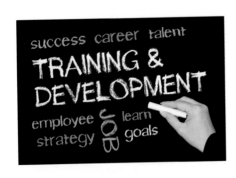

If, between your appraisals and reviews, you have received positive feedback, your appraisal should be positive. If you have been reprimanded, for example for time-keeping or performance, then you should expect this to be addressed in your appraisal.

Your appraisal will:

- prepare you for the future, set clear achievable targets and personal goals
- review past performance
- establish where you are now.

Your appraisal should help you to identify your strengths and the areas in which you need to develop. When you and your manager review your past performance you should expect discussions to take place on the following areas, which may be graded.

HANDY HINT

Always remember that the appraisals and reviews are a two-way process and you should be actively involved with agreeing your past performance and your future targets.

Activity

Using the 'Areas to grade during the appraisal process' table, grade yourself on each area and list any areas you need to improve.

Areas to grade during the appraisal process

Areas to grade	Staff grade (your self-assessment)	Manager grade (your manager's assessment of you)
Time-keeping and punctuality		
Attendance		
Appearance		
Ability to work effectively in a team		
Ability to use own initiative		
Relationships with other staff members		
Performance in job role		

Grade 1 – Excellent   Grade 2 – Good   Grade 3 – Satisfactory   Grade 4 – Unsatisfactory

Prior to the meeting you should check if you have met all your previous targets, and, if not, plan to discuss why these have not been achieved. Some targets may not have been met because your job role changed and the target was no longer relevant, or because the salon did not allow you time off for training. Other targets may not have been met because you have not put in enough effort and you should prepare to discuss the reasons for this during the meeting.

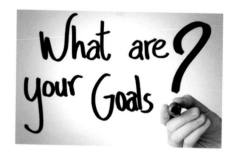

The next stage of the process will be reviewing your current performance against your job description and discussing any areas that you have worked well in or found difficult.

Stage two of the review is to establish:

- where you are now
- what you have achieved
- how you have developed
- whether or not you are ready to take on more responsibility
- whether or not you need more training.

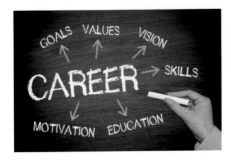

When you are preparing for the meeting, think about:

- what you want
- your personal goals
- what further training would help you to progress
- whether you find any areas difficult
- what your manager or the salon could do to make you more effective at work.

The final part of your appraisal is to plan for the future, your targets and goals. This will also include what your manager wants you to do to help the salon achieve its objectives and increase profitability.

You should both agree on your future development plan and set some targets. These are often referred to as SMARTER targets.

- **S**pecific to your job role and clearly defined
- **M**easurable in achievement
- **A**greed by both parties
- **R**ealistic to achieve and relevant to your role and ability
- **T**ime-bound – the targets should be achieved by a particular date
- **E**valuated – a date will be agreed to evaluate progress
- **R**eviewed – a date will be agreed to review the outcomes or retarget if necessary

During your appraisal it is important that you're positive and you listen to what your manager has to say; make some notes if you want to, and ask questions if you do not understand something. At the end of the appraisal you should receive a written copy of what has been discussed and agreed to keep for your own records.

Using and updating your own personal plan

You may need a review meeting to discuss the progress of your targets and generally assess your position in the salon. These meetings could be formal review meetings or discussions at monthly or bi-monthly intervals.

At these meetings you should discuss with your manager your progress, any identified training needs, and any issues that you have or areas that need to be addressed.

You should continually identify your emerging strengths but also areas to develop in order to progress and encourage personal growth and development. The feedback you receive at these meetings could arise from your manager, your peers and also from client comments from a variety of situations, such as your appraisal, training sessions or your day-to-day work.

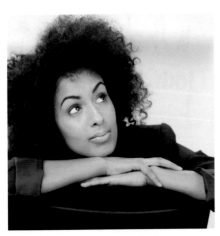

Think about your personal plan

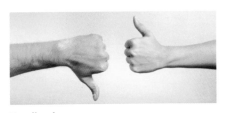

Feedback

If you fail to meet any set targets, not only may you feel demotivated, demoralised and lose your reputation, but there could be further implications too.

You personally could undergo disciplinary proceedings, you may be demoted or miss out on commission or bonuses. If you receive a negative appraisal, you may receive negative comments from colleagues, especially if team targets have not been met because of you.

Your manager sets targets for you in order to maintain and achieve the salon objectives; failure to achieve your targets will have an effect on the salon as a whole. There may be a loss of profits, the business might fail or, if it's a **limited company**, its share price may fall. The team's morale could be lowered because of resentment and the salon could lose clients.

Limited company

A company that has shareholders.

Activity

Work targets may be set as an incremental target once achieved. If you were given three targets and each one was worth £250 on top of your salary, once achieved how much more money would you would now earn a year?

Often these targets are pro rata, which means if you work five days you would get £250 but you would only achieve ⅗ of this if you worked three days a week. How much would these three targets be respectively if you achieved them but only worked two days, three days or four days a week?

Managing your time effectively

To enable you to manage your time effectively, you must be aware of the service times for all your salon appointments and check the salon appointment bookings regularly throughout the day.

Always try to plan your day ahead, work out what your daily priorities are and focus on these. If you are very busy, avoid wasting time on less urgent tasks that can wait until tomorrow or be delegated to someone else.

It may help you to create a to-do list or chart for the day's activities, highlighting your jobs in order of priority. A week-per-page diary would enable you to plan tasks for less busy days. For example, if you need to maintain the stock levels and complete an order, you should do this as soon as you can and before a busy Saturday when stocks will get even lower.

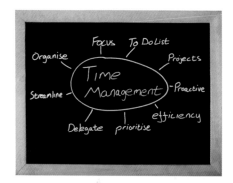

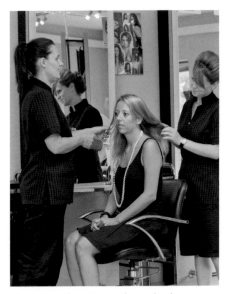

Work together to produce the best results for your client

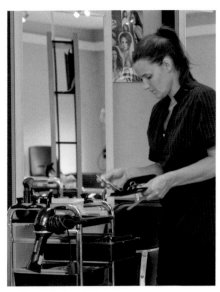

Prepare for the day ahead

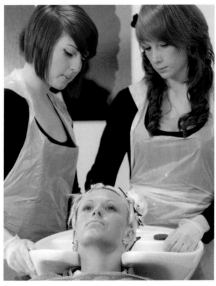

Assist each other and ask your peers for advice if needed

Timely performance of hairdressing services

Activity

Complete the table below comparing the average salon allocated time for services against your salon's service times.

Service	Guide for commercially viable time	Salon commercially viable time
CH1 – Style and finish hair		
Blow dry above the shoulders	30 minutes	
Blow dry below the shoulders	30–45 minutes	
CH2 – Set and dress hair		
Above-shoulder wet set	30 minutes	
Below-shoulder wet set	45–60 minutes	
Below-shoulder dry set	30 minutes	
CH3 – Cut hair using basic techniques		
Wet cut	30 minutes	
Restyle	45 minutes	
CB2 – Cut men's hair using basic techniques	30 minutes	
CB3 – Cut facial hair to shape using basic techniques	15 minutes	

Activity (continued)

Service	Guide for commercially viable time	Salon commercially viable time
CH4 – Colour and lighten hair		
Semi-permanent colour	20–30 minutes	
Quasi-permanent colour	20–30 minutes	
Regrowth tint	30 minutes	
Full-head colour	30–45 minutes	
Pulled-through highlights	30–60 minutes	
Woven highlights	60–90 minutes	
CH5 – Perm and neutralise hair		
Full-head perm wind	45 minutes	
Partial-head perm wind	30 minutes	
CH6 – Plait and twist hair		
Full-head cornrows	60–90 minutes	
Partial-head flat twists	30–45 minutes	
Plait	15–30 minutes	
CH7 – Temporarily attach hair to enhance a style		
Clip-on or grip-in method	Up to an hour	
Bonding or fusing method	Up to 2 hours or more	

Activity

If you spent all day completing below-the-shoulder blow drys, how many could you do in one day? Using your salon price list, how much money would you bring into the salon? Compare this with a whole day of wet cuts.

VALUES & BEHAVIOURS

Refer to the values and behaviours chapter for more information on completion of services in a commercially viable time.

Working with others

Salon teamwork is very important. It provides a professional working environment and promotes team spirit and harmonious working conditions. Through team meetings and effective communication the salon staff should all agree on ways of working together to help achieve the salon's objectives. It is also vital that you use your time at work effectively to enable you to carry out your daily duties.

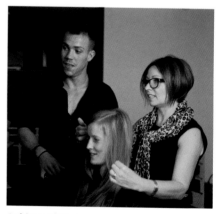

Asking advice

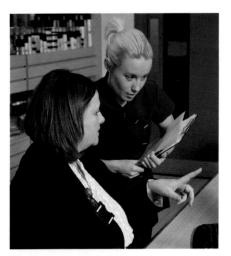

Always be polite when asking colleagues to help you

HANDY HINT

Working harmoniously relies on everyone working together as one. It is very important that everyone communicates clearly with each other so that every one has a clear understanding of what is required.

HANDY HINT

Sometimes, when you face a disagreement with a colleague, you just have to agree to disagree. The workplace is diverse and everybody is different, has different views and expresses them differently.

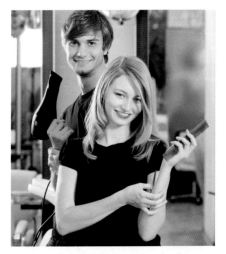

Try to anticipate the needs of others to keep the salon running smoothly

Working harmoniously with others

It is essential that everyone is polite and respectful to each other in the workplace. You will not get on with everyone you work with, but you must act professionally at all times. If your clients think that you don't work well within your team, they may feel uncomfortable and the salon may get a bad reputation. Sadly, some salons already have a reputation for being 'catty' and 'spiteful'; help to change this reputation, don't add to it. Be friendly and courteous at all times.

When you're working with your colleagues and one of you needs assistance, be polite and open, have trust that you will support each other for the salon's benefit and those working in it. Be enthusiastic when helping others and show that you are flexible and a real team player.

As you become more experienced and confident in your role, you will be able to anticipate the needs of others and promptly offer support even before they ask.

Co-operative ways

The day-to-day salon business requires all staff to be supportive of one another and to work in collaboration. Always find co-operative ways of working such as anticipating the needs of others and sharing information which could help your team members. Offer your full support and, if necessary, show that you are willing to help resolve disagreements.

Difficulties in working with others

Working all day in a busy and sometimes strained atmosphere can be demotivating. If you encounter relationship problems you must deal with them effectively to prevent the situation from escalating. You might need to be assertive at times to get your point across so as not to be ignored. However, you should always treat people in the same manner as you would wish to be treated.

Activity

Imagine a colleague has upset you at work. Their lack of organisation has caused the salon to run behind and you are now working extra late on a Saturday night to catch up. How would you explain to this person why you are upset with them whilst making sure you were calm and not rude? Practise this explanation with a colleague – being assertive but remaining polite and professional.

Disagreements

If you have a disagreement with a work colleague, try to follow the following guidelines.

1 If you have a disagreement with a colleague, try to sort it out sooner rather than later. Show a willingness to resolve the disagreement and communicate your concerns clearly, without added drama or malice.

2 If you and the individual can't resolve the situation on your own, then you need to refer the problem to your manager and ask for help.

3 A meeting at the end of the day between the two of you and your manager could be the best way forward to air your views.

4 During the meeting, ensure that you remain calm and avoid raising your voice. Issues often arise from misunderstandings, so when it's your colleague's time to talk, it is essential that you listen to the other person's view and don't interrupt them. As you have asked your manager for help, be sure to listen to their view of the situation.

5 When it is your turn to speak, diplomatically and constructively air your grievance, and make suggestions about how the situation could be resolved.

6 If you need to challenge your colleague or ask further questions to aid your understanding of the situation, use open and closed questions that are relevant and show that you are listening to their views by using effective body language, such as maintaining eye contact, nodding in agreement and smiling.

7 If the situation doesn't have an amicable outcome, you may need to refer to the company handbook and the grievance procedure.

A relaxed and friendly environment to work in is more motivating, helps to maintain the team spirit and ensures good communication between staff. Clients will feel happier visiting a friendly salon, and the professional image is maintained.

Reacting positively to reviews and feedback

It is important that you react positively to all feedback, even to comments that are not positive about your performance! Feedback helps you to learn and identify your strengths and your areas to develop. Reacting positively to all feedback is important for you to grow and realise your full potential.

You may receive feedback from the following:

■ Clients – they will regularly feed back on their satisfaction on their hair, but you can guarantee that at some point in your career, you

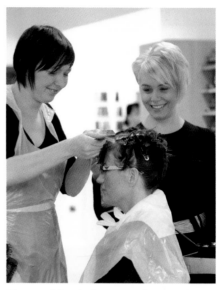
Always strive to be a good team player

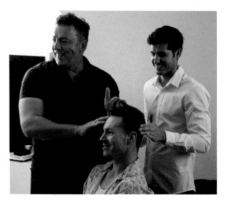
Helping colleagues promotes a harmonious working environment

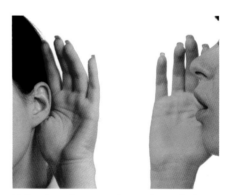
Listen to other people's points of view

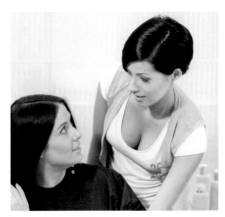

Question and listen

will receive some criticism from clients about their hair and the end result not meeting their expectations.

■ Your peers – they will feed back on your day-to-day performance and if you're not pulling your weight in the salon and being a team player, they will criticise your performance.

■ Other stylists – they will offer feedback on your function within the team and the impact your performance has on the salon and their job role.

■ Your manager – they will also feed back to you and critique your performance, letting you know if they are happy with your standards of work and behaviour.

Questioning and listening skills

You will need to find out lots of information when working in the salon: information from your clients about their hair and their needs; information from colleagues – how you can help and support them and what they need you to do; and information from your manager to ascertain what tasks and services they require you to carry out through out the day.

Here's how to have great questioning and listening skills:

■ ask open questions to gain detail

■ ask closed questions to confirm requirements

■ listen carefully to instructions and detail

■ ask questions to clarify any uncertainty

■ confirm your understanding.

Develop and maintain personal and team effectiveness at work – review

Identify personal strengths and weaknesses

During your assessment you will need to be able to identify your own strengths and weaknesses, and discuss them professionally with your manager, supervisor or perhaps a trainer – a person relevant to you, your salon and your training and development plan.

You'll need to find out additional information from your 'relevant' person or persons to confirm instructions and clarify any instructions that are not clear to you.

You'll also need to seek feedback from these people to ascertain how you can improve your performance. Here's how to excel:

- seek feedback on your performance
- identify your strengths and weaknesses
- clarify and confirm any instructions.

Produce and follow a self-development plan with targets

Once you have identified your strengths and weaknesses, you will need to produce a self-development plan, set your own targets and follow the plan over a period of time.

To produce a self-development plan:

- regularly review developments in hairdressing and related areas
- agree realistic work targets with your relevant person
- use the results of your reviews to develop your future personal development plan
- ask colleagues to help; take opportunities to learn
- seek help from relevant people when you are unable to obtain learning opportunities at work.

Develop working relationships with clients and colleagues

You'll also be assessed on how you develop your working relationships with your clients and other colleagues.

You will need to:

- agree ways of working together to achieve objectives
- ask for help and information from your colleagues, when necessary
- respond to requests for assistance from colleagues
- anticipate the needs of others and offer assistance within your capabilities
- make effective use of your time throughout your working day
- report problems likely to affect salon services to the relevant person
- resolve misunderstandings with your colleagues.

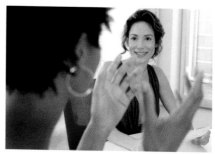

Your working relationships are vital to personal and business success.

Answers in the back of the book.

1   Which one of the following best describes a contract of work?

  a   A written document stating staff hours of duty

  b   A legal document setting guidelines for job roles

  c   A legal document setting health and safety policies

  d   A written document stating when holidays are to be taken

2   Why is it important to know about other people's job roles within the salon?

  a   To check up on them

  b   For effective team work

  c   To ask for help when needed

  d   To enable them to give help

3   **Statement one**

  It is important to work within your own responsibilities to minimise accidents.

  Statement two

  If a member of staff carries out a job without being trained, mistakes could occur.

  Which one of the following is correct for the above statements?

  a   True   True

  b   True   False

  c   False   True

  d   False   False

4   Which two of the following are methods of identifying your own strength and weaknesses?

  1   Providing a CV to the employer

  2   Checking appraisal documents

  3   Self reflection

  4   Peer review

  a   1 and 2

  b   2 and 3

  c   3 and 4

  d   4 and 1

5   **Statement one**

  An appeals procedure is carried out if a member of staff needs to complain.

  Statement two

  A disciplinary procedure is carried out if a member of staff has misbehaved.

  Which one of the following is correct for the above statements?

  a   True   True

  b   True   False

  c   False   True

  d   False   False

6   What does CPD stand for?

  a   Certificate of professional development

  b   Continuing professional development

  c   Certificate of progress to date

  d   Continued progress diary

7   Which one of the following best describes an appraisal?

  a   A regular review to identify training needs and progress

  b   A weekly review to set targets and change job roles

  c   A regular discussion with the salon team

  d   A weekly meeting with all staff

8   What does the 'T' in SMARTER targets stand for?

  a   Tools

  b   Time bound

  c   Talking

  d   Thought about

9 Which two of the following are ways of managing time effectively?

1 Being aware of salon service times

2 Making sure lunch break are taken

3 Checking the time every hour

4 Planning the day's activities

a 1 and 2

b 2 and 3

c 3 and 4

d 4 and 1

10 Which one of the following best describes how to cooperate with others?

a Always following the salon rules

b Always solving disagreements within the team

c Being supportive to the team and anticipating their needs

d Being experienced and more confident than others in the job role

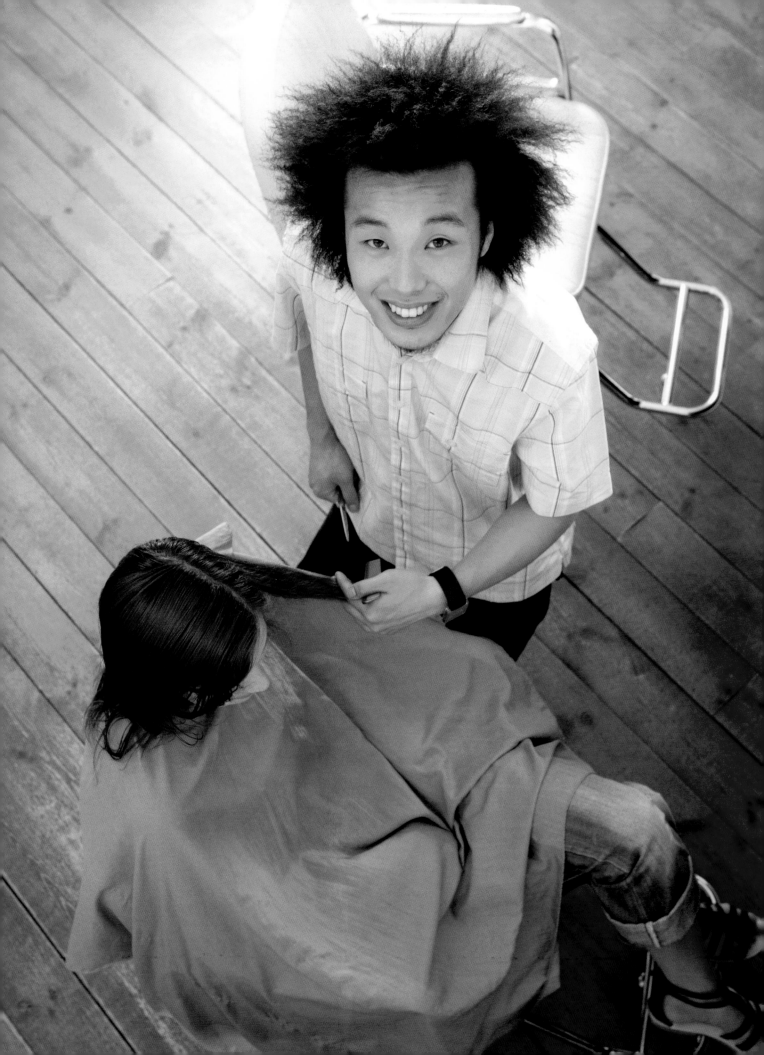

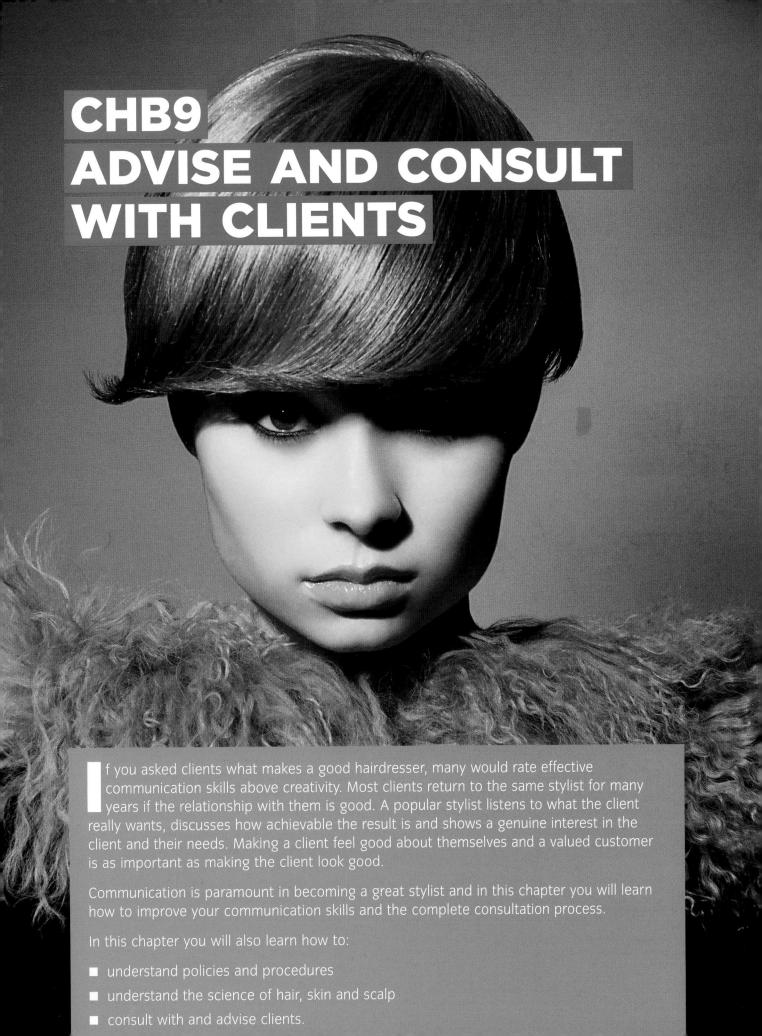

CHB9
ADVISE AND CONSULT WITH CLIENTS

If you asked clients what makes a good hairdresser, many would rate effective communication skills above creativity. Most clients return to the same stylist for many years if the relationship with them is good. A popular stylist listens to what the client really wants, discusses how achievable the result is and shows a genuine interest in the client and their needs. Making a client feel good about themselves and a valued customer is as important as making the client look good.

Communication is paramount in becoming a great stylist and in this chapter you will learn how to improve your communication skills and the complete consultation process.

In this chapter you will also learn how to:

- understand policies and procedures
- understand the science of hair, skin and scalp
- consult with and advise clients.

Policies and procedures

Health and safety

When carrying out a consultation with your client you'll need to understand the relevant policies and procedures.

HANDY HINT

Keep yourself up to date with the latest updates on health and safety Acts by visiting www.hse.gov.uk.

HEALTH & SAFETY

Refer to the health and safety and salon policies chapter for more information on health and safety legislation.

Health and safety legislation

The subsequent Acts must always be followed and can be found in detail in the health and safety chapter:

- The Health and Safety at Work Act
- The Reporting of Injuries, Diseases and Dangerous Occurrences Regulations (RIDDOR)
- The Health and Safety (First Aid) Regulations
- The Regulatory Reform (Fire Safety) Order
- The Manual Handling Operations Regulations
- The Control of Substances Hazardous to Health (COSHH) Regulations
- The Electricity at Work Regulations
- The Environmental Protection Act
- The Management of Health and Safety at Work Regulations
- The Health and Safety (Information for Employees) Regulations.

Working time directives

The UK law states that workers are not expected to work more than 48 hours per week on average, unless they choose to. This average is calculated over a 17-week period. If you are aged 18 or over, you can choose to opt out of the 48-hour limit for a certain period of time or indefinitely. This must be voluntary and stated in writing – you can choose to cancel your 'opt-out' at any time. Employers can ask you to opt out, but if you choose not to, they must not sack you or treat you unfairly.

HANDY HINT

For more information on working hours and your legal rights, visit the government website – https://www.gov.uk/maximum-weekly-working-hours.

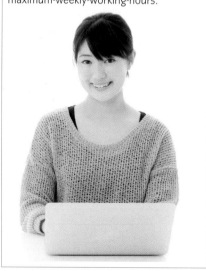

If you are 16–17 years old you can only work eight hours a day and 40 hours per week; these hours are not averaged out and you cannot opt out.

Activity

If you are an apprentice, visit https://www.gov.uk to identify your working rights and hours of work.

Personal hygiene, protection and appearance

Always ensure your personal hygiene does not put others at risk of harm – never attend work if you are contagious, always protect open cuts and wounds, and follow your salon policy for work wear and appearance.

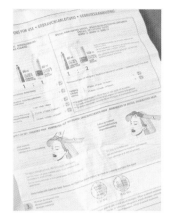

Protect open cuts and wounds

Salon procedures and manufacturers' instructions – tests

You have a duty of care to all your clients and when carrying out tests on the hair, skin or scalp to follow the manufacturers' instructions as well as your salon policies.

Colour manufacturer's instructions

Maintaining confidentiality and privacy

Your salon will have a policy on where and how you store your clients' details and personal data. Breaking the salon rules of confidentiality can result in damage to your professional image, loss of clients and possible legal action. Your salon's competitors may also gain access to company information that could be detrimental to the business and salon trade.

When **conversing** with clients avoid discussing personal aspects of your life or gossiping about others. Never provide one client with personal details about another client or staff member, including personal information such as addresses and contact details.

Converse

Talk.

Data Protection Act

The Data Protection Act protects the client's personal details by ensuring that:

- only authorised staff have access to client details
- you record the details accurately and keep them up to date
- you use them only for official use
- you destroy any out-of-date details securely
- the salon is registered with the Data Protection Registrar if the details are held on a computer system.

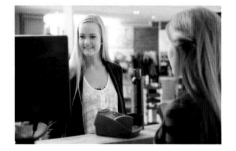

Client data should be kept secure in line with the Data Protection Act

Importance of not discriminating

It is important that all clients are treated equally and made to feel welcome in the salon. Sometimes when working with clients with different needs it can be difficult to know how to assist a client or how to communicate with them. Not all disabilities can be seen. Ask your client how you can help them; if necessary adjust how you communicate with them and ensure you do not discriminate against clients with illness or disabilities.

HANDY HINT

Some general disabilities categories include: autism, chronic illness, hearing loss or deafness, intellectual disability, learning disability, memory loss, mental illness, physical disability, speech and language disorders and vision loss and blindness. Ensure that no client feels left out.

Activity

In pairs or small groups, discuss how you would be made to feel if you were discriminated against because you had a disability.

Activity

Under the Equality Act 2010, disabilities are one of the nine protected characteristics – research this Act to identify the remaining eight protected characteristics.

HANDY HINT

If you need any guidance on your rights as a consumer, contact www.adviceguide.org.uk/consumer.

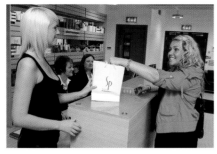

Selling salon products is covered under the Sale of Goods Act

Legal responsibilities when selling and promoting retail products

When you are promoting services and retail products you should do so in a manner that promotes goodwill and is in the clients' interest, not based around your commission or salon targets.

You must ensure that you follow the legal requirements of the following Acts which were created to protect the buyer:

- Cosmetic Products Regulations
- Sale of Goods Act
- Consumer Contracts Regulations (formerly Distance Selling Regulations)
- Trade Descriptions Act
- Consumer protection legislation.

These laws can be found in more detail on https://www.gov.uk/consumer-protection-rights.

Cosmetic Products (Safety) Regulations

The Cosmetic Products (Safety) Regulations were put in place to safeguard public health. They cover any substances that are to be placed on external human skin (including the epidermis and hair system):

- to clean – such as shampoo
- to perfume
- to change appearance – such as hair colour
- to correct body odour
- to protect – such as styling products
- to keep hair or skin in good condition – such as conditioner.

So the regulations relate to everything from hair colouring products to hand cream and deodorants.

Under these regulations the following restrictions have been put in place:

- Products and substances must have been safety-assessed by a qualified professional.
- Ingredients must be clearly labelled.
- Warnings must be displayed such as: 'not intended for use on persons under 16 years of age', 'may contain nuts', 'do not use to dye eye-lashes'.
- Instructions on use and how to dispose of the substance and container must be supplied.

The container must include:

- the country of origin
- the best before date
- the weight and measurements
- the batch number.

Sale of Goods Act

When you go shopping, a law called the Sale of Goods Act covers everything you buy. This means that when you buy a product it should be:

- as described
- fit for purpose
- of satisfactory quality.

As described

This means that the item you buy should be the same as any description of it. A description could be what the seller has said to you about the item or something written in a brochure.

Fit for purpose

What you buy should be able to do the job that it was made for. Goods should also be fit for any specific purpose that you agreed with the seller at the time of sale. For example, if you are looking to buy a shampoo and ask the seller how many shampoos it will give you, then the advice you are given has to be correct.

Satisfactory quality

Goods that are of satisfactory quality are:

- free from minor defects (problems)
- of a good appearance and finish
- strong and safe.

> **WHY DON'T YOU...**
> Look at three different substances in the salon and check to confirm the bottles or packaging abides by the requirements of the Cosmetic Products Regulations.

> **HANDY HINT**
> Customers have exactly the same rights to refunds when they buy items in a sale as when they buy them at full price.

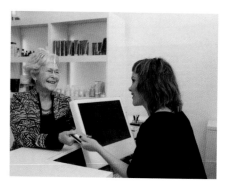

Only sell products that are as described, fit for purpose and of satisfactory quality.

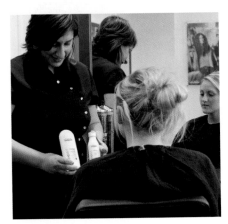

Product consultation

Geographical

Relating to physical location.

HANDY HINT

You must tell the customer if they will be responsible for paying for the return of goods if they cancel. If you don't, they're not liable for the costs.

Consumer Contracts Regulations (formerly Distance Selling Regulations)

Buying goods and services online, via mail order or over the phone can be convenient and often cheaper than buying from a shop or salon directly. These are all covered under the Sale of Goods Act. However as clients can't see or touch the products being sold they have extra consumer protection provided by the Consumer Contracts Regulations.

From 13 June 2014 the Consumer Contracts Regulations in UK law applies to all purchases made at a distance.

Under these regulations, you must:

- provide a description of the goods or services being sold
- list the price of the goods or services being sold, including all taxes
- explain the delivery arrangements and cancellation rights of the consumer
- display information about the seller including their **geographical** address.

Under the regulations clients are protected in the following ways:

- They have a right to cancel as soon as the order is made and up to 14 days after receipt of goods. They don't have to provide a reason.
- If goods are faulty and they are sent a replacement item they do not want, then the retailer must pay the postage costs. They have up to six years to make a claim (five years in Scotland).

Trade Descriptions Act

The Trade Descriptions Act prevents salons from misleading their customers as to what they are spending their money on. What you must know is that the Trade Descriptions Act makes it an offence for a trader to apply, by any means, false or misleading statements, or to knowingly or recklessly make such statements about goods and services.

Generally speaking, this means you have rights as a consumer for what you purchase to do what it says it will.

Consumer protection legislation

This legislation is aimed at protecting the public by:

- prohibiting the manufacture and sale of unsafe goods
- making the manufacturer or seller of defective products responsible for any damage caused
- allowing local councils to seize unsafe goods and suspend the sale of any suspected unsafe goods
- prohibiting misleading price indications.

The Consumer Protection Act ensures the safety standards of consumer goods and goods used in the workplace. Under this Act anyone who suffers personal injury, damage to personal property or death can take legal action against:

- producers
- importers
- own-branders.

Completing client records

After carrying out hair and skin tests you should record the outcome and gain client consent for the service to be carried out. For legal, health and safety purposes you should always complete a client record card at the end of all chemical and treatment services. This will help you in case of legal action, as well as provide information for future services.

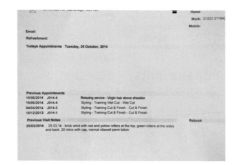

Client record card

Effective communication

When identifying what your client wants, you will need to question your client using client-friendly language, avoiding jargon and too many technical terms. Ask plenty of questions to identify accurately what they would like the outcome to be and to clarify both of your understandings.

Why effective communication is important

Effective communication is important to the salon business to ensure that the client receives the services they desire and that they are happy with the end result. Unhappy clients share their experiences with other people whereas happy clients return to the salon; repeat trade is vital for a successful business.

Using effective consultation techniques

You will need to adapt your style of communicating and consulting to suit the different needs and expectations of your clients. Clients' personalities vary immensely and although it is fair to say most people enjoy visiting the salon, a few compare it to visiting the dentist!

You will encounter clients who are angry, confused, behave unconventionally and have different needs and expectations; you must be able to adapt to these different situations. This can include what you say, the amount you say and how you say it. You will have to adapt your manner and tone of voice, remain calm and patient and use non-technical and jargon-free terminology.

You may find that you communicate differently with men and women; topics of discussion may vary immensely and personalities too.

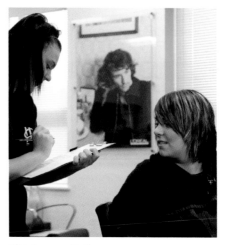

Client consultation

To ensure you follow the laws of equality and diversity, always treat clients equally, avoid flirtatious behaviour and be professional at all times. Some of your clients may have disabilities such as sight, hearing or speech difficulties and you must adapt to the needs of these clients and be careful not to cause offence.

Type of client	Adaptation to be made
Clients with visual impairments and/or disabilities	Clients with a visual impairment or those with a physical disability may benefit from being escorted and or guided through the salon. Always offer your arm to such clients when moving through the salon and check for any obstacles ahead. Be mindful that a client with a visual impairment may take a little while to adjust to different light conditions. You may need to adapt your terminology and clarify what you say, as you will not be able to rely on visual aids to confirm the requirements of your clients.
Clients with hearing impairments	Clients with a hearing impairment may struggle to hear you over the background noise in the salon. Try to lower the noise level in the salon and speak clearly so the client can read your lips. Do not shout or exaggerate your words as this can affect your voice patterns and lip movements. Stop speaking if you have to turn away from them. Keep to the subject matter and pronounce your words clearly to aid the client's understanding.
Clients with speech impediment	Clients with a speech impediment may need time to be able to express what they want to say. Always show your clients respect and patience, and remain relaxed and calm. Listen carefully to your clients and never finish their sentences for them. Ask them to repeat anything you do not understand.
Clients who are not fluent English speakers	Clients whose first language is not English may need you to speak a little slower. Shouting in English does not translate itself into another language; you need to remain calm and listen carefully. Ask your clients to repeat any areas you do not understand. It is important that you do not guess their needs just because you are too embarrassed to ask them to repeat themselves.

HANDY HINT

Refer to the Values and Behaviours chapter for more information on communicating with clients of varying ages and with people from different cultures or religions.

HANDY HINT

Your speaking and listening skills are valuable English skills that are required in the workplace and help you to communicate effectively with your clients.

The giving and receiving of accurate information is a very important part of communicating with your client and colleagues as this aids the understanding process. It also enables all staff members involved with the service requirements to know their roles and responsibilities.

Questioning and listening skills

Your questioning techniques should include asking relevant open and closed questions to identify what your clients want. Listening to their responses helps you to confirm the desired outcome.

Body language

When you communicate, you do so verbally and non-verbally. Body language is a method of non-verbal communication and can be positive as well as negative. It can give away secrets about whether you are telling the truth, listening to your client and interested in what your client is saying. Also look at your client's body language. If your client is showing signs of uncertainty, you need to ask more relevant questions to clarify the situation and put them at ease.

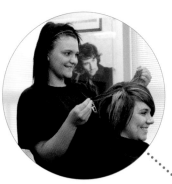

Smiling indicates you are happy and approachable

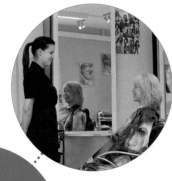

Eye contact indicates you are listening

WHY DON'T YOU…
Casually glance around your salon and look at everyone's body language. Make some notes and discuss your findings with a colleague.

POSITIVE BODY LANGUAGE

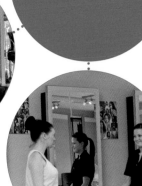

Open palms indicate openness and honesty

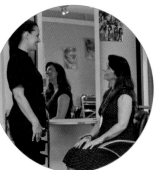

Good open body posture indicates you are alert and ready for work

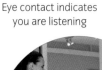

Keeping a little distance shows respect for personal space

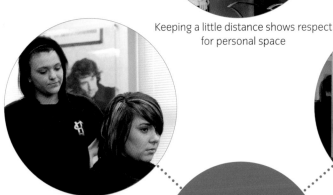

Poor posture looks unprofessional and indicates tiredness

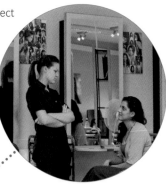

Crossed arms, closed-in body posture indicates defensive behaviour and a closed mind

NEGATIVE BODY LANGUAGE

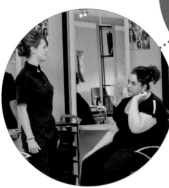

Scratching behind the ear or rubbing the back of the neck indicates that the listener is uncertain

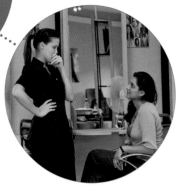

Talking with your hand in front of your mouth indicates to your client that you are not being honest or truthful

> **HANDY HINT**
>
> You should always clarify your client's understanding of the consultation process and what has been agreed. Encourage them to ask questions about areas they do not understand.

> **HANDY HINT**
>
> Use visual aids such as colour charts or style magazines to confirm client requirements.

> **HANDY HINT**
>
> Don't set up your client for disappointment – always discuss whether the desired look is going to be achievable and state the likely outcome before the service commences.

> **HANDY HINT**
>
> Aftercare for each service is covered in more detail in each technical unit – see CH1, CH2, CH3, CH4, CH5, CH6, CH7, AH2, CB2, CB3 and CHB11.

> **HANDY HINT**
>
> Knowing your salon's pricing structure will help you to guide a client on the total cost of the service and it will give you confidence in advising on services and products.

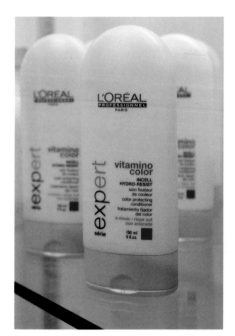

Aftercare products

Encourage your client to ask questions

Always give your client time to consider what has been discussed and ask any questions to gain clarity on what is being discussed and agreed.

Providing advice and recommendations

At the end of the consultation you should inform your client of the maintenance and aftercare that will be required. You should confirm the service, what products you are going to use and how long you expect the service to take. Discuss the cost, but remember, if you have encouraged the client to buy some new products, the total cost may change.

Recommendations

As you are the expert and your client has come to you for advice, it is important to advise your client on how to maintain their look, the time interval between services, present and future services, and additional products and services.

However, when you are discussing aftercare and home maintenance with your client, remember to maintain their trust and keep their details confidential.

You should record any retail products sold and the service details on the client record card, ensuring that it is accurate, up to date and easy to read. Make sure you follow the Data Protection Act.

Calculate your client's bill

At the very end of the service you must calculate the total bill, including any retail products sold. Your salon will have established the costs involved for each service including products, materials, salon utilities and business overheads, the stylist's time and expertise. Your calculation, based on these, results in the service costs charged to your client.

> **Activity**
>
> Using your salon pricelist, calculate the following service bill:
>
> - half head of woven highlights
> - short hair cut and finish
> - colour-saving shampoo and conditioner.

Science of hair, skin and scalp

Hair characteristics and classifications

When carrying out a consultation with a client (for any service) you will need to consider the hair's characteristics and classifications to identify whether the desired look would be achievable.

Hair characteristics

Hair characteristics include density, texture, elasticity, **porosity**, condition and hair growth patterns.

> **Porosity**
>
> Having small holes. Porous materials absorb liquids.

Hair characteristic	Impact on services
Density 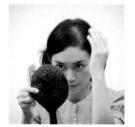 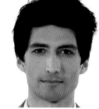 Sparse Abundant **Sparse** Thin or scarce.	Hair density refers to the amount of hair and is described as **sparse**, average or abundant. Sparse hair often means the hair is fine and there is not a lot of it covering the head. The scalp may be visible through the hair, less product will be required and the types of hair styles that will suit this density of hair will need to be considered. Abundant hair means the client has a full head of hair; this may be fine or coarse in texture but there is lots of it. Abundant hair requires more products, more drying time; it will take longer for services to be carried out. Cutting techniques will need to be considered as the hair may need to be thinned out.
Hair texture 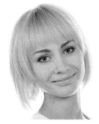 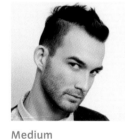 Fine Medium 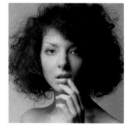 Coarse	Hair texture refers to the thickness of each strand of hair and is described as fine, medium or coarse. Fine hair has a small circumference and fewer layers of cuticle scales. Medium hair is greater in circumference than fine hair with an average number of layers. Coarse hair has a large circumference and the most layers of cuticle scales. Fine hair will absorb chemicals much faster than coarse hair because there are fewer cuticle scales. Coarse hair can often be resistant to chemicals. A porosity test can be carried out on all hair textures to check whether these cuticle scales are rough and open, or smooth and closed. 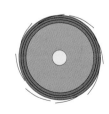 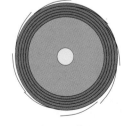 Very fine hair Average hair Very coarse hair

Hair characteristic	Impact on services
Elasticity 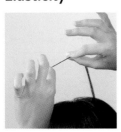	Elasticity of hair refers to how weak or strong the hair is and whether the cortex layer has been damaged. When working with hair that has weak elasticity you will need to consider whether the hair is strong enough to take additional chemicals or whether to advise on an alternative product, such as a semi-permanent colour. You will also need to consider the choice of styling products and decide on how much tension can be applied to the hair when cutting and styling.
Porosity 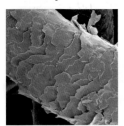 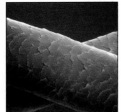 Porous hair Resistant hair	Porosity of hair refers to the cuticle layers – if the cuticles are damaged and open then hair is porous, they can also be normal/non-porous or closely compacted/resistant. Porous hair will absorb chemicals much faster and may not be able to handle any additional chemicals. As the cuticles are open the hair will tangle more easily and you must consider this when combing or styling the hair. Resistant hair may be resilient to some colouring or perming products and suitable techniques will need to be considered. Hair may be coarser and it will take longer to dry as it holds onto the moisture.
Condition 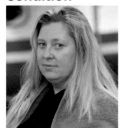 Chemically damaged hair	The condition of your client's hair can vary greatly; it may be normal, naturally dry, oily or damaged (by chemicals, environment, heat or lifestyle). If hair is damaged you'll need to identify how it has been damaged and advise clients on how to prevent further damage and improve their hair condition. Consider whether the hair is able to have any further chemical services or whether a course of treatments is required. Damaged hair is likely to be either porous or have weak elasticity – or both.
Hair growth patterns 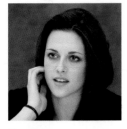 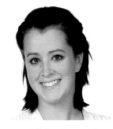 Cowlick Widow's peak 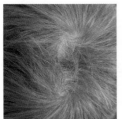 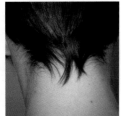 Double crown Nape whorl	Hair growth patterns consist of cowlick, widow's peak, double crown and nape whorl. Cowlick – found at the front hairline, this hair stands straight or lies at an odd angle and affects whether a fringe can be worn and how it is worn. Widow's peak – also found at the front hairline, the hair grows into a point near or at the centre of the front hairline. This can affect choice of hairstyles and fringe options. Double crown – found at the crown area. There can be a single crown whorl instead. This affects how the hair will sit around the crown area. The length of the crown hair must be considered when cutting and styling. Nape whorl – found at the nape area, the hair grows into a whorl direction and can affect shorter hairstyles. Sometimes one side of the nape hairline sits differently from the other, so always check both sides of the nape before cutting hair short, or styling hair into up-dos.

Hair classifications

As a guide, hair classifications refers to hair types that are straight, wavy, curly or very curly.

Hair type	Definition	Further information	Impact on services
Straight hair – type 1 Asian hair	Fine/thin straight hair tends to be very soft, shiny and oily, and it can be difficult to hold a curl. Medium hair generally has lots of volume and body. Coarse straight hair is normally extremely straight and difficult to curl.	Asian hair is very straight and grows directly up from the hair follicle. It is round shaped and has about 11 layers of cuticle scales. The more cuticle scales the hair has, the more resistant the hair will be to chemicals and to styling. Straight hair is often more oily in condition than other hair types, because oil from the sebaceous glands can travel more easily along the hair shaft.	Difficult to curl and may affect the styling of hair. May be resistant to chemicals such as colour and perming products. When cutting the hair, straight hair can show cutting marks on the hair.
Wavy hair – type 2 Caucasian hair	Fine/thin wavy hair has a definite 's' pattern and you can normally accomplish various styles. Medium wavy hair tends to be frizzy and a little resistant to styling. Coarse wavy hair is also resistant to styling and normally very frizzy; tends to have thicker waves.	**Caucasian** or European hair is generally referred to as wavy; this is because of the way the hair grows out of the hair follicle. The hair shaft is oval with around four–seven layers of cuticle scales. In straight and wavy hair, the follicles are more or less vertical to the surface of the scalp. The angle of the hair follicle determines the natural wave pattern of the hair. **Caucasian** Description of people of Northern European origin with lighter skin tone.	Can be great hair to work with, but coarse wavy hair can make styling more challenging at times. When cutting the hair use products which may help with any frizziness and aid control. Coarse hair may be a little resistant to chemical processes.

Hair type	Definition	Further information	Impact on services
Curly hair – type 3	Loose curls – the hair tends to have a combination texture. It can be thick and full with lots of body, with a definite 's' pattern. It also tends to be frizzy. Tight curls – the hair also tends to have a combination texture, with a medium amount of curl.	Caucasian or European hair can be naturally curly, as well as the hair of people with mixed race or dual heritage. Curly hair has hair follicles that grow from the scalp almost parallel to the surface of the scalp.	The styling of curly hair needs products and control with styling tools. Hair will appear shorter once cut, so less tension will be required. Hair may be delicate and take quickly to colour and chemical processes.
Very curly hair – type 4 African type hair	Soft curly hair tends to be very fragile, tightly coiled and has a more defined curly pattern. Wiry hair also tends to be very fragile and tightly coiled; however with a less defined curly pattern, it has more of a 'z' pattern shape.	African type hair is very curly and grows out of the follicle at an acute angle. The hair shaft is kidney shaped with around seven to eleven layers of cuticle scales. As the hair's oil cannot travel so easily along the hair shaft, the curlier the hair, the drier the hair tends to be.	Very curly hair needs lots of control when styling and products designed for curly hair. Hair will tangle easily and spring up when cutting. Hair is fragile and care must be taken with chemical processes.

Straight hair	Wavy hair			Wavy-curly hair		Tight-curly hair	Kinky-curly hair	Kinky hair	Z-pattern hair
1	2A	2B	2C	3A	3B	3C	4A	4B	4C

Hair types

The shape of the hair shaft is determined by the shape of the hair follicle: people with straight or wavy hair have typically round or oval-shaped hair follicles; people with curly or very curly hair have follicles which are kidney-shaped or elliptical. How your hair is shaped is determined by the follicles and follicles vary in size, shape and thickness due to genetics.

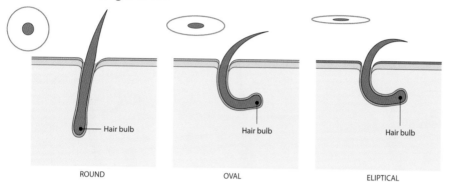

Shapes of hair shafts

The more kidney-shaped/elliptical the shaft is, the curlier the hair. The cross-sectional shape also determines the amount of shine the hair has. Straighter hair is shinier because sebum from the sebaceous gland (a kind of oily substance that is responsible for protecting your hair from becoming dry, brittle and cracked) can travel down the hair more easily. The curlier the hair, the more difficulty the sebum has travelling down the hair and therefore the drier or duller the hair looks.

Structure of hair and skin

Before you can begin to fully understand how and why you analyse the hair, skin and scalp, you must first understand the structure of the hair, skin and scalp.

Hair

Hair covers the entire body except for the palms of our hands and soles of our feet. Body hair is called **vellus hair**; the hair on the head is referred to as **terminal hair**.

The hair shaft

The hair shaft is made up of three main layers, two of which it is vital you are familiar with: the **cuticle** and cortex layers. These two layers play a huge part in all areas of hairdressing and can affect the outcomes of services and products available for use.

The cuticle layer

The outer layer of the hair is called the cuticle and is made up of many layers of transparent overlapping scales which protect the hair. The cuticle scales lift when chemicals are added to the hair to allow

VALUES & BEHAVIOURS

When referring to a client's skin colour and hair type you must ensure you use terminology that will not offend. Clients with dual heritage are often referred to as 'multi-racial', 'mixed race' or 'bi-racial' and these terms are deemed as politically correct and non-offensive. Clients with African type hair often self-identify as 'black'.

Vellus hair

Fine, downy hair that appears all over our bodies except the palms of the hands and soles of the feet.

Terminal hair

The hair on our heads, underarms and genital areas of the body.

Cuticle

Outer layer of the hair.

penetration of the chemicals into the layer underneath. Heat can also open the cuticle layer. Ideally the cuticle scales should be closed and lie smoothly from root to tip. Shiny, healthy hair that reflects light does so because the cuticle scales are closed and smooth, and therefore non-porous. Dull, **lacklustre**-looking hair appears flat and absorbs the light because the cuticle scales are damaged or open, and the hair is therefore porous.

Lacklustre

Lacking in shine and body.

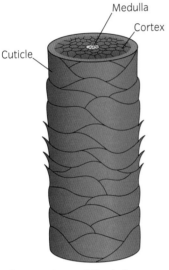

The structure of the hair

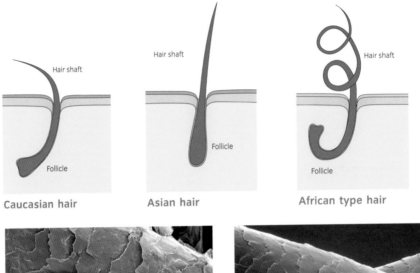

Caucasian hair   Asian hair   African type hair

> **HANDY HINT**
>
> Cuticle scales are often described as 'fish scales' or 'overlapping roof tiles'; they overlap from root to point.

> **HANDY HINT**
>
> Different hair types have varying layers of cuticle: Caucasian hair types have four to seven layers, African hair types have seven to eleven and Asian hair types have up to eleven layers.

Cortex

Layer of the hair under the cuticle.

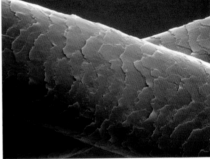

Microscope view: damaged cuticle absorbing light

Microscope view: smooth cuticle reflecting light

The cortex layer

The **cortex** is the section under the cuticle and the most exciting layer of the hair. Your natural hair colour is determined in the cortex: it is here that artificial colouring takes place. It is this layer that holds the bonds which hold your hair in place to determine whether your hair is naturally very curly, curly, wavy or straight. When hair is temporarily or permanently changed from curly to straight or straight to curly, this takes place here in the cortex. The cortex is the main body of the hair, giving the hair its strength and elasticity.

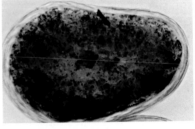

Microscope view: colour molecules in the cortex

THE CITY & GUILDS TEXTBOOK

The medulla layer

The **medulla** is the least interesting layer of the hair and does not play any real part in hairdressing. It is the central layer of the hair but it is not always present. Little is known about what the medulla is for or its significance. In a single strand of hair the medulla may fade in and out, be present the whole way through or not be there at all. In thicker hair it appears to be present more often than not.

> ### Activity
>
> Draw and label the three layers of the hair and list two or three facts about each layer.

The skin and scalp

The hair on our heads helps to protect our scalps and keeps us warm. The skin and scalp have three main layers, each with a role to play.

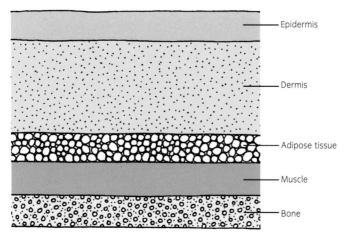

Epidermis

Dermis

Adipose tissue

Muscle

Bone

Cross-section of the body's tissues

The epidermis layer

The outer layer of the skin is called the **epidermis**. There are a few nerve endings but no blood supply to this layer. The epidermis protects us from bacteria and temperature changes and are regularly replaced. House dust is partly made up of the epidermis that our bodies have shed. Our whole body is covered with the epidermis which varies in thickness; it is thickest on the soles of our feet and thinnest on our eyelids.

The epidermis is made up of five layers: the top three contain dead cells, one layer contains old cells and the bottom layer is constantly producing new cell growth.

- The ***stratum*** *corneum* is the outer top layer and provides us with a waterproof 'coat'. This 'horny' layer flakes and dries out easily. We remove the dead skin cells from here when we exfoliate.

Medulla

Central layer of the hair.

HANDY HINT

To help you remember the three layers of the hair you can think of a pencil. The cuticle is like the varnish/paint on the outside of a lead pencil and this area sometimes gets a little flaky. The cortex is like the main body of the pencil, which gives it its strength, and the medulla is like the lead.

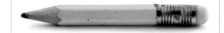

Epidermis

Outermost layer of the skin.

Stratum

Layer.

Mitosis

Cell division.

- The *stratum lucidum* is a clear layer present only in thick skin, helping to protect it from the force of friction.

- The *stratum granulosum* is a granular layer which contains most of the skin's protein called keratin.

- The *stratum spinosum* is the prickle cell layer. These cells are formed as new cells grow and the old ones are pushed up to create a new layer. The cells interlock and are capable of **mitosis** under friction or pressure, eg on our feet or on the palms of our hands.

- The *stratum germinativum* is the base and deepest layer of skin. It is the primary site of mitosis which produces new cell growth. This can take 28–30 days to move through the five layers of the epidermis before it is shed. This layer contains a pigment called melanin which gives the skin its natural colour.

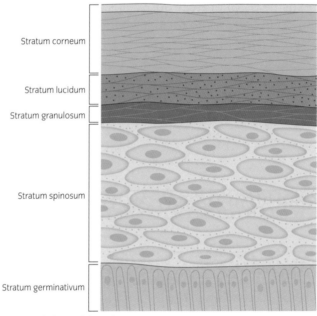

Strata of the epidermis

The dermis layer

Dermis

Middle layer of the skin.

The **dermis** attaches the epidermis to the subcutaneous layer and passes nutrients between the two layers. It is this layer that provides strength and elasticity to the skin.

The subcutaneous layer

Subcutaneous layer

Fatty tissue layer.

Arrector pili muscle

Muscle attached to the hair follicle at one end and dermal tissue on the other.

Sebaceous glands

Glands in the skin that secrete oil.

The **subcutaneous layer** is fatty tissue that is attached to the dermis layer. Its functions are to keep us warm and supply nutrients via the blood supplies. All the nerve endings, hair follicles, **arrector pili muscles**, sweat and **sebaceous glands** travel through here to the dermis. It is much thicker on the body than on the head.

The main activities of the skin structure take place within the dermis and subcutaneous layer.

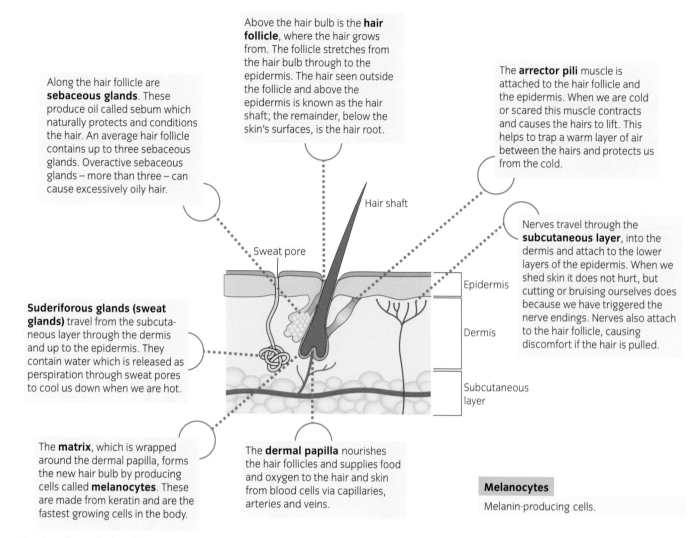

Along the hair follicle are **sebaceous glands**. These produce oil called sebum which naturally protects and conditions the hair. An average hair follicle contains up to three sebaceous glands. Overactive sebaceous glands – more than three – can cause excessively oily hair.

Above the hair bulb is the **hair follicle**, where the hair grows from. The follicle stretches from the hair bulb through to the epidermis. The hair seen outside the follicle and above the epidermis is known as the hair shaft; the remainder, below the skin's surfaces, is the hair root.

The **arrector pili** muscle is attached to the hair follicle and the epidermis. When we are cold or scared this muscle contracts and causes the hairs to lift. This helps to trap a warm layer of air between the hairs and protects us from the cold.

Hair shaft

Sweat pore

Suderiforous glands (sweat glands) travel from the subcutaneous layer through the dermis and up to the epidermis. They contain water which is released as perspiration through sweat pores to cool us down when we are hot.

Nerves travel through the **subcutaneous layer**, into the dermis and attach to the lower layers of the epidermis. When we shed skin it does not hurt, but cutting or bruising ourselves does because we have triggered the nerve endings. Nerves also attach to the hair follicle, causing discomfort if the hair is pulled.

Epidermis

Dermis

Subcutaneous layer

The **matrix**, which is wrapped around the dermal papilla, forms the new hair bulb by producing cells called **melanocytes**. These are made from keratin and are the fastest growing cells in the body.

The **dermal papilla** nourishes the hair follicles and supplies food and oxygen to the hair and skin from blood cells via capillaries, arteries and veins.

Melanocytes

Melanin-producing cells.

Section through the skin

The growth cycle of hair

The hair grows in three stages: we call these cycles. Our hair grows on average 1.25cm per month (½ inch). We have thousands of hairs on our heads, all at different stages of the hair growth cycle; we each lose on average 100 hairs per day.

■ Anagen – in this stage of the growth cycle the hair follicles are active and the hair is growing. Up to 80% of our follicles are in this stage at any one time. The blood and oxygen from the capillaries form the hair follicle in the dermal papilla and can grow for up to seven years or stop growing after as little as one-and-a-half years. Clients trying to grow their hair may find it stops when it reaches a certain length; this could be due to the limited hair growth in their anagen cycle.

- Catagen – during this part of the cycle the hair growth slows down for a couple of weeks. The follicle starts to shrink and detaches from the dermal papilla.

- Telogen – during this phase the hair is resting; it can last for 10–12 weeks.

- New anagen – towards the end of the resting cycle, new activity and cell division take place in the dermal papilla and the anagen cycle begins again. The new hair growth pushes the old hair further up the hair follicle, which is often then completely removed from the follicle when the hair is brushed or combed.

HANDY HINTS

To help you remember the order of the three stages of hair growth, use the word ACT – Anagen, Catagen and Telogen.

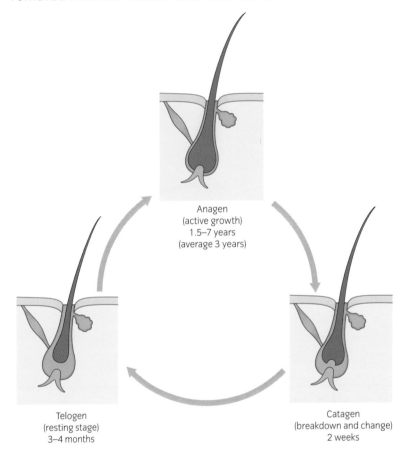

Anagen
(active growth)
1.5–7 years
(average 3 years)

Telogen
(resting stage)
3–4 months

Catagen
(breakdown and change)
2 weeks

Assessing factors that may limit or affect services

Hair tests

You must carry out tests before and during all services. These tests must be completed following the manufacturers' instructions to ensure that you follow health and safety guidelines. You must record the results on the client record card and you must seek guidance from the relevant person if any adverse reactions occur. Remember to work within the limits of your authority and report all **adverse** reactions.

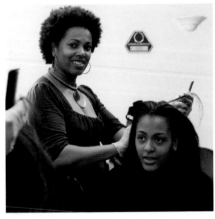

Assessing the hair prior to service

Adverse

Unfavourable, poor, difficult or not suitable.

The following table sets out the necessary tests. Additional tests are required for relaxing and perming services – see chapters AH2 and CH5.

Test	When to carry out the test	How to carry out the test	Why is it important to carry out the test?	Expected results of the test	Consequences of not carrying out the test
Porosity test	Before any service on dry hair	Take a few hairs and slide your fingers up the hair shaft from point to root.	To test the cuticle layer to identify if the cuticles are smooth or rough	Hair cuticles will feel smooth if the hair is non-porous, or rough or raised if the hair is porous.	Damage to client's hair might occur or the desired outcome might not be achieved.
Elasticity test	Before any service on wet hair	Take one or two hairs and mist them slightly with water. Then stretch the hair a couple of times between your finger and thumb.	To test the strength of the cortex	As a guide, normal straight/wavy hair, when wet, should stretch about 30% more than its original length and then return when released.	Damage to client's hair might occur or the desired outcome might not be achieved.
Incompatibility test	Before chemical services, if you suspect **metallic salts** or henna products are present in the hair If the client has previously had a **thioglycollate** lotion applied to the hair	Take a small cutting of the client's hair and place it in a solution of 20ml liquid 6% peroxide and 1ml of perm solution, the chosen relaxer cream, or a solution of 20:1 liquid peroxide and ammonium hydroxide. Leave for up to 30 minutes or for the manufacturer's recommended development time.	To identify whether any henna or metallic salts are present which would react with professional chemical products	If metallic salts are present the hair may change colour, the solution may bubble and fizz and/or give off heat. If the service is for rerelaxing hair, remember that thioglycollate used in perming is *never* compatible with hydroxide and will cause breakage.	Damage to and/or disintegration of client's hair could occur.

Thioglycollate

Perm salt – a chemical compound.

Metallic salts

These can be found in products which contain lead compounds or a variety of other metals depending on the shade of colour required.

HANDY HINT

Before you carry out any chemical services, remember to ask the age of your client and check ID. This will ensure you are following your MFIs and confirm that client is aged 16 years or older.

Test	When to carry out the test	How to carry out the test	Why is it important to carry out the test?	Expected results of the test	Consequences of not carrying out the test
Strand test	During the colouring or lightening service	Wipe off the colour or lightener from a few strands of hair.	To see whether the colour result has been achieved, or if the lightener development is sufficient	If permanent colour is developed, then the desired result should be achieved. If the bleach is regularly checked, the level of lift should be achieved without damage to the hair. Further development may be required if the colour result has not been achieved.	Damage to and/or disintegration of client's hair could occur if colour left on for too long. The desired outcome may not be achieved if the colour is not left on long enough.
Development test (curl or curl reduction)	During the perming or relaxing service	Wipe off or rinse the product from a few stands of hair. Check for sufficient degree of curl or straightness.	To see whether the curl or relaxing result is sufficient	If desired level of curl/relaxing has been achieved, the result is positive. If it has not been achieved, further development time may be required.	Damage to client's hair could occur if relaxer or perm solution is left on too long. The desired outcome may not be achieved if the solution is not left on long enough.
Skin test	24–48 hours before 'most' colours or perming services	Always follow the manufacturers' instructions as these may vary. As a guide only: Clean an area in the inner elbow or behind the ear. Then apply the chosen product to the area and leave it exposed to dry.	To test for an allergic reaction or sensitivity to the product	A positive reaction is red skin and/or sore areas that may weep and itch. A negative reaction is no change to the skin area.	An allergic reaction, anaphylactic shock, contact dermatitis or damage to the client's skin could occur.

Test	When to carry out the test	How to carry out the test	Why is it important to carry out the test?	Expected results of the test	Consequences of not carrying out the test
Density	During the consultation and analysis of the hair before proceeding with a relaxing service.	Take a 2.5cm²/1in² cross-section of the scalp and see how many hairs are growing from this area.	To see if the hair is sparse (thin), regular (medium) or abundant (thick)	The number of hairs in the section will tell you the density of the hair. This knowledge will help you to use the correct strength of relaxer cream to carry out the service.	If the hair is sparse, the relaxer may take rapid effect and overprocess – avoid pulling the hair during application and preparation. If the hair is abundant, then this will have an impact on the time taken to apply the relaxer cream.
Texture	During the consultation and analysis of the hair before proceeding with a relaxing service	Isolate individual hairs from the head and compare the diameter to that of your own or a colleague's hair.	To find out the diameter of each hair so you can assess to establish how much relaxer can be absorbed and which strength of product to use.	Thick (coarse) hair – process longer; may be more resistant to processing. Medium hair – does not pose any special problems or concerns. Fine hair – more fragile, easier to process, and more susceptible to damage from chemical services than coarse or medium hair.	If thick (coarse) hair is not processed for long enough, you may not achieve the desired degree of straightening. Processing fine, thin hair for too long can cause damage and even breakage.

HANDY HINT

You must always carry out any relevant tests on the hair and skin to ensure that the service and products to be used are compatible with the client's requirements. Not carrying out the tests could result in damage to the client's hair and skin, which could lead to legal action.

HEALTH & SAFETY

Remember thioglycollate and hydroxide chemicals are not compatible and will cause the hair to break.

HANDY HINT

Factors are anything that could influence or affect the hairdressing service.

HANDY HINT

You should always refer to a client's records to check if there are, or have been, any factors that may affect the service.

Activity

Research all of your salon's colour manufacturers' instructions. Note which colours need a skin test and how to carry out the skin test. Check for any age restrictions too.

Activity

Practise some of these hair tests on your colleagues.

Importance of identifying factors

You must ensure that the hair, skin and scalp are suitable for the service required and that the products, tools and equipment you use are the most appropriate for your client. Identifying which techniques and services you offer in order to create the desired result will depend on the outcome of the hair tests and from identifying relevant factors.

Factors affecting hair services

Factors that can affect hair services include:

- adverse hair, skin or scalp condition
- incompatibility of previous services and products used
- client's lifestyle
- test results.

Adverse hair, skin and scalp conditions

If hair is physically or chemically damaged, further services could make the condition of the hair deteriorate or cause breakage. Physical damage can be caused by overuse of electrical heat appliances or excessive brushing. Chemical damage can be from colouring, bleaching and perming the hair, but also from chemicals like chlorine if your client is a regular swimmer.

Adverse skin and scalp conditions such as psoriasis, cysts, impetigo, scars and moles, infections and infestations can all affect whether a service can be carried out, especially if the client's condition is infectious. Some non-infectious conditions do not affect the service but extra care must be taken to avoid causing discomfort or aggravating a condition.

Incompatibility of previous services and products

There may be factors that affect potential services because treatments and products have already been used on the hair. For example, tint will not lift tint, so if a client wants a full head tint but already has tint on their hair, the desired look might not be achieved.

Although it is rare, some products will react with other products on the hair and could cause the hair to break and disintegrate. Metallic salts that are found in a few hair colouring products available in high street shops will react with the chemicals in professional brands.

Some clients' hair may not be suitable for further chemical treatments, for example if the hair is in poor condition as a result of previous services or products.

Activity

In pairs, discuss which services could cause barriers to future services and may not be compatible with the client's requirements.

Lifestyle

Your client's lifestyle must be considered for most services to identify if your client will be able to maintain their hair between visits.

It would be wrong to recommend a vibrant fashion colour service to a client whose workplace would not allow it. Equally, if your client has a shy personality, a vibrant fashion look that draws attention to them would not be suitable.

A mother with a hectic lifestyle might not have the luxury of the time needed for a high-maintenance hairstyle; a quick-style look may be what is really required. A keen swimmer should not be advised on colouring or relaxing services that would affect the condition of the hair in chlorinated water.

Test results

The results of all hair and skin tests need to be considered. If a client has had an allergic reaction to a colour then alternative services need to be discussed. A client whose hair has been identified as porous, weak or incompatible will also need to be offered alternative services and further discussions on what service is most suitable for their hair.

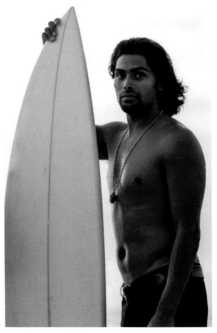

Outdoor activities can be hard on the hair!

Activity

Identify factors that you could deal with by yourself and where you would be able to advise the client on the best outcome. Then identify factors that you would need to refer to the appropriate person.

Adverse hair, skin and scalp conditions in detail

Adverse hair conditions

Adverse hair condition or defect	Description	Cause	Symptoms	Possible treatment
Fragilitas crinium Microscope view of split ends	Split ends	Physical damage or chemical treatments	Dry, split ends, damage to cuticle and cortex at the end of the hair shaft	Regular use of surface conditioners and deep-penetrating conditioners improve the condition. Cutting the hair removes the split end.
Trichorrhexis nodosa Microscope view of trichorrhexis nodosa	Swollen, hardened areas of the hair shaft	Physical damage or chemical treatments	The hardened swelling can break off and cause the hair to split.	Regular use of surface conditioners and deep-penetrating conditioners improve the condition. Cutting the hair may help to remove the damaged area.
	 Microscope view of broken hair caused by trichorrhexis nodosa			
Monilethrix Beaded hair	Beaded hair shaft	A rare hair defect that is hereditary and caused by an uneven production of keratin	Very weak hair that may break off near the root. The hair feels bumpy where the 'beads' are formed.	Treat with caution and care. Conditioners and treatments may help. Refer to a GP.

Adverse skin and scalp conditions

Adverse skin and scalp conditions are varied, but most can affect which services you can offer your client. A client with **psoriasis** can have a cut and blow dry but you may decide that colouring treatments are best avoided. Other adverse conditions of the skin and scalp could be:

Psoriasis

A skin disease that can make the skin red, itchy and scaly in patches.

- moles
- scars
- cysts
- infections and infestations.

How to recognise hair, skin and scalp problems

Adverse hair, skin and scalp condition	What you will see	Infectious or non-infectious	How the condition may limit the service
Alopecia	Bald patches (alopecia areata) and in extreme cases total baldness (alopecia totalis)	Non-infectious condition	When working on a client who has alopecia areata you will need to consider the hair length and layers to aid disguising the hair loss. Where possible avoid chemical treatments while the client has this disorder.
Barber's itch (sycosis barbea)	Folliculitis – inflammation and infection of the hair follicles on the hairy parts of the face	Yes, bacterial infection can be spread by infected shaving tools	Do not carry out service until condition has cleared up. Refer to GP if it does not clear up after improved hygiene.
Boils/abscesses	Raised, inflamed pus-filled spots	Potentially infectious condition	Do not carry out facial hair-cutting treatments – refer to GP.

Adverse hair, skin and scalp condition	What you will see	Infectious or non-infectious	How the condition may limit the service
Impetigo	Yellow crusty spots on the skin	Infectious condition caused by a bacterial infection	No services can be carried out. Refer to GP.
Folliculitis	Inflammation of the hair follicles	Infectious. A bacterial infection, which can be caused by harsh physical or chemical actions	No salon services to be offered. Refer to GP.
Eczema	Red inflamed itchy skin, sometimes split and weeping	Non-infectious. Can be caused by physical irritation or allergic reaction. Genetic factors can also cause eczema	Refer client to GP or dermatologist. Salon services can be carried out but avoid chemicals on any broken skin.
Psoriasis	Silvery yellow scales and thickening of the skin	Non-infectious skin/scalp condition	Psoriasis can cause discomfort to the client and the scales of skin overlap the hair and may cause uneven haircuts. If skin is open and weeping do not carry out any services.
Dandruff/ pityriasis capitis	Dandruff – dry or oily scaling scalp, yellow in appearance and can smell	Can be infectious if it's a fungal infection. The condition is an over-production of skin cells or a fungal infection. Can also be stress-related or caused by irritants	Dry dandruff can be treated in the salon with a medicated shampoo but if the dandruff is caused by fungi, then treatment should not be carried out in the salon.

Adverse hair, skin and scalp condition	What you will see	Infectious or non-infectious	How the condition may limit the service
Scars	Healing tissue that has become thickened and raised	Non-infectious. Scar tissue is caused when damaged skin heals	During the healing process this area may be tender, delicate and open to infection. Once healed, proceed with normal services.
Keloid	Overgrown area of scar tissue that encases the original wound. More common on people with darker skin	Non-infectious	Generally normal services can resume, but extra care should be taken with tools and equipment in case the area is sensitive or protrudes slightly.
Cysts	A small pea-sized, non-cancerous lump that is filled with pus or fluid	The most common cyst is a non-infectious sebaceous cyst	These are often painless and rarely affect services. However they can be painful when knocked, so take care with clippers, combs and tools, etc. Avoid services if the cyst has become infected.
Cold sores (herpes simplex)	A cold sore – on the facial area or lip	Yes – viral infection	Do not carry out facial hair-cutting treatments – refer to pharmacy for treatment.
Moles	Dark coloured skin lesions either under or on the skin	Most moles are non-infectious and are usually made of cells called melanocytes. Others occur from a **subdermal** growth. **Subdermal** Under the skin.	Normal services can be carried out, although take care not to catch the mole with hairdressing tools, as this will cause discomfort to your client and the mole could then be susceptible to infection.

Adverse hair, skin and scalp condition	What you will see	Infectious or non-infectious	How the condition may limit the service
Ingrowing hair	Also known as razor bumps – hairs that grow inwards and cause a mild infection or discomfort	Non-infectious as long as the blocked follicle has not become infected	Service can continue if not infected. Recommend exfoliating treaments and products.
Ringworm/tinea capitis	Ringworm – red ring surrounding a grey patch of skin, sometimes seen with broken hairs	Infectious	Fungal infection – no services can be offered or provided. Refer client to their GP.
Scabies	A very itchy rash in the folds of the skin, normally the midriff or inside of arms and thighs	Infectious	Infestation of an itch mite, burrowing into the skin and laying its eggs. Treatments cannot be carried out in the salon.
Head lice/ pediculosis capitis Microscope view: nits Microscope view: louse	Head lice and nits (eggs)	Contagious – risk of infestation and cross-contamination	The head louse feeds off the blood in the scalp and lays its eggs on the hair close to the warmth of the scalp. No salon services to be offered. Refer client to GP/pharmacy.

Activity

Using your salon's list of services, identify which products you could use and which services you could recommend to clients who have the following adverse hair, skin and scalp conditions:

- allergic reaction to permanent tint
- metallic salts identified during an incompatibility test
- weak elasticity
- alopecia areata
- infected scalp cyst
- scalp moles
- impetigo.

Reporting infections and infestations

If your client has an infection or infestation, you will need to report this to your supervisor diplomatically. You do not need to report any conditions that are not contagious.

Activity

From the chart showing adverse hair, skin and scalp disorders identify which of these you would need to report to your supervisor.

Activity

Research other infectious and non-infectious conditions, such as furunculosis, sycosis, tinea pedis, herpes simplex and herpes zoster.

> **HANDY HINT**
>
> 'Infectious' means 'contagious' so these ailments can be passed from one person to another. Infestations are parasites living on the body in large numbers and are also contagious. Salon services, therefore, must not be carried out on clients with infectious conditions.

> **HANDY HINT**
>
> Any infectious condition on the skin would affect the service offered to the client.

Consult with and advise clients

An effective consultation must take place before every hairdressing service. This includes services such as shampooing and conditioning treatments, cutting hair and facial hair, styling, setting, colouring and perming.

Prepare for consultation service

You should complete the consultation process in a relaxed environment and your client must have plenty of time to express their views and wishes. It is not unusual for consultations to take up to 20 minutes for new clients, as this gives you both time to clearly understand what is required and whether or not it is achievable. When carrying out a consultation on a regular client it is important to confirm whether your client wants a repeat service or if they are looking for a new service or style.

> **HANDY HINT**
>
> Some consultations might be carried out a few days before the service is booked; this enables you to carry out the relevant hair and skin tests.

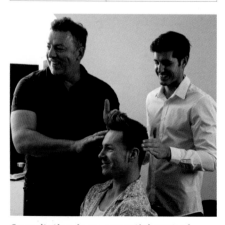

Consultation is an essential part of every service

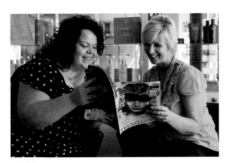

Salon magazines can help clients and stylists agree a look

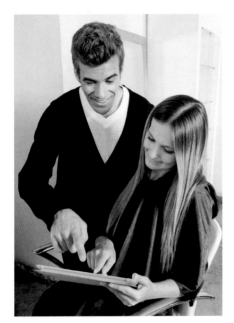

Tablets and smart phones are great visual aids

Use visual aids

If your client is requesting a new style, cut or colour, you should use visual aids to help you both get a clearer picture of the desired look.

Many salons now use smart phones or tablets to search the internet for images to use as a visual aid. The internet or use of styling magazines helps the stylist or client describe what the finished result should look like. With the image in mind you can discuss with the client how feasible the outcome will be. Remember, as the expert, it is up to you to suggest alternative ideas if the style will not suit the client's face shape, hair type or texture, or even their lifestyle. Always be prepared to suggest other positive options.

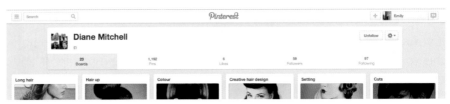

Pinterest is a great place to keep your personal 'look book'

The use of colour charts is very important when discussing a colouring service with your client. Most manufacturers have colour charts with removable samples that you can drape through the client's hair and against their skin to check that the colours suit the client's skin tone and their existing hair colour.

Personal hygiene, protection and appearance

Your personal hygiene is important and must be maintained throughout the working day. Ensure you shower every day, use deodorant and wear clean, presentable clothes to meet salon, organisation and industry standards.

Consult client records

Before making any recommendations to your client your must refer to their record cards (when available) and identify any factors likely to affect future services.

These may consist of:

- adverse hair, skin and scalp conditions
- incompatibility of previous services and products used
- client's lifestyle
- test results.

Salon pricing structure

You'll need to know your salon's pricing structure to be able to accurately calculate the likely charges for a client's service. Many salons have a variable pricing structure, taking into account the experience of the stylist and charging accordingly. For example, a service carried out by an artistic director may cost more than the same service by a newly qualified stylist.

Calculating likely charges

Always ensure you charge the correct price; if your salon charges separately for a cut and blow dry after a colour service make sure you add all services to the total bill.

Activity

Using your salon price list, work out the costs for four different services, adding 20% to the bill for an artistic director and reducing the bill by 10% for a newly qualified stylist. Add a different retail product to each bill.

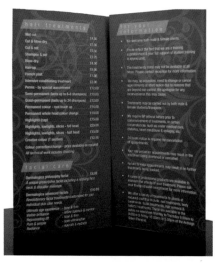

Know your salon's pricing structure

HANDY HINT

Always check the total bill with a senior staff member if you are unsure of the costs.

HANDY HINT

Always *listen* to what your client is asking of you. Allow them time to express their wishes before suggesting your ideas and recommending services.

Perform consultation techniques

The consultation is the most important part of any service. To be able to meet your client's expectations you need to know exactly what they want from the service.

During the client consultation you need to ascertain your client's wishes and identify whether the desired result is achievable.

Ask relevant questions in a way your client will understand

Open questions demand more than one-word answers and therefore help you to get information and details from the client to help you understand their vision. These questions might start with 'why' or 'how'. This will also help you improve your English communication (speaking and listening) skills.

Some useful open questions are:

- What service would you like today?
- Why would you like this particular service/technique?
- What result would you like your colour service to achieve?
- When did you last visit the salon?
- How do you manage your hair at home and what do you do to your hair on a daily basis?
- What products do you use on your hair at home?

Closed questions are questions that can be answered with either 'yes' or 'no' or one-word answers.

WHY DON'T YOU...

Practise using some open and closed questions with your colleagues to help gain more information or clarify a point.

WHY DON'T YOU...
Listen to the other stylists in your salon carrying out consultations with their clients.

HANDY HINT

Always ensure you ask relevant questions and listen to their responses in order to find out all the information required to carry out the desired service.

The following are examples of closed questions:

■ Are you having a colour service today?

■ Would you like a cup of coffee while you wait?

Towards the end of the consultation, closed questions can be very useful, as these help to confirm that you and your client are sharing the same vision.

For example:

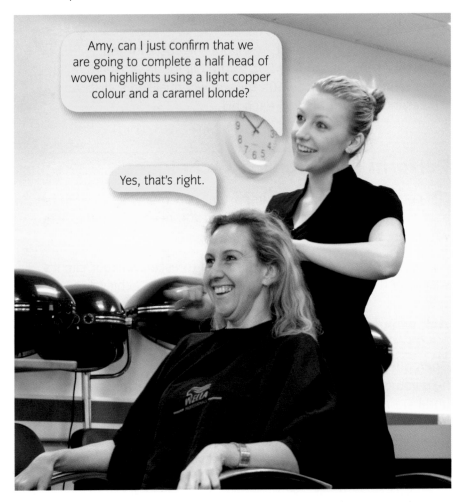

Amy, can I just confirm that we are going to complete a half head of woven highlights using a light copper colour and a caramel blonde?

Yes, that's right.

Activity

Use the example 'open' questions above.

Try to list up to:

• six questions you could ask your client if they were booked in for a styling or dressing service

• eight questions you could ask your client if they were booked in for a cutting service

• ten questions you could ask your client if they were booked in for a colour service.

HANDY HINT

As you gather information from your client and answers to your questions, encourage your clients to ask any questions, particularly if they are unsure about any areas discussed.

Carry out visual checks and necessary tests

As well as questioning your client it is important that you carry out visual checks on the hair, scalp and skin to check for any lumps, bumps or abrasions, infections and infestations, and adverse skin or scalp disorders. You must also carry out any relevant hair or skin tests to ensure you can proceed with the chosen service.

Identify and report any problems

If you identify any problems during the questioning of your client and the routine checks and hair tests, you should report these to the relevant person in your salon.

The main problems that are likely to need reporting are infections and infestation, and hair skin and scalp disorders, but excessively damaged hair, reactions to skin tests or incompatibility tests may need reporting too.

Activity

List as many problems as you can that you think would need to be reported, such as different infections, infestations or scalp disorders. Try to list at least five. If you need more guidance you could read 'Adverse hair, skin and scalp disorders in detail' earlier in the chapter.

> **HANDY HINT**
>
> When reporting your concerns to your manager or supervisor, you must be discreet and professional at all times, to ensure your client is not made to feel uncomfortable.

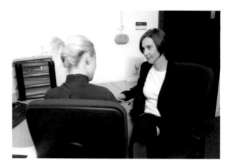

Report any concerns discreetly

> **HANDY HINT**
>
> Throughout the whole consultation you must communicate in a friendly manner, using client-friendly language and in a way that promotes goodwill and trust.

Provide clients with advice and recommendations

Identify and confirm clients' wishes

You should observe your client's behaviour and body language to ensure the client looks comfortable with what has been discussed and agreed. You can identify the intentions of the client by listening to the manner in which they speak to you, their tone of voice and the vocabulary used. Always confirm that your client understands and agrees with the service requirements.

> **HANDY HINT**
>
> To clarify and confirm what has been discussed, use closed questions as these are more likely to require clear 'yes' or 'no' answers from your client.

Make recommendations to the client

Once you have listened to the client's wishes and discussed the best outcomes for their hair, you should make your recommendations. Your suggestions should be based on what will produce the best results taking into consideration their hair characteristics and classifications.

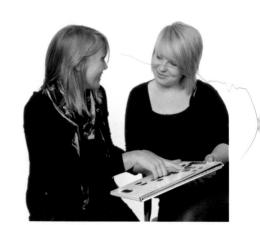

Make recommendations to your client

Explain how hair characteristics may impact on services

The following hair characteristics may affect the service:

- hair density
- hair texture
- hair elasticity
- hair porosity
- hair condition
- hair growth patterns.

You must explain to your client if their hair is too damaged to be permanently coloured, too fine to achieve a chosen style, etc. so that they understand why their expectations cannot be met. Try to offer an alternative solution so that your client is not too disappointed.

Activity

Consider how the above characteristics would affect the following services:

- restyle
- woven highlights with lightener.

These characteristics are covered in more detail above, under the heading 'Science of the hair, skin and scalp'.

How hair classifications affect the service

Hair classifications will affect various hair services, from drying and styling, setting and dressing, cutting to colouring and perming the hair.

Activity

How would the following hair classifications affect the following services?

- an Asian client with very straight hair requesting a setting service
- a European client with wavy fine hair requesting a highlighting service
- a male client with African type, tightly curled hair requesting a short haircut
- a mixed-race client with curly hair requesting a smooth blow-dry service.

Agree services, products and outcomes

At this stage of the consultation you are armed with plenty of information: what the client wants, the condition of the hair, skin and scalp, the hair's characteristics and whether achieving the desired result is likely to be **attainable**. Now is the time to agree the service you are going to carry out, what products you are going to use and what the expected outcomes are.

As your experience and confidence as a stylist grow and develop, you will become more skilled at presenting a valid argument and expressing your ideas clearly and professionally. Your clients are relying on your professional opinion on what is best for their hair. Your vocabulary should change to suit your client groups and their needs. For example, you should adapt your vocabulary when communicating with a child, someone of the same age group as you with similar interests, or an older person.

In order to move the consultation process forward or bring it to a suitable end, summarise what you have discussed and agreed together. Any points that need further development should be re-addressed but remain focused on the purpose of the discussion and the required outcomes.

Once you and your client have agreed the service to be carried out, you need to inform them of the likely cost of the service – you do not want your client to be in for a nasty shock at the end of the service or for them to sit there throughout the service worrying about what it is going to cost. You should also advise them of how long the service is likely to take and the duration of the salon visit – you don't want to be halfway through a colour when your client advises you that they need to pick up the children from school! Always ensure your client is happy with the recommended and agreed service and products, the costs advised and that they have time for the service to be carried out.

Future advice and recommendations

At the end of the service you should always provide aftercare advice to ensure they can maintain the look in between salon visits, recommending any products or equipment to the client to assist with home maintenance. Explain to them how long the look is likely to last and advise them as to when they should rebook for their next cut or colour. During the service you may have discussed future services or products to use. Recap on these suggestions at the end of the service and suggest that your client books their next appointment before leaving the salon.

Attainable

Realistic or possible.

HANDY HINT

Ask another stylist to help you with your consultation if you are unable to do this on your own.

WHY DON'T YOU...
Practise consultation techniques with a colleague to help build your confidence.

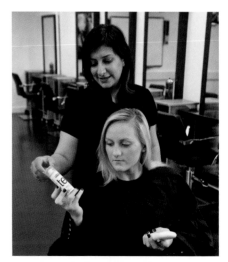
Recommend aftercare products

Answers in the back of the book.

1 Which of the following is **not** a working time directive according to UK law?

  a 16- to 17-year-olds can only work for 8 hours per day

  b It is against the law to work for more than 48 hours per week

  c 16- to 17-year-olds are not allowed to work longer than 40 hours per week

  d Employees aged 18 or over can opt out of the average 48 hours per week rule

2 Not all disabilities can be seen. Which one of the following may not be obvious, but still needs to be considered when ensuring equality and diversity?

  a A client in a wheelchair

  b A client with a broken leg

  c A client with mental illness

  d A client with a contagious skin condition

3 Which one of the following regulates the selling of goods online?

  a Consumer Contracts Regulations

  b Trade Descriptions Act

  c Cosmetic Products Regulations

  d Consumer Protection Legislation

4 Which one of the following legislations requires the seller to give details of their geographical location?

  a Consumer protection legislation

  b Cosmetic Products Regulations

  c Trade Descriptions Act

  d Consumer Contracts Regulations

5 Which one of the following is the best way of communicating with a client with a hearing impairment?

  a Using images and shouting

  b Raising the voice and smiling

  c Facing them whilst clearly speaking

  d Asking another team member to help

6 Talking with the hand in front of the mouth indicates

  a Tiredness

  b Dishonesty

  c Uncertainness

  d Defensiveness

7 Which one of the following hair classifications is type 4b?

  a Medium texture and frizzy

  b Very straight and fine

  c Very curly and fragile

  d Medium texture and wavy

8 Which one of the following best describes a Northern European with a light skin tone?

  a Asian

  b Caucasian

  c Puerto Rican

  d African Caribbean

9 Which one of the following best describes the cuticle?

  a Overlapping, coils inside the hair

  b Overlapping, translucent scales

  c The centre of the hair

  d Polypeptide chains

10 The anagen stage usually lasts for between

  a 1.5 and 4 years

  b 1.5 and 5 years

  c 1.5 and 6 years

  d 1.5 and 7 years

CHB11 SHAMPOO, CONDITION AND TREAT THE HAIR AND SCALP

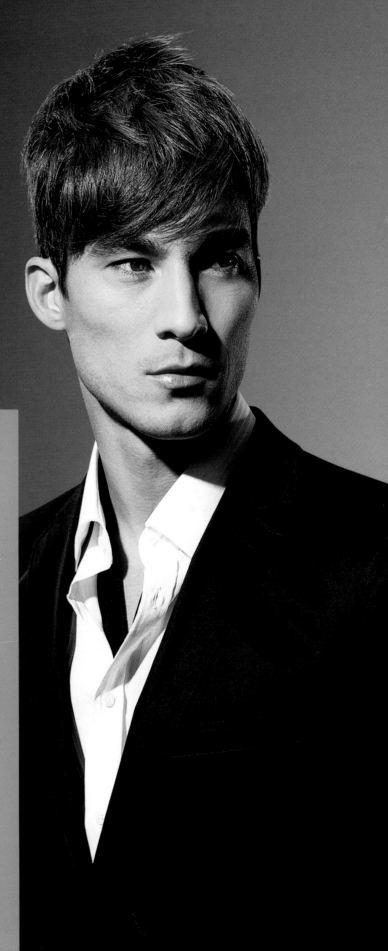

The shampoo and conditioning process is often a favourite with clients, because of the massage techniques used and the resulting clean, conditioned feel of the hair. It can be relaxing and therapeutic if the scalp is massaged correctly and the client is positioned comfortably at the basin. The hair and scalp must be checked for any damage or disorders and the most suitable products recommended. The client's enjoyment is a key factor, but treating the hair is the most important reason for shampooing and conditioning.

After reading this chapter you will:

- know how health and safety affects shampooing, conditioning and treating the hair and scalp

- understand the basic science and techniques used in shampooing, conditioning and treating the hair and scalp

- understand which products and equipment to use to shampoo, condition and treat the hair and scalp

- be able to provide shampooing, conditioning and scalp treatment services.

Health and safety

HEALTH & SAFETY

Refer to the health and safety and salon policies chapter for a recap on the health and safety legislation you must follow when shampooing, conditioning and treating the hair and scalp.

Your responsibilities for health and safety

The shampoo and conditioning service is often the first part of any service, so it is important to give a positive impression of yourself and your salon. Always follow the health and safety acts and behave in a manner that will not put you or your client at risk of injury or harm. Mop up any spillages that occur at the shampoo area and always protect your client throughout the service.

Activity

How many of the ten pieces of health and safety legislation listed in the health and safety chapter can you list and remember?

Personal hygiene, protection and appearance

You must always ensure you are fit and ready for work, maintaining your personal health and hygiene at all times. Don't attend work if you have a contagious condition, such as influenza, a common cold or an eye infection. Ensure you cover any open wounds and refer any potential cross-infection, hazards or risks to your manager.

During the shampooing and conditioning service, you will be leaning over your client, so it is of great importance that your personal hygiene is maintained and you do not have any body odour. You must shower or bathe every day, use deodorant and wear clean clothes. Brush your teeth regularly and always represent the industry and salon's image with clean, well-groomed hair.

HANDY HINT

Always protect your hands with hand cream and/or barrier cream to prevent dermatitis.

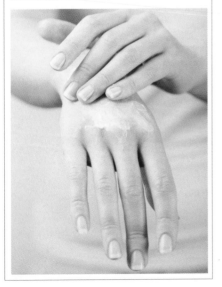

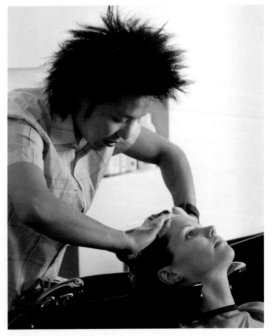

Ensure your personal hygiene is tip top

Hazards and risks

It is important that you always act in a manner that does not put you or your client at risk of injury or harm.

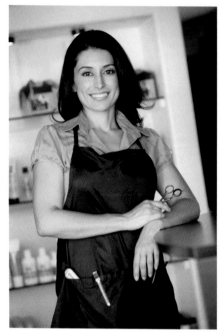

Work safely

Activity

Complete the 'prevention' column in the activity below. Can you list any other potential hazards and risks?

Hazard	Risk	Prevention
Water on the floor	People could slip over	
Shampoo and conditioner	Product could get into the client's eyes	
Shampoo and conditioner	Dermatitis	
Hot water	Could burn self or client	
Infection/ infestations	Cross- contamination	

Safe working practices and safety considerations

Working safely, cleanly and tidily minimises the risk of harm and injury to yourself and others and prevents cross-contamination. It also ensures that a professional image is observed by the client and visitors.

Safe and professional methods of working when you complete shampoo and **conditioning treatments** include carrying out the relevant hair tests. You must carry out a porosity test to identify whether the cuticle scales are open or closed and whether the hair is porous or non-porous. If the cuticle scales are open, the hair is porous and will need more conditioner and maybe even a treatment. You must also test the strength of the cortex with an elasticity test, and weak hair will need treating.

Protective clothing

You must always protect your client during a shampoo or conditioning treatment with a fresh, clean gown and towel, using a shoulder cape for clients with longer hair to prevent moisture from damp hair soaking through to their clothes. The shoulder cape will also protect the client from accidentally getting wet if you have not

Conditioning treatment

A process to improve condition – in this instance we mean a penetrating conditioner that improves the condition of the cortex.

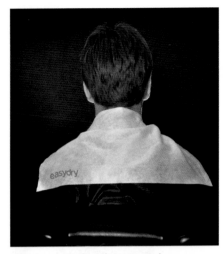

Client gowned and protected

taken adequate care during the shampoo process. You should wear appropriate personal protective equipment (PPE): gloves to prevent dermatitis and an apron to protect your clothes.

Positioning your client and yourself

To ensure the comfort of your client, sit them upright with their back and neck supported at the basin area.

During the shampoo process you will need to lean over the client, and if shampooing from a side basin you will also need to twist your body slightly. Make sure your balance is evenly distributed; stand with your feet slightly apart and avoid stretching and twisting where possible to prevent back problems and fatigue. You can sometimes be standing over the basin for as long as 15 minutes, for example when shampooing long hair or applying conditioning treatments, and this is a long time to spend leaning over. You need to ensure that you stand correctly to avoid risk of injury.

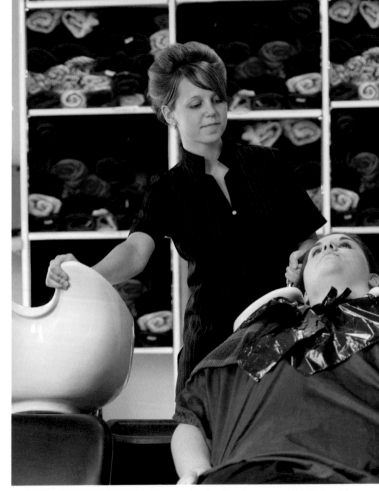

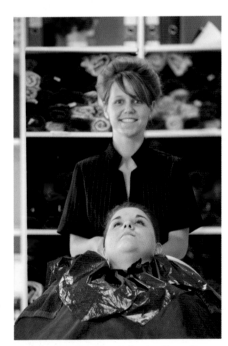

Standing correctly at the basin reduces the risk of fatigue

Excessive twisting and leaning at the basin can cause back problems

Working methods and sustainable practices

Activity

Complete the chart below and identify what you can do in your salon to promote environmental and sustainable working practices.

How to support the environment	What can you do in your salon?
Reduce and manage waste	
Reduce energy consumption	
Use disposable items	
Use organic hair products	
Use products with environmentally friendly packaging	
Offer responsible domestic products such as Fairtrade tea and coffee	
Reduce your carbon footprint	

Using electrical equipment

When you use electrical equipment near water or on wet hair, be aware of the potential hazards and follow the Electricity at Work Regulations. Always ensure your equipment is in good working order and fit for use, to prevent the risk of harm or injury to you or your client. Use equipment correctly, following the manufacturers' instructions (MFIs).

Using products safely

When you use shampoos and conditioning products, you must do so safely and economically. Always ensure that you follow COSHH regulations – controlling the substances that could be hazardous to your health. Always store substances correctly, handle them carefully, use them correctly and dispose of them in a non-harmful way. Make sure you follow the manufacturers' instructions, the local by-laws and your salon policies. Using too much product is wasteful and the salon will lose profit; excessive use of products can overload the hair, affecting further services. Always read the MFIs to ensure you use the correct amount and achieve the best results.

HEALTH & SAFETY

Refer to the health and safety and salon policies chapter for a recap on protecting the environment and maintaining sustainable working practices.

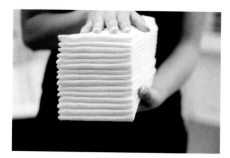

Disposable hair towels

HANDY HINT

Always replenish stock without causing a disruption to the client's service and report shortages to the relevant person.

HANDY HINT

Complete the service within a commercially viable time and make effective use of your time to ensure the salon runs smoothly throughout the day.

HANDY HINT

Promote environmental and sustainable working practices whilst carrying out a shampoo and conditioning service by turning off the tap in between shampoos and not wasting water.

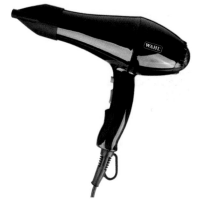

Be aware of the potential hazards of using electrical items near water or wet hair

Hygiene considerations

Dermatitis

A common workplace disease is contact dermatitis. This can leave you unfit for work and in the worst case scenario you may need to leave the industry. Dermatitis can be recognised by inflamed skin that may be red and sore and may weep and crack. To avoid developing dermatitis, you must rinse and dry your hands thoroughly after every shampoo and conditioning treatment, and wear gloves when necessary. Using moisturising hand cream can also help.

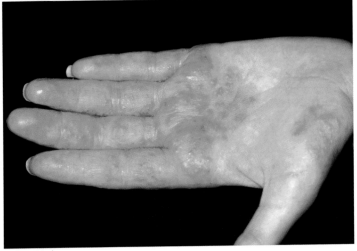

Dermatitis

Preventing cross-infection and infestation

If you have encountered an infection or infestation, remove all infected waste immediately and dispose of it in the dedicated salon bin, boil wash the towels and gowns, and sterilise tools thoroughly. Always follow your salon's policies and procedures for dealing with infections and infestations. If you encounter an unrecognised scalp disorder, you must refer this to a senior staff member to prevent possible cross-infection and infestation.

Working safely and hygienically

You must keep your work area clean and tidy at all times. Ensure the basin area is clean, free of waste and ready for your client's service. Clean basin areas and work surfaces with detergent and water, disinfect the basin and your equipment using either suitable chemical liquids or a UV light, and sterilise tools in an autoclave.

HANDY HINT

Cover any open wounds to prevent cross-contamination.

HANDY HINT

Poor standards of health and hygiene can cause offence to others, lead to cross-contamination and present a poor salon image.

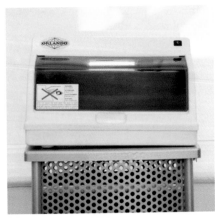

UV light cabinet

VALUES & BEHAVIOURS

Refer back to the sterilisation section in the values and behaviours chapter for more information on how to clean, sterilise and disinfect equipment.

Activity

In pairs or small groups, list six ways in which you can work safely and hygienically.

Importance of questioning clients

Your language and communication skills are very important in hairdressing, and the way in which you ask questions and the types of questions you ask your clients will affect the information you receive. It is important that you ask suitable questions to establish whether your client has any contra-indications to the service.

Contra-indications

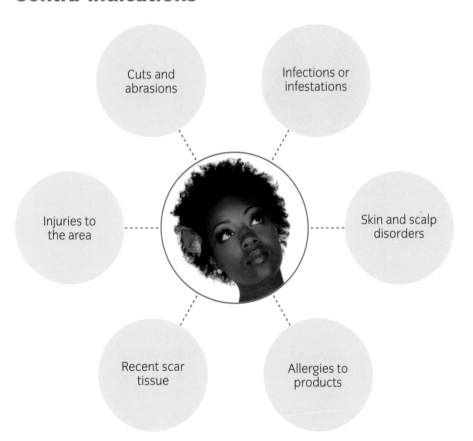

Cuts and abrasions

Infections or infestations

Injuries to the area

Skin and scalp disorders

Recent scar tissue

Allergies to products

Activity

List three to five open questions that you could ask to obtain relevant information from your client about their hair and scalp condition or any contra-indications.

Hair and scalp conditions

As the stylist it is your responsibility to identify which products should be used to suit the client's requirements, the following service, and their hair and scalp condition.

HANDY HINT

Refer to chapter CHB9 to remind yourself about hair and scalp conditions, and their likely causes.

Common hair conditions

Hair condition	Identified by?	Likely cause and products to use
Damaged 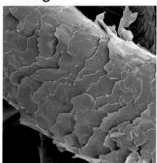 Microscopic view: damaged cuticle 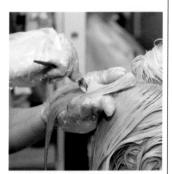 Chemical damage 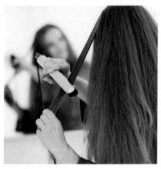 Heat damage	Porosity testing and identifying damaged cuticles. Elasticity testing and identifying weakness to the hair's cortex. The hair may also be dull in appearance and lacklustre as the light is being absorbed and not reflected due to the damaged cuticles.	Chemical damage – too many harsh chemical treatments leave the hair dry and porous and the cuticle scales open and rough. The cortex may be weak with poor elasticity. This can affect further services and may cause the hair to tangle easily. Use a moisturising shampoo for coloured or chemically treated hair and a penetrating conditioning treatment to strengthen the cortex and smooth the cuticle scales. 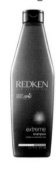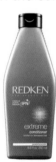 Heat damage – the continued daily use of hairdryers, straightening irons or curling tongs can damage the cuticle scales and remove moisture from the cortex layer, destroying the bonds. Excessive heat from appliances, incorrect usage and/or failure to use heat protector products when styling can cause the hair to be porous, with the cuticle scales open and rough and decreased elasticity in the cortex. Use a moisturising shampoo and surface conditioner. A penetrating conditioning treatment may also be required. 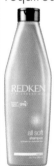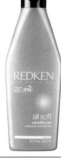

Hair condition	Identified by?	Likely cause and products to use
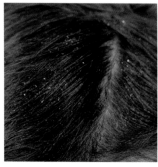 Environmental damage		Environmental damage – the sun and wind can affect the hair's condition, causing colours to fade and the cuticle scales to open, resulting in porous hair. Chlorine and seawater can also affect the hair. Use a moisturising shampoo and surface conditioner. A penetrating conditioning treatment may also be required. You should advise your client about wearing a hat and protecting their hair against the effects of the environment. 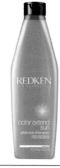 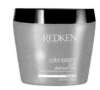
Product build-up 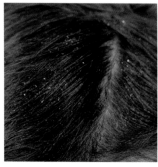	The hair may look oily, flaky or 'crunchy' with excess products visible on the hair. The hair may also appear dull and lacklustre; this is because the cuticles are filled with products and the light is being absorbed rather than reflected.	The overuse of some products, applying too much or using an incorrect product can cause a build-up on the hair. An unsuitable shampoo may also prevent the products from being effectively removed from the hair. Oil-based products, such as wax, do not mix with water and need a good detergent to break them down. Excessive hairspray, sprayed too closely to the hair, can often leave a coating on the hair that is difficult to remove. Product build-up can create a barrier to the subsequent service. A thorough shampoo process with a clarifying shampoo will be required, as this shampoo will deeply cleanse the hair and scalp. A light surface conditioner is recommended after shampooing. 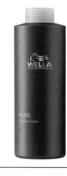 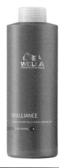

Hair condition	Identified by?	Likely cause and products to use
Normal hair 	Hair should appear shiny and cuticles smooth.	For normal hair, use a shampoo suitable for the scalp condition or a normal shampoo and surface conditioner.
Oily hair 	Hair will appear wet-looking at the root area and slightly along the hair shaft. Oily hair can also 'clump' together rather than lie as single hairs.	Oily hair may be caused by an oily scalp (seborrhoea) or can simply be because the hair needs to be cleansed. Excessive use of oil-based products may also cause hair to look oily. The course of action required will depend on the cause. Straight fine hair can get oily quite quickly because the hair's sebum travels easily along the hair shaft.
Dry hair 	The hair may appear dull in appearance and lacklustre as the light is being absorbed and not reflected due to the dryness of the hair and the cuticles may be raised slightly.	For damaged dry hair – see the section above on damaged hair. Very curly hair is often naturally dry, as the sebum cannot travel along the shaft as easily as it can on straighter hair shafts. A moisturising shampoo and conditioner is required, but if the hair is fine as well as very curly, be careful not to overload the hair and cause it to be weighed down with product.

Common scalp conditions

Scalp condition	Identified by?	Likely cause and products to use
Dandruff (pityriasis capitis) 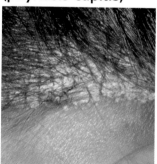	Dandruff can be yellow in appearance and often smell if caused by fungi, or appear dry, white and flaky if it's stress-related dandruff.	You must identify whether the dandruff is caused by fungi or stress, as treatment will vary. For fungus-related dandruff you can refer your client to their GP for prescription treatments. For stress-related dandruff, caused by an overproduction of skin cells, then a medicated shampoo can be used. Use a conditioner to suit the hair condition and a leave-in scalp treatment to aid dandruff control. 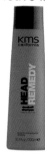
Oily scalp (seborrhoea) 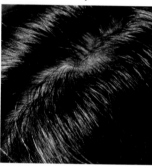	The scalp area will look shiny in appearance and slightly damp-looking. Excessively oily scalps can also smell quite pungent.	You must identify whether the hair and scalp area are oily because: ■ the hair is due to be shampooed ■ of a poor shampooing service/the hair and scalp are insufficiently cleansed ■ the client has been sweating (for example from exercise) ■ the client has overactive sebaceous glands. If the hair is in need of a good cleanse, use a shampoo for oily hair and a surface conditioner on the mid-lengths and ends only. If the client has seborrhoea, use a shampoo for oily hair, a surface conditioner or penetrating treatment on the mid-lengths and ends and a leave-in scalp treatment to aid seborrhoea control. 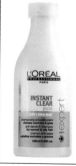 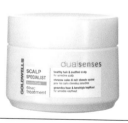

Scalp condition	Identified by?	Likely cause and products to use
Dry scalp 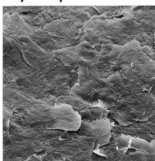 Microscope view	A dry scalp looks whiter than normal and has white flakes close to the scalp.	There are many causes of dry scalp, such as: ■ a natural moisture imbalance ■ change in seasons and temperature ■ reactions to products and chemicals ■ diet ■ health issues and underactive sebaceous glands. Use a moisturising shampoo and a dry scalp treatment. You may need a surface conditioner or treatment on the mid-lengths and ends of the hair too. 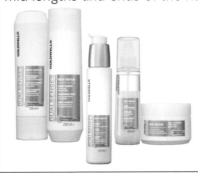
Product build-up 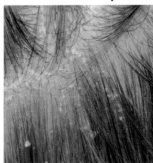	The root area may look oily, flaky or 'crunchy' with excess products visible on the scalp. The roots could also look dry, as some products dry and flake and give the illusion that the scalp is dandruff affected.	Products can coat the scalp, as well as the hair, making it feel sticky or oily. High-maintenance styles can sometimes be the causes of product build-up as excessive amounts of products may be required to support the style. Use a clarifying shampoo to cleanse the scalp and then repeat the shampoo process with a normal shampoo and a surface conditioner if required. 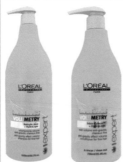

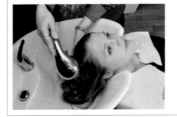

Scalp condition	Identified by?	Likely cause and products to use
Normal	A healthy scalp is a lighter version of the normal skin tone, without any dry or oily patches present.	For normal scalp conditions, use a normal shampoo and a light surface conditioner if required.

How contra-indications can affect the service

Contra-indications, such as skin and scalp disorders or product allergies, can affect the treatment being carried out, the type of product that can be used and the massage technique used. You must ask your client appropriate questions to find out the information required, if you cannot see a visible contra-indication. You should look at and feel the hair and scalp and listen to your client's responses to be sure which treatment is most suitable.

The following table shows the contra-indications that you must consider and the **implications** these may have for the service.

HANDY HINT

For more information on contra-indications, see chapter CHB9.

Implication

A likely effect or consequence.

Contra-indication	Possible implications for the service
Infections, infestations, and skin and scalp disorders	If your client has a disorder that is infectious, it will prevent the treatment being carried out. If it is non-infectious, check that the scalp is not tender, adapt the massage movements and be gentle.
Product allergies	Always ask if your client has experienced any reactions to previous treatments. Ask about other known allergies, such as allergies to nut products or aloe vera, as these are common ingredients in shampoos and conditioning treatments. If your client has a known allergy, check the ingredients on the container and use alternative products if required.
Recent scar tissue	If there is evidence of scar tissue, check that it has healed and is not tender or open. Use gentle massage movements over the scar tissue area.
Injuries to the area	If your client has had a recent bump to the head, it may not be visible through the hair but could cause the client discomfort if the massage is too firm. Use gentle massage movements.

Contra-indication	Possible implications for the service
Cuts and abrasions	If the cuts are open, then the treatment should not be carried out. If they are healed but sore and tender, be aware of where they are on the head and use gentle massage movements. Avoid scalp treatments containing alcohol, as these may cause a stinging sensation to the wound.

When asking your clients about the above contra-indications, always record their responses to your questions clearly and accurately on their client record card.

These details can be referred to for the client's next treatment. Should any problems arise which lead to legal action, you will have a clear record of the service and treatment you carried out and evidence of the client's responses.

Activity

List the information that should be recorded on a client's record card. Practise completing a record card recording all the information from your list. Double check your spellings, punctuation and grammar, and write neatly and accurately.

Science of shampooing, conditioning and scalp treatments

How shampoo and water act together to cleanse the hair

Oil and water don't mix! We know this from washing greasy roasting dishes in the kitchen, where we have to use plenty of washing-up detergent. Shampoos work in the same way as washing-up detergents.

Water is made from both hydrogen and oxygen atoms (H_2O). There is strong cohesion (sticking together) between water molecules, causing a skin-like surface to the water. This is commonly known as **surface tension** and can be seen by the way water forms droplets and the way they pool together.

Water and oil don't mix

Surface tension

The skin-like surface layer of a liquid.

Activity

Completely fill a glass with clean, fresh tap water until it is overflowing. You should be able to see that the water's surface is dome shaped and the level is higher than the glass! This is due to the surface tension of the water. Gently lay a small metal paperclip on the surface of the water. It should float on the surface of the water, again because of the surface tension. Now add another small metal paperclip that has been coated lightly in detergent. What happened when you added the second paper clip?

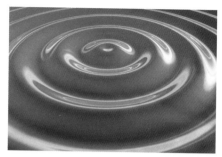

Ripples form on surface tension

Shampoos are made from cleansing agents called surfactants (the name surfactant is derived from 'surface', 'active' and 'agent'). A surfactant is an agent that actively reduces the surface tension. Surfactants contain molecules that are attracted to water at one end and oil at the other.

A surfactant molecule has a hydrophilic (water-loving) 'head' and a lipophilic (oil-loving) 'tail'. (We also refer to this lipophilic tail as hydrophobic – a water-hating tail.) A surfactant molecule dissolves in both oil and water and joins them together, enabling the breakdown of oils within water.

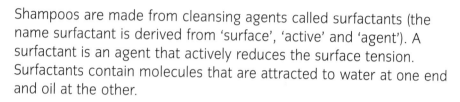

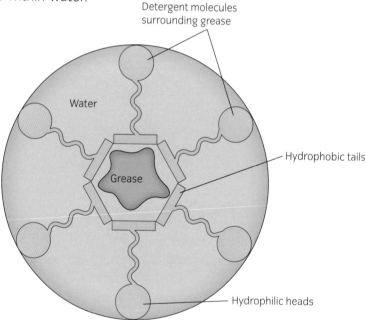

Surfactant (detergent) in water, surrounding grease

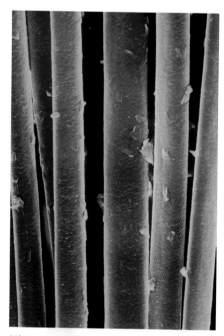

Microscope view: grease and dirt on the hair

When you apply a shampoo and water mix to the hair, you create lather. The hydrophilic head of the surfactant is drawn to the water, while the hydrophobic tail is drawn to the oil and grease on the hair and scalp.

The oil and grease contain dirt and skin particles. The lathering action of the 'head' and 'tail' of the surfactant creates a push and pull effect on the oil and grease, lifting it from the hair shaft. The more oil and grease there is to bond with the surfactant molecules,

HANDY HINT

If the hair does not lather on the first shampoo, it indicates that oil still remains within the hair and therefore further shampoo applications are required.

the less the shampoo will lather. This is why a second shampoo always lathers more richly, because the majority of the oil and grease has already been removed by the initial shampoo.

When you use fresh water to rinse away the shampoo's lather, which now contains the oil and grease from the hair, it leaves a clean, oil-free hair shaft.

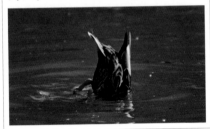

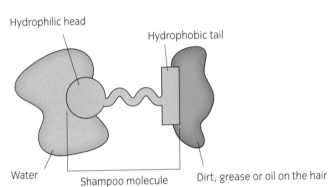

Hydrophilic head attached to the water and hydrophobic tail attached to the grease and dirt

Activity

Fill a glass almost to the top with fresh tap water and add a couple of tablespoons of oil (cooking oils work best as you can see the colour difference). What happens? Now add a small squirt of detergent and watch through the side of the glass and look at the oil pattern on the top. What happens? Give it a stir, wait a while, and see what happens next.

Now try it in a different order. Fill a glass with water, add detergent, then add the oil. What happens?

How products affect the hair

Our hair and skin are acidic and have a natural pH of 4.5–5.5. Therefore the day-to-day shampoos and conditioners we use must be pH-balanced to our hair and skin – also pH 4.5–5.5. This ensures that the hair and skin's natural moisture is maintained and the cuticle scales are closed.

The pH scale has a range of pH 0–14. Acid products (pH 0–6.9) close the cuticle. Alkaline products (pH 7.1–14) open/lift the cuticle scales.

Acid products, pH 0–pH 6.9:

- pH 0–1 – strong acids, which would destroy and dissolve the hair completely
- pH 1.5–4 – mild acids, which would cause the outer cuticle layer to shrink and harden while the body of the hair would swell (and eventually the hair could disintegrate)

- pH 4.5–5.5 – weak acids, found in shampoos and conditioners that are balanced to the hair and skin's natural pH.

pH-neutral (pH 7):

- water
- soapless shampoos – shampoos used to cleanse and clarify the hair before a perm are pH 7, which lifts the cuticle scales slightly to aid the perming process.

Alkaline products, pH 7.1–14:

- pH 7.1–7.9 – weak alkali, which slightly lifts the cuticle scales
- pH 8–10 – mild alkali, which swells the hair and causes the cuticle scales to open, allowing penetration into the cortex
- pH 10–14 – strong alkali, which causes a **depilatory** action, destroying and dissolving the hair completely.

Depilatory

Causing hair removal.

The diagram below shows the effects of acid and alkali products on the hair shaft.

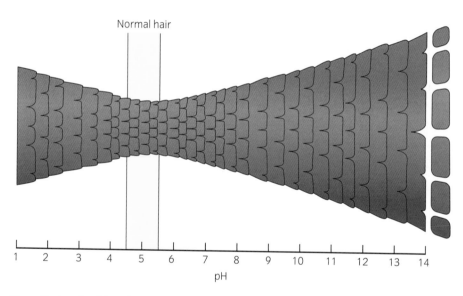

The effects of acid and alkali products on the hair shaft

You would most commonly use alkaline products when you need to lift the cuticle scales so that chemicals can **penetrate** the cortex layer.

Penetrate

Enter into.

HANDY HINT

Alkali perm solutions are pH 7.5–9.5.
Permanent colouring products are pH 8–9.5.

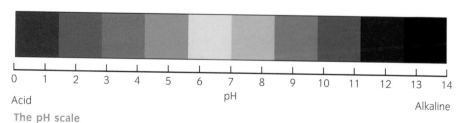

The pH scale

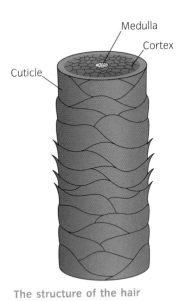

Medulla

Cortex

Cuticle

The structure of the hair

Accelerator

Appliance used to apply heat to the hair and speed up a service, for example a steamer, rollerball or climazone.

HANDY HINT

Heat and hot water open the cuticle scales while cold and cool water close the cuticle scales.

HANDY HINT

You must always carefully check the water temperature on your hands or wrists before you apply it through the hair.

HANDY HINT

If the hair is coated with oil-based products, you could apply the shampoo directly onto the hair, prior to wetting it during the shampoo process. This will give the hydrophobic tails in the shampoo molecule a chance to break down the oils and attach themselves before the water is added.

HANDY HINT

To help you remember which products lift or close the cuticle scales:

A**C**ID	ALKALINE
L	**I**
O	**F**
S	**T**
E	**S**
S	

The 'C' in 'a**C**id' helps you to remember they 'Close' the cuticle scales.

The 'L' in 'a**L**kaline' helps you to remember they 'Lift' the cuticle scales.

How heat affects hair during conditioning treatments

Temperature affects the cuticle scales in a similar way to acid and alkaline products. Heat aids the opening of the cuticle scales and is often used to reduce the processing time of chemical services. Heat is used to open the cuticle scales during a penetrating treatment so that the product can enter the cortex to strengthen the hair and aid repair.

Excessive heat, either from an **accelerator** used during a treatment, or from very hot water, can cause damage to your client's hair and scalp. Hot water should be avoided when shampooing oily scalps as the heat can activate the sebaceous glands and produce more sebum.

Effects of water temperature

It is essential that you consider the temperature of the water to maintain your client's comfort. While very hot water may scald, cold water is unpleasant and will cause discomfort.

After shampooing and conditioning, a cooler rinse may benefit the client by closing the cuticle scales.

Product build-up and its effects

Some products are more difficult to remove from the hair and can build up over time. Daily applications of products build up in between shampoos and can then coat the hair and the cuticle layer. Product build-up can cause hair to lose its shine and look lacklustre, as the light is being absorbed into the cuticles rather than being reflected. A build-up of products will coat the hair, causing a barrier, which may affect styling and chemical services too.

Products and techniques

Once you have consulted with your client and carried out the relevant hair tests, you are ready to choose the most suitable products for the client's hair and scalp condition, to prepare the hair for the service and to achieve the best result. You'll need to make sure you use the most suitable massage techniques for the hair and scalp type and to ensure client comfort.

Types of shampooing and conditioning available

Shampooing cleanses the hair and scalp, and prepares the hair for the following service. Conditioner provides shine by smoothing the cuticle scales, which improves the handling of the hair and makes combing and brushing easier.

The table below shows ingredients that are most suitable for certain hair and scalp conditions, and which type of conditioner should be used.

Hair and scalp condition	Likely ingredients used for shampoos and conditioners and how they affect the hair and scalp	Type of conditioning treatment
Normal	Rosemary, soya, aloe vera and jojoba oils are often key ingredients in all shampoos and conditioners. These ingredients help to maintain the hair's condition and moisture levels. Shampoo for normal hair Rinse-out conditioner for normal hair	Surface conditioner (rinse-out or leave-in) Leave-in conditioner
Dry	Coconut oil, jojoba oil, honey and almond or brazil nut oil are some of the main ingredients found in shampoos and conditioners to help treat dry hair and scalps. These products are naturally moisturising and nourish the hair.	Moisturising surface conditioner (rinse-out or leave-in) Penetrating conditioner (rinse-out or leave-in)

Hair and scalp condition	Likely ingredients used for shampoos and conditioners and how they affect the hair and scalp	Type of conditioning treatment
Dandruff-affected	Tea tree oil, zinc pyrithione and selenium sulphide are the main ingredients used to treat dandruff. Ginger, eucalyptus, lavender and sage may help to soothe the scalp. Shampoo for dandruff-affected hair	Scalp treatments (rinse-out or leave-in) Scalp treatment
Oily	Lemon, camomile, egg and citrus fruits are the main ingredients used to help break down the oils and scalp treatments (rinse-out or leave-in) slow down the production of sebum from the sebaceous glands. Shampoo for oily hair/scalp	Scalp treatments (rinse-out or leave-in) Scalp treatment

Activity

List the range of shampoos, conditioners and treatments available in your salon for dry, normal, oily and dandruff-affected hair and scalps.

Activity

Create a poster for your clients providing information about one or two of the products listed above. Make sure you check your spellings and that your grammar and punctuation are also correct. Make it colourful and appealing for your clients.

Potential effects of using incorrect products

Shampoos and conditioners are available for every hair type and scalp condition. If you use the incorrect shampoo or conditioner the hair and scalp could dry out. Using products that are too moisturising on an oily scalp could make the condition worse.

Importance of following instructions

You must always refer to the MFIs:

- for the correct use of products
- to check how much to use
- to find out how to apply the product
- to check whether heat is required
- to know how to remove the product from the hair.

If an inappropriate shampoo or conditioner is used, the product could coat the cuticle and cause a barrier to the following service. When shampooing the hair prior to a perm you should use a pre-perm shampoo, as it is pH neutral and lifts the cuticle scales, ready for the perm solution to enter the cortex. Never condition the hair and smooth the cuticle scales before a perm, as this will create a barrier to the perm solution.

Always ensure that you use the correct shampoo and conditioning product for the hair and scalp condition.

- Fine hair – excessive conditioner or deeply moisturising products can cause fine hair to become limp and lank.
- Oily scalps – using a moisturising shampoo will coat the hair with a layer of moisture and could activate the sebaceous glands, producing more sebum.
- Dry hair and scalps – using a shampoo for oily scalps may cause the hair to feel drier with rough cuticle scales. The product is designed to break down the natural oils needed for the hair, which may cause irritation to dry scalps.

HANDY HINT

For clients with fine hair, you will need less product and use more gentle movements, as the head is not protected as much as with dense hair. For dense hair you may need to use more product to cover the head and enable the shampoo to remove oil, dirt and debris from the hair.

HANDY HINT

When massaging, do not rub the hair as this will cause friction on the cuticle scales and tangle the hair. Ensure the hair is free from excess moisture so that when the client sits up they will not get wet and uncomfortable. Ask the client to sit up, and support their head and back as they rise.

HANDY HINT

Using the incorrect shampoo/conditioner can create a barrier by coating cuticle scales and preventing penetration of chemical services. They can also cause irritation to the scalp or the hair to become lank.

HANDY HINT

After chemical processes you must always use a pH-balancing conditioner to smooth and close the cuticle scales, and lock in the moisture to prevent the hair from drying out and becoming brittle.

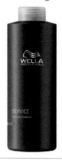

HANDY HINT

Avoid wastage and use products cost-effectively – use only the amount you need for the length and density of your client's hair.

HANDY HINT

At the end of the shampoo service, squeeze out and remove excess water from the hair before you apply the conditioner. This will prevent the conditioner from being diluted.

HANDY HINT

After the conditioning process, remove any excess water from the hair to prevent the hair from dripping and causing the client to get wet.

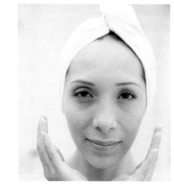

Massage techniques

There are a variety of different massage techniques that can be applied during the shampooing and conditioning process.

Shampooing massage techniques

Technique	When to use and purpose of massage	How to perform massage
Effleurage	During shampooing – it is particularly good for long hair to prevent tangles.	Effleurage massage is a gentle stroking massage movement used to apply the products to the hair.
Rotary	During shampooing – this massage movement benefits the client by stimulating the blood supply and relaxing the client. For clients with long hair, ensure that you remove your hands from the head regularly and comb through with your fingers, as continued rotary movements could cause tangles.	Rotary massage is a firm circular movement using the pads of the fingers over the surface of the scalp.
Friction	During shampooing for normal to dry scalps only – it is stimulating, rather than relaxing, and is not always carried out. It is only done for a few minutes, working from the front to the back. This method enables the sebaceous glands to be stimulated and the fast, firm, plucking movements help to stimulate the blood flow. This method must not be used on oily scalps or long hair.	A vigorous rubbing and plucking movement using the finger pads.

Conditioning massage techniques

Technique	When to use and purpose of massage	How to perform massage
Effleurage	During conditioning – used to apply the products to the hair and is particularly good for long hair to prevent tangles.	Effleurage is a gentle stroking massage movement.
Petrissage	During conditioning – this can be very relaxing for the client, but must be avoided on oily scalps. For long hair, your hands must be removed from the head regularly to prevent tangles, and you should return to the effleurage technique in between to detangle and soothe the scalp.	Petrissage is a slow, firm, deep, circular kneading massage movement, which stimulates the scalp and the sebaceous glands.

Tools and equipment

Before shampooing, you should use a bristle brush through the hair to remove tangles and loosen products. After shampooing, you can detangle the hair with a wide-toothed comb before applying a surface conditioner. While the surface conditioner is on the hair, comb through again with a wide-toothed comb. A brush shouldn't be used on wet hair because it can cause the hair to overstretch and break.

You can apply a penetrating treatment to the hair with a tint brush, then comb the product through. Long hair should be clipped up to prevent moisture from the hair soaking through the towel to the client's clothes. Always follow your MFIs to ensure that the correct product is chosen to achieve the best result and that you use an adequate amount. If heat is recommended to allow the treatment to open the cuticle scales and penetrate into the cortex, use the appliance safely.

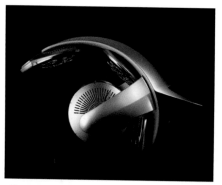

Climazone

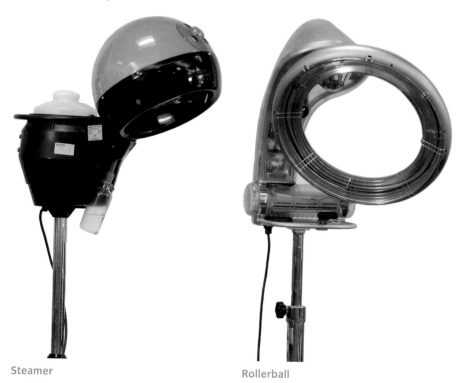

Steamer

Rollerball

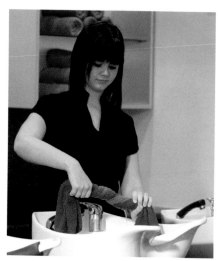

Heated damp towels

Steamers can be used to add heat to open the cuticle scales. This method uses moist heat.

Climazones or rollerballs can be used to apply dry heat to the hair to open the cuticle scales.

Heated damp towels can also be used as a moist heat method for hot oil treatments.

Detangling hair from point to root

The cuticle scales overlap each other and lie flat from root to point when closed. When you detangle the hair after shampooing and conditioning you should always use a wide-toothed comb. Start combing at the ends of the hair (points), in a downwards direction, and start each new stroke further up so that you work progressively up towards the root area. This ensures that you work with the direction of the cuticle scales.

Keeping your knowledge up to date

It is important that your knowledge of the salon's product range, both at the shampoo area and available for retail, is sound and up to date. You should be advising your client of the most suitable shampoos, conditioners and treatments available in the salon and to purchase for use at home.

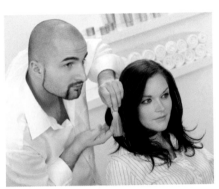
Providing advice to a client

Providing aftercare

The products you use in the salon to shampoo and condition the hair and scalp should be explained, demonstrated and recommended to your client for use at home. When advising your clients about retail products you must give clear and accurate information about why you are recommending these products, and their benefits. Openly and constructively discuss the condition of the client's hair and scalp and how these retail products will help to improve or maintain the condition.

When giving aftercare advice, use positive body language that promotes an open and trusting relationship. Use eye contact and check the client's body language to identify any areas of uncertainty. Use open and closed questions to really understand your client's needs for home haircare.

You will need to know your salon's available brands of products to be able to give the most effective aftercare advice to your client. Give them advice for maintaining the condition of their hair and scalp between salon visits, and include how the products should be used and how often.

Always consider your client's lifestyle. Does your client have time for further salon treatments, or would they be best suited to maintain the condition of their hair at home? Would your client prefer the convenience of surface conditioners, rather than having to find 20 minutes to develop a penetrating conditioner and heat some towels to aid the process?

HANDY HINT

When providing aftercare you should do the following to communicate effectively:

- provide clear and accurate information
- give feedback and advice that is open and constructive
- use positive body language
- use open and closed questions.

THE CITY & GUILDS TEXTBOOK

If your client's hair had product build-up, you should suggest alternative products that will still suit their particular hairstyle, but will work more effectively with the hair and scalp. If your client wants to keep working with their current styling product, offer advice on how the client could improve the removal process; perhaps suggest that your client uses neat shampoo on the hair, if wax products have been used. Neat shampoo will attach to the oil-based product prior to wetting the hair and enable a more thorough removal.

Clients with damaged hair should be given advice on how to detangle the hair, and how to comb and brush their hair correctly to avoid further damage.

For clients who are off on holiday, offer advice on hair protection from the sun and wind, and perhaps the benefits of wearing a hat.

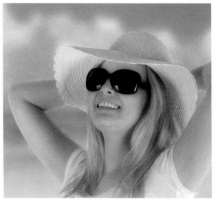

Protect hair from environmental damage with a hat

Activity

What advice would you give the following clients?

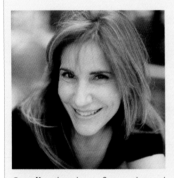

Caroline has long, fine, coloured hair and is going on holiday next week in the sun.

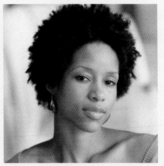

Leticia has very curly short dry hair and dandruff caused by an allergic reaction to chemicals.

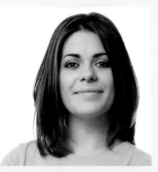

Claire has oily, medium-length hair that is a little dry at the ends from previous colour treatments.

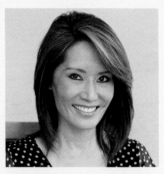

Gita has a dry scalp, medium-length red-tinted Asian hair, and swims regularly.

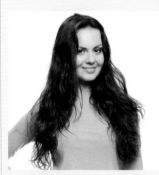

Anita has long, abundant hair that is very dry on the mid-lengths and ends.

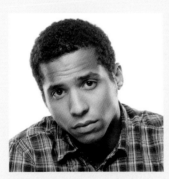

Kelvin loves his sport and washes his hair regularly.

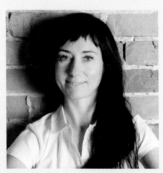

Suzie enjoys going for a spin on her motorbike, but her long hair suffers in the wind.

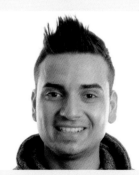

Paul has oily-looking hair and uses a lot of wax products to support his hairstyle.

Activity

How long does your salon allow for:

- a shampoo and surface conditioning service on above-shoulder-length hair?
- a shampoo and surface conditioning service on below-shoulder-length hair?
- a shampoo and penetrating conditioning service on below-shoulder-length hair?
- a shampoo and scalp treatment on above-shoulder length-hair?

Based on your answers to the previous activity, in one hour and 30 minutes how many of the following could you do?

- Shampoo and surface conditioning service on above-shoulder-length hair
- Shampoo and surface conditioning service on below-shoulder-length hair.

In two hours and 30 minutes how many of the following could you do?

- Shampoo and penetrating conditioning service on below-shoulder-length hair
- Shampoo and scalp treatment on above-shoulder-length hair.

Shampooing, conditioning and scalp treatment services – review

Prepare to shampoo, condition and treat the hair and scalp

In order for you to be ready and prepared for the service, you need to ensure your own personal hygiene and appearance are up to salon standards and meets with client expectations. You should prepare your hands for the service ahead and use barrier or hand cream.

Work safely and hygienically

Ensure that you:

- maintain your responsibilities for health and safety
- wear personal protective equipment if required
- consider your posture and your client's body position for health and safety, and comfort
- keep your work area clean and tidy
- minimise risks of damage to tools
- use clean resources and minimise the risk of cross-infection

- promote environmental and sustainable working practices and minimise waste

- ensure your personal hygiene, protection and appearance are up to salon standard

- minimise risk of injury to self and others and follow manufacturers' instructions

- use your time effectively and complete the service in a commerically acceptable time.

Consult with clients and select products and tools

Ask your clients questions to identify whether they have any contra-indications to hair and scalp treatments. When you have identified the best service to provide for your client's hair and scalp condition, you can select the correct products and set up your tools and equipment for the service.

Carry out shampooing, conditioning and treatment services

Before you shampoo the client's hair, always ensure you protect your client's clothing, and gown them for the service.

Make effective use of your time

You must work effectively and manage your time successfully. Ensure the basin area is well prepared, clean and tidy, with a supply of fresh towels and gowns. If you are using a trolley and applying a treatment at the workstation, you must ensure that you have the trolley to your favoured side of working, to suit whether you are left- or right-handed.

Make sure that there is sufficient stock of shampoos and conditioners and that treatments are available. If you notice you are running low on resources, such as towels and gowns, you must inform the relevant person or reload the washing machine/dryer to ensure a plentiful supply. If stock, such as shampoos, needs re-ordering, inform the relevant person or note it on the stock list.

The shampoo and conditioning service

You will be assessed carrying out a shampoo service and whilst applying either a surface conditioner and or a treatment conditioner.

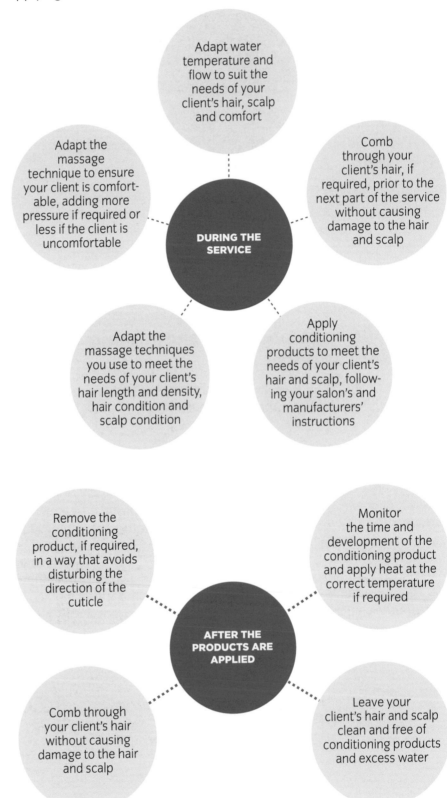

DURING THE SERVICE

Adapt water temperature and flow to suit the needs of your client's hair, scalp and comfort

Comb through your client's hair, if required, prior to the next part of the service without causing damage to the hair and scalp

Apply conditioning products to meet the needs of your client's hair and scalp, following your salon's and manufacturers' instructions

Adapt the massage techniques you use to meet the needs of your client's hair length and density, hair condition and scalp condition

Adapt the massage technique to ensure your client is comfortable, adding more pressure if required or less if the client is uncomfortable

AFTER THE PRODUCTS ARE APPLIED

Remove the conditioning product, if required, in a way that avoids disturbing the direction of the cuticle

Monitor the time and development of the conditioning product and apply heat at the correct temperature if required

Leave your client's hair and scalp clean and free of conditioning products and excess water

Comb through your client's hair without causing damage to the hair and scalp

Provide advice and recommendations

Always:

- advise your client on the correct detangling techniques
- advise on suitable shampoos and conditioning products
- advise on appropriate time intervals between services
- advise on present and future products and services.

Step by steps

In this part of the chapter we look at how to shampoo the hair and scalp using the correct massage techniques.

Shampoo the hair and scalp using massage techniques

Once you have decided on the correct tools, equipment and products required to achieve the desired result, you can begin the shampoo process. You'll need to use the effleurage massage technique to apply the product to the hair. Effleurage is a gentle stroking movement, using the palms of your hands. Once the product is applied, you would use rotary massage movements to cleanse the hair. Rotary is a quick, small circular movement used to loosen the dirt from the scalp and hair. Your hands are positioned in a claw-like manner and you use your finger pads to work around the head in a methodical way to cleanse the whole head.

> **HANDY HINT**
>
> Brush dry hair before shampooing to detangle, but use a wide-toothed comb when the hair is wet. Always comb or brush the hair following the direction of the cuticles. Start towards the points of the hair in a downwards direction and then start each new stroke further up so you work up towards the roots.

> **HANDY HINT**
>
> Always check that the hair is not caught between the basin and your client's neck as you position your client. Push the hair back so that water does not drip on your client's face. Ensure that the water is directed away from your client's face. For the client's comfort, ensure you use your finger pads and not your fingernails on the scalp.

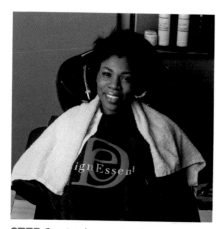

STEP 1 – Apply a protective gown. Take a disposable towel and fold a small lip across the long edge at the top, double lining the collar area for extra protection. The doubled side provides a firm edge for tucking.

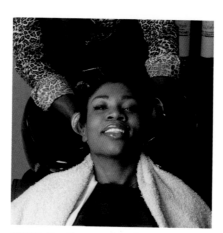

STEP 2 – Support the client when moving back into the backwash, adjust the basin and check that the client is comfortable. Ensure all the hair is in the backwash.

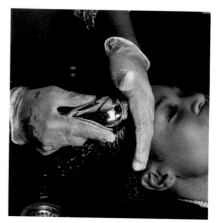

STEP 3 – Wet your hands and shake off any excess water. Gently wet the hairline to gather in all the hair. Protective gloves may be worn.

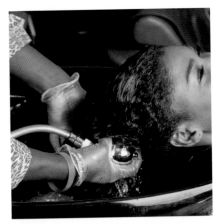

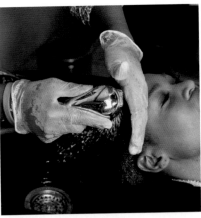

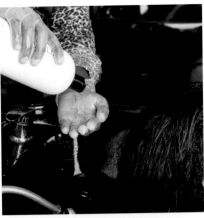

STEP 4 – Apply water to the crown first. Apply the water on and off the scalp and check client is happy with the temperature. Ensure that all the hair is saturated including hairlines and lengths.

STEP 5 – Using your hand as a guard move the water flow nearer to the hairline, stroking away excess water as you work. Continue until both sides are evenly damp. Lift the head and check the underneath for saturation. Evenly soak the back of the head by cupping one hand along the hairline and applying water with the other to prevent the water from soaking the client.

STEP 6 – Brush away or wring the excess water from the hair before applying the shampoo. Depending on the manufacturer's instructions, use approximately a 3cm (1¼in) diameter of shampoo in the palm of the hand.

HANDY HINT

The same process is used for a male client. With shorter hair be aware that the saturated hair can spring back and splash the client.

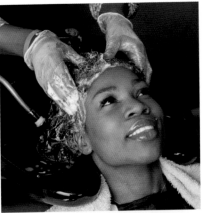

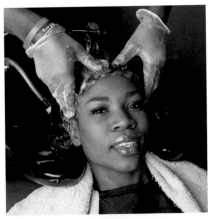

STEP 7 – Massage the product in your hands and with your palms flat, work from the front hairline to apply the shampoo with an effleurage technique. Make sure you apply the product to all of the hair, especially around the hairlines and throughout long hair. Lift the head to apply shampoo to the underneath.

STEP 8 – Use your fingers and thumbs and a rotary technique to work the shampoo into the hair. Start from the front hairline to the top of the head.

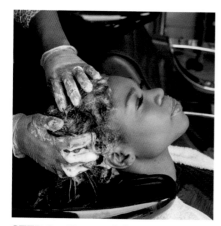

STEP 9 – Then work from the centre front hairline into the side hairlines. Then work behind the ears into the nape and up through the centre of the head. (If the hair is short you could also use the friction massage technique through the sides and back.)

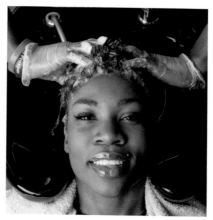

STEP 10 – Rinse the product from your hands, check the water temperature and rinse the hair, guarding the face, ear and neck areas. Repeat if necessary.

Condition the hair and scalp using massage techniques

Having completed the shampooing procedure, you can now apply a surface conditioner.

Before applying surface conditioner, ensure the hair is free from excess moisture, as the water will dilute the product.

HANDY HINT

Surface conditioners add moisture to the surface of the hair and smooth the cuticle scales. Penetrating treatments can help to repair the hair's structure and strengthen the cortex. Scalp treatments treat scalp conditions.

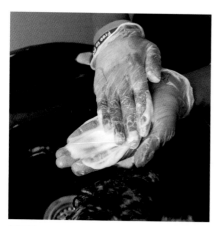

STEP 1 – Apply conditioner to the palms of your hands and rub together.

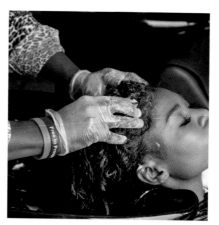

STEP 2 – Apply conditioner using an effleurage technique to work the product into the hair. This will relax your client and will stimulate the blood supply. Apply a petrissage massage technique to the sides and work in to the top. Apply the same technique down the centre ensuring coverage of lengths, hairline and the nape.

HANDY HINT

Care must be taken when using petrissage massage movements on long hair to avoid tangling the hair and causing discomfort to your client.

Do not use petrissage massage movements on oily scalps as it will activate the sebaceous glands and make the hair greasy.

For long hair and oily scalps only use effleurage massage movements. For oily scalps use a surface conditioner on the mid-lengths and ends only.

HANDY HINT

Hair stretches when wet, so always use a wide-toothed comb so that you don't damage the hair and to prevent the hair from snagging.

HANDY HINT

Ensure the water flow follows the direction of the cuticle scales to help smooth them.

HANDY HINT

If you notice there is still conditioning product in the hair, rinse the hair again, otherwise it may cause a barrier on the hair, making it lank and limp.

HANDY HINT

Surface conditioners and penetrating treatments can be used alongside a scalp treatment, as one conditions the hair and the other treats the scalp.

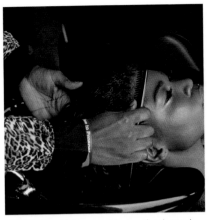

STEP 3 – Using a wide-toothed comb, comb through the conditioner from the ends to the tips and then rinse thoroughly.

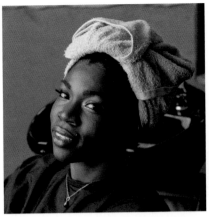

STEP 4 – Apply a folded towel over the front hairline, wrap it down over the ears, under the back and pass one side over the other. Wrap up and over and secure into the fold.

Scalp and penetrating conditioner treatments

Most scalp treatments come in the form of tonics and are applied directly to the scalp. If the product is very watery, then apply it at the basin and ensure your client keeps their head back. If it is sprinkled onto the hair, it can be applied at the workstation. These products are not washed out of the hair and can be applied after a surface or penetrating conditioner.

Before applying penetrating conditioner, ensure the hair is free from excess moisture, as the water will dilute the product. Section the hair from the centre to each side. Each section should be approximately 2cm (¾in) in depth apart.

The treatment can also be applied to mid-lengths and ends only, if this is more suitable for the scalp. If you are applying the product to the scalp, and when you have coated the product through the entire surface of the hair, use petrissage massage movements to stimulate the blood flow to the scalp.

Steamers are the preferred method of applying heat with penetrating treatments as they add moisture and are kinder to the hair.

Always accurately monitor the time, following the MFIs.

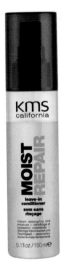

Scalp treatment

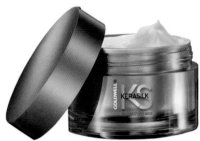

Penetrating conditioner mask

Answers in the back of the book.

1 Which one of the following is a risk associated with the shampooing service?

a Scalp burns

b Using shampoo

c Hot water

d Water on the floor

2 Which one of the following is the best way of minimising risks due to contact with shampoo?

a Drying hands

b Rinsing hands

c Wearing a plastic apron

d Wearing non-latex gloves

3 Which one of the following is the most likely consequence of incorrect positioning of the client at the basin?

a They could get wet and be uncomfortable

b The stylist may suffer from allergies

c Contact dermatitis

d Slippery surfaces

4 Which one of the following is the best way of supporting the environment when working in the salon?

a Reusing all products

b Recycling all products

c Disposing of all products

d Reducing the use of all products

5 Which one of the following describes the risk of contracting contact dermatitis when shampooing hair?

a The risk is low

b The risk is high

c There is no risk at all

d It's not a risk, it's a hazard

6 Which one of the following is not a contra-indication to shampooing?

a Oily scalp

b Skin disorders

c Cuts and abrasions

d Allergies to products

7 Which two of the following describes product build-up on the hair?

1 Dull hair

2 Flaky deposits on hair

3 Smooth cuticle scales

4 Excessively oily hair

a 1 and 2

b 2 and 3

c 3 and 4

d 4 and 1

8 Which one of the following states how the name 'surfactant' is derived?

a Surface additive alkali

b Surface active agent

c Salt acidic agent

d Salt active alkali

9 A detergent molecule is partly hydrophilic. What is the meaning of the term and which part is hydrophilic?

a Water loving; the head

b Water loving; the tail

c Water hating; the head

d Water hating; the tail

10 Which of the following is the best conditioner to recommend for a client with dry, damaged hair?

a A surface conditioner

b A penetrating conditioner

c A scalp treatment conditioner

d A conditioner containing zinc pyrithione

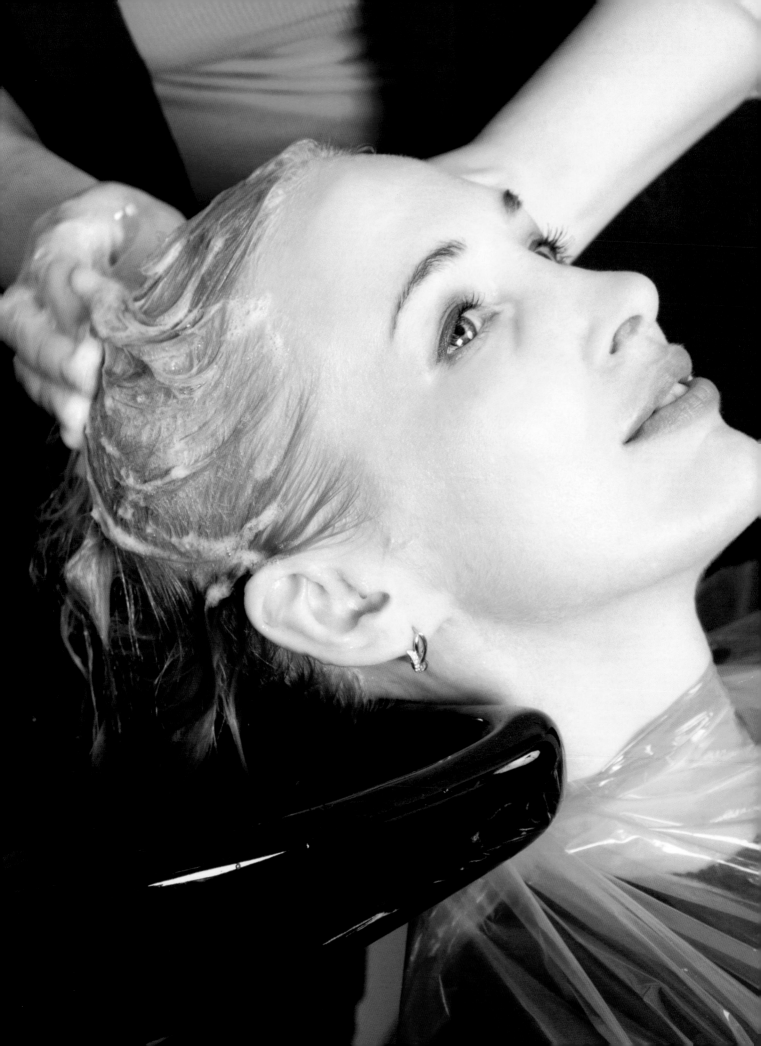

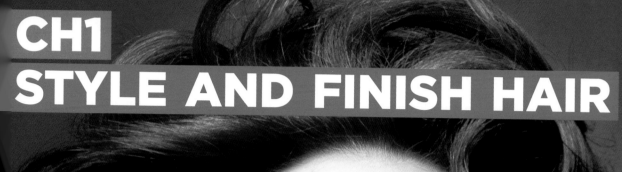

CH1
STYLE AND FINISH HAIR

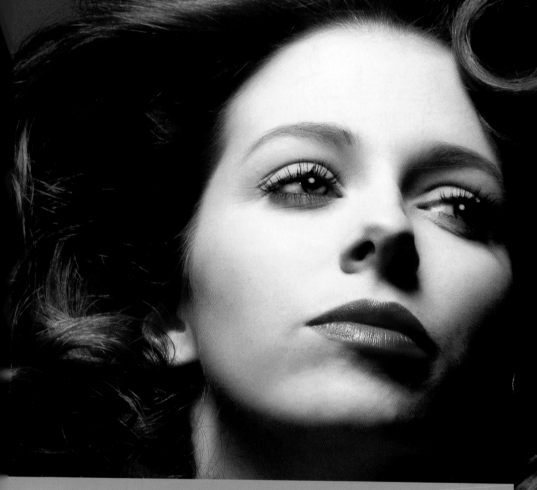

The style and finish of the hair usually complete the overall service. If the hair has been cut, coloured or permed before styling, the styling and finishing procedure presents the fabulous end result. It is essential that the overall finish is satisfactory to your client and they have been advised on how to maintain their style between salon visits.

This chapter gives you the underlying knowledge and understanding of the basic skills required to style and finish hair, which can be built on as you gain confidence and experience.

After reading this chapter you will:

■ know how health and safety affects styling and finishing services

■ understand the factors that influence styling and finishing services

■ know the tools, equipment, products and techniques used to style and finish hair

■ be able to provide styling and finishing services.

HEALTH & SAFETY

Refer to the health and safety and salon policies chapter for a recap on the health and safety Acts you must follow when styling and finishing hair.

HEALTH & SAFETY

Refer to the health and safety and salon policies chapter for a recap on protecting the environment and maintaining sustainable working practices.

VALUES & BEHAVIOURS

Refer to the values and behaviours chapter for more information on maintaining effective, hygienic and safe working practices, and the importance of adhering to instructions.

HANDY HINT

Always replenish stock without causing a disruption to the client's service and report shortages to the relevant person.

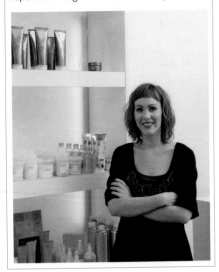

VALUES & BEHAVIOURS

Refer to the values and behaviours chapter for more information on appearance, personal hygiene and behaviour.

Health and safety

During a styling and finishing service you will be working with electrical equipment on wet hair and using substances that could be hazardous to your health if inhaled, ingested or absorbed.

Always take care when using electrical items and using products, and follow the instructions of the manufacturer, the supplier and your salon.

Your responsibilities for health and safety

Working methods and sustainable practices

There are hundreds of different styling and finishing products available on the market to help the stylist and client maintain great-looking hair. They are all marketed differently to attract various client groups to their designs. The instructions on the product advise you and the client how to use the product effectively and how much of the product should be used. Always read the manufacturer's instructions (MFIs) to ensure you use the correct amount to achieve the best result, to prevent overloading the hair and to protect the environment.

Personal hygiene, protection and appearance

It is important that you meet your organisation and industry standards of appearance and ensure your personal hygiene is well maintained.

Activity

- List four things you should do to maintain your personal hygiene.
- What protection (PPE) is available for you to use when styling and finishing hair?
- Describe your salon's dress code.

Client protection and preparation

To prepare your client for a styling service you would gown and protect them in the same way as you would for a shampoo service. Shampooing and conditioning the hair prior to starting the blow dry or finger dry prepares the hair for the service. Styling products are then applied to towel-dried hair.

Hazards and risks

Complete the risks of the listed hazards and add one or two hazards to the list.

Hazard	Risk
Electrical equipment	Working with wet hair or if equipment is simply faulty, this could lead to an electric shock
Substances – styling and finishing products	
Trailing wires	

Safe working practices

Using products safely

When using styling and finishing products, you should ideally wear gloves during application, wash and dry your hands regularly, and use hand cream afterwards to avoid contact dermatitis.

When using styling and finishing products you must do so safely and economically. Always ensure you follow COSHH regulations.

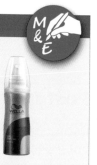

Wella Curl Craft wax mousse comes in a 200ml container. If you waste 8ml of this product on every client and use this on 12 clients a week, how much product would you waste every week? Work out how many full containers of Curl Craft wax mousse you will have wasted over a three-month period.

> **HANDY HINT**
>
> Dermatitis can be recognised by inflamed skin, which may be red and sore, and the skin can weep and split.

> **HANDY HINT**
>
> Using too much product is wasteful and the salon will lose profit; excessive use of products can also overload the hair, affecting the end result.

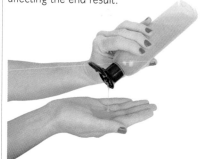

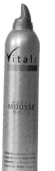
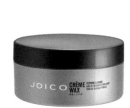
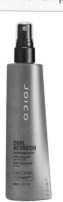
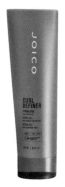
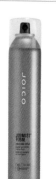
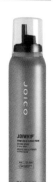

Styling products

HANDY HINT

Ineffectively maintained tools and equipment can lead to poor health and safety, poor hygiene, risk of cross-infection and infestation, and a negative salon image.

HANDY HINT

Incorrect application of heat can cause damage to the hair and a loss of elasticity, damage to the cuticle scales and an increase in porosity. You could also discolour the hair, or cause client discomfort.

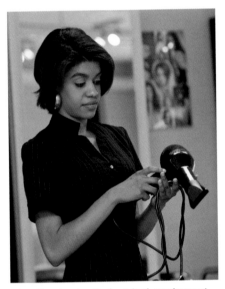

Visually check all electrical equipment before use

Health and safety

In the health and safety chapter, refer to the 'Environmental and sustainable practices' section to ensure you dispose of styling and finishing products and faulty electrical equipment correctly and in a manner that will protect the environment.

Using your tools and equipment effectively and safely

Always ensure your equipment is in good working order and fit for use. Use equipment correctly, following the MFIs to minimise damage to the tools and prevent any risk of injury to you and your clients. Maintain the condition of your tools and prevent a reduction in their performance by cleaning them regularly and keeping them free from product build-up and hair. Before plugging in and switching on your hairdryer, check that it is safe to use and the air vent filter is attached and clean.

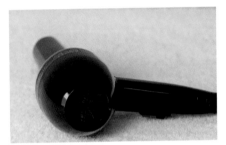

Check hairdryer air vent filter before use

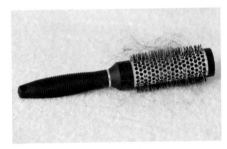

Clean your tools regularly

When using your electrical equipment, be aware of potential hazards and follow the Electricity at Work Regulations. You must visually check your appliances for cracks in the main body and plug and kinks in the wires. Always label, remove and report faulty electrical equipment.

Posture and positioning

During the styling and finishing service make sure that you maintain a good posture and keep your back straight with your legs slightly apart for an even balance. A good posture will help to prevent back injuries and fatigue. Keep your trolley to the correct side of you – right-hand side if you're right-handed and left-hand side if you're left-handed. This will help you work effectively and methodically, as well as preventing you having to stretch over for tools and equipment.

For the comfort of your client ensure that they have their feet supported on a footstep, if the stylist chair is raised, or on the floor. Sit them upright with their back against the chair. It's important that your client is comfortable throughout the service and evenly balanced, so that you can produce a balanced hairstyle.

THE CITY & GUILDS TEXTBOOK

Preventing cross-infection and infestation

Working safely, hygienically and tidily minimises risk of harm and injury to yourself and others and prevents cross-contamination. It gives the client an image of professionalism while their hair is being styled.

Safe and hygienic working practices

You must always protect your client during the styling service with a fresh, clean gown and towel. You should wear gloves when applying styling and finishing products, to prevent dermatitis and maintain healthy hands, and an apron to protect your clothes.

Clean and tidy work area

You must keep your work area clean and tidy at all times. Make sure that your trolley and workstation are prepared for the required styling service and that you are ready for the client to arrive. Sterilise your styling tools and equipment to ensure they are hygienic and ready for use. Clean your workstation and surfaces with detergent and water, disinfect your equipment with suitable disinfectants or a UV light, and sterilise tools in the autoclave.

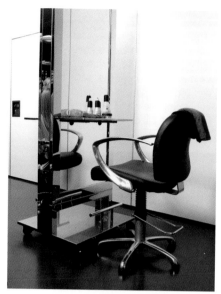

Professional work area, clean and tidy

HANDY HINT

Poor standards of health and hygiene can cause offence to others, cross-contaminate and present a poor salon image.

VALUES & BEHAVIOURS

Refer to the sterilisation section of the values and behaviours chapter for more information on how to clean, sterilise and disinfect styling equipment.

Importance of questioning clients

During the consultation you will need to use your English skills to ask your client questions to identify their needs, and analyse the hair by visually checking and feeling it, to identify any factors that may affect the service.

You'll need to ask your client the following types of question:

- What is their conception of the finished look?
- What products do they generally use on their hair and why?
- What time or lifestyle factors affect the time they spend on their hair between salon visits?
- Have they been happy with their previous style and do they wish to change or alter anything?
- Have they had any specific problems maintaining their style?
- What styling equipment do they use at home?
- Does the client have any allergies?

You'll need to visually check and feel the hair to identify:

- the condition of the hair and scalp
- the length, style, type, texture and density of the hair

HANDY HINT

Use open and closed questions to obtain all relevant information required. Open questions that start with 'what', 'why', 'how' and 'when' usually require more in-depth and specific answers while closed questions require 'yes' or 'no' or one-word answers.

HANDY HINT

You must carry out a porosity test to identify if the cuticle scales are open, and the hair therefore porous, and an elasticity test to test the strength of the cortex.

WHY DON'T YOU...

Listen to the stylists in your salon consulting with their clients.

VALUES & BEHAVIOURS

Refer back to the values and behaviours chapter for more information on maintaining customer care, personal and professional ethics, identifying and confirming the client's expectations and keeping he client informed and reassured.

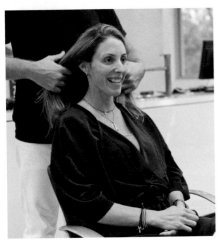

Stylist visually checking the hair prior to the service

- any growth patterns
- the client's head and face shape
- any scalp problems
- how long the service will take.

Once you have this information from your client you will be able to provide them with advice and recommendations on what products to use to maintain the look or suggest any additional services that may benefit the client.

Activity

Think of any other questions that you could ask your client about their hair or their requirements.

During this process, record any answers about allergies and the hair's condition on a record card in case you need to refer back to the information in the future, or if there are any problems and you need evidence of the client's comments. You must write clearly and ensure all spellings and details are correct.

Factors affecting styling and finishing services

The following factors need to be considered when styling and finishing hair:

- hair characteristics
- hair classifications
- hair length and haircut
- hair growth patterns
- head and face shape.

Hair characteristics

The table shows the types of hair characteristics that can affect the style, causing you to have to adapt your choice of products and their quantities, and your choice of tools and equipment.

THE CITY & GUILDS TEXTBOOK

Factor	Effect on the style	Effect on product choices	Effect on tool choices	Effect on equipment choices
Texture Fine hair	With fine hair you will need to consider the length of the hair; longer lengths may look thinner and be more suited to a shorter cut style.	Fine hair will need less product. Use products which support the style and give the hair body and volume – even for smooth straight styles.	Fine hair will need brushes to give root lift and support the style.	Finger drying with a diffuser may work well if the hair has natural body and movement, or a brush blow dry for lift. Tonging may help give longevity to curls but take care with the heat settings on fine hair.
Coarse hair	Coarse hair can have a tendency to look rough and dry, and smoother styles may be difficult for the client to maintain between salon visits.	Coarse hair will need more product that smooths the hair and gives it shine, such as a serum.	Coarse hair will need a bristle brush to smooth the hair, but will not require much root lift.	Coarse hair generally benefits from smoothing and blow drying rather than finger drying as the hair is smoothed around the hair brush. Straighteners can be used to smooth the coarse look of the hair.
Density Sparse hair	**Sparse** hair should be treated in the same way as fine hair. **Sparse** Thinly scattered.			
Abundant hair	**Abundant** hair will take longer to dry and may make the style look big, so the style needs to be considered. **Abundant** Great in amount or number.	Abundant hair will need more products and those that do not provide any volume or lift but help to smooth the hair.	Thoroughly dry the root area and take smaller sections of hair; blow dry towards the ends. Avoid brushes that promote volume and root lift.	Always rough dry abundant hair before sectioning and blow drying to make effective use of your time and reduce the excess moisture. Use straightening irons to help flatten thick hair.

Factor	Effect on the style	Effect on product choices	Effect on tool choices	Effect on equipment choices
Porosity Porous hair can tangle and break easily	If hair is porous, avoid longer styles or longer layers. Hair will tangle and might break. Suggest shorter styles and/or conditioning treatments.	Avoid 'sticky' products that offer strong hold as the hair will tangle easily. Suggest smoothing products, such as serums. Use heat protectors with heated appliances.	Avoid using non-bristle brushes, as these may cause the hair to snag and break. Use smoothing brushes and wide-tooth combs.	Suggest minimal use of heated appliances, as these will cause further worsening of porosity. Nozzles may be suitable, attached to the dryer to encourage the airflow down the hair to help smooth the cuticles. Avoid too much direct heat.
Elasticity Elasticity test	For hair with poor elasticity, avoid longer styles and suggest shorter lengths and/or conditioning treatments to improve the condition of the hair's cortex.	Choose products, tools and equipment for hair with poor elasticity as you would for porous hair.		
Condition	Hair that is in bad condition will have either poor porosity or poor elasticity and possibly both. Suggest shorter lengths and/or conditioning treatments to improve the condition of the hair's cortex.	If hair is in bad condition, choose products, tools and equipment as you would for porous hair.		
Hair growth patterns Cowlick	A cowlick affects the fringe area; you may need to advise of a more suitable style.	When working with a cowlick, use a stronger styling product on the fringe area and a hairspray to hold.	Use a brush to smooth and control the cowlick, or work with it when finger drying the hair.	Use a nozzle when blow drying to aim the airflow in the direction you want the cowlick to go. Try using straighteners to hold the cowlick in place, taking care with the heat near the skin.

Factor	Effect on the style	Effect on product choices	Effect on tool choices	Effect on equipment choices
Nape whorl	Nape whorls don't cause a problem to longer styles. Consider how nape whorls work with shorter styles, and avoid cutting into the nape area.	Use a strong finishing product on a nape whorl if it tries to defeat you. A little hairspray may help too.	Use a flat brush and dry into the neck to avoid root lift near the nape whorl.	Use a nozzle on the hairdryer to aim the airflow downwards and dry the nape whorl flat. Straighteners will not help you if the hair is short – you will burn the client's neck.
Double crown	Try to work with double crowns, as they can cause the hair to stick up. Play with the hair and see in which direction it settles the best; use this to recommend to your client the best direction for the style.	Use a strong-hold styling product around the crown area and hairspray to hold the finished look.	Use a radial brush and direct the airflow to the root, bending the hair into the desired direction.	Use a nozzle with the hairdryer to aim the airflow in the desired direction. If aiming for a funky, messy image, work with the double crown and use it in a finger dry.
Widow's peak	With a widow's peak, you should avoid fringes and aim for styles where the front section is styled backwards or slightly to one side.	Use products to hold and support the hair over or to one side.	Use a radial brush to direct the root area over or to one side.	Use a nozzle on the hairdryer to aid the direction of the airflow. Diffusers can be used to finger dry and **manipulate** the hair into the desired direction. Straighteners can be used – take care near the skin and forehead. **Manipulate** Handle skilfully.

Hair length and haircut

Factor	Effect on the style	Effect on product choices	Effect on tool choices	Effect on equipment choices
Hair length 	Longer hair requires more maintenance. Longer layers will need to be supported with suitable products and styling tools. More blow drying is likely to be required on longer hair styles, and possibly the use of straightening irons or tongs to give long-lasting effects.	Supporting products, such as hairsprays and root lift products may be required. Use heat protectors with any heated appliance. Use serums on the ends of the hair. More product will be required for longer hair.	A variety of brushes may be required to obtain root lift. Large round/radial brushes will help to obtain lift and smooth the hair.	A good, professional hairdryer would be beneficial to you to speed the drying process time. Straightening irons or curling tongs may be used to enhance the longevity of the style. Nozzles may help when blow drying to smooth the hair and help direct the heat where it is needed.
Haircut 	The haircut is very important, as this is the how the hair has been cut for the style; you must work with it, not against it. Identify if you are blow drying or finger drying the hair to achieve the best finished result.	Suggest and use products to support the hairstyle. Identify whether you need root lift and volume, or a smooth and straight finish. Use products to suit length and condition of hair.	Use a radial brush for lift and volume, or a flat brush to smooth and avoid lift.	Does the result require a brush and hairdryer blow dry, or can you use a diffuser and finger dry? Would a nozzle help you to smooth the hair? Would the style benefit from straightening or tonging for **longevity**? **Longevity** Ability to last longer.

Hair classifications

Factor	Effect on the style	Effect on product choices	Effect on tool choices	Effect on equipment choices
Straight hair – type 1 Fine/thin hair	Hair tends to be very soft, shiny and oily; it can be difficult to achieve a curl.	Use products that will aid body and hold. Avoid oily products and do not overload the hair.	Use tools that will grip the hair and hold it in place whilst styling, as it will resist curling.	May benefit from using heated styling equipment such as tongs if curl and body are required. Tongs
Medium density hair	Hair can have lots of volume and body and can be wonderful to work with.	Use products to suit style.	Use tools to suit style. Paddle brush	Use equipment to suit style.
Coarse hair	Hair can be extremely straight and difficult to curl.	To curl straight, coarse hair, use products with strong hold and curl-enhancing products. Serums will help add shine when using straighteners. Heat protector spray	Use tools that will grip the hair and hold it in place whilst styling, as it will resist curling. Medium radial brush	May benefit from using heated styling equipment such as tongs if curl and body are required.

Factor	Effect on the style	Effect on product choices	Effect on tool choices	Effect on equipment choices
Wavy hair – type 2 Fine/thin hair	Hair can normally be styled easily and has a definite 'S' pattern.	Use products to suit style.	Use tools to suit style.	Use equipment to suit style.
 Medium density hair	Hair tends to be frizzy and a little resistant to styling.	Use styling products to smooth frizz and also give hold and movement to the hair. Serum	Use tools that will grip the hair and hold it in place whilst styling, as it will resist styling.	May benefit from using heated styling equipment such as tongs or straightening irons to provide longevity to the style.
 Coarse hair	Hair tends to be very resistant to styling and normally very frizzy. The waves are often quite thick.	Use products to smooth frizz and control the waves, whilst providing hold.	Use tools that will smooth the frizz and grip the hair holding it in place whilst styling, as it will resist styling.	May benefit from using heated styling equipment such as tongs or straightening irons to provide longevity to the style. Straightening irons
Curly hair – type 3 Loose curls	Hair tends to have a combination texture – it can be thick with lots of body, but can sometimes be frizzy.	Use products to smooth frizz. If working with the curls use curl-enhancing products or smoothing products if a sleeker style is required. Curl-enhancing product	If working with the curls, use a diffuser and control the curl with a finger dry. If aiming for a smoother look, use a medium to large radial brush to smooth the curls.	If curling, tongs may help even out the curls. If smoothing, straightening irons will provide longevity to the smoother style.

Factor	Effect on the style	Effect on product choices	Effect on tool choices	Effect on equipment choices
Tight curls	This hair can also have a combination texture. Hair tends to have a medium number of curls.	Use products that will work with the curls and even out the textures – serums, heat protectors, creams and wax would work well. *Anti-frizz product/ moisturiser*	If working with the curls, use a diffuser and control the curl with a finger dry. If aiming for a smoother look, use a large radial brush to smooth the curls.	If smoothing the hair, straightening irons will provide longevity to the smoother style – but ideally work with the curls and not against them, as continued straightening of curly hair will cause damage.
Very curly hair – type 4 **Soft hair**	Hair tends to be fragile, tightly coiled and has a defined curly pattern.	Use products that will protect the hair from heat and further damage, but also help to control the curls.	Take care with tools, avoid pulling on the hair and work with the curls wherever possible. Use diffusers to style the hair. *Diffuser*	As the hair is fragile, avoid wherever possible the use of heated styling equipment.
Wiry African type hair	Hair tends to be very fragile and tightly coiled and has more of a 'Z' pattern shape.	Use products that will protect the hair from heat and further damage, but also help to control the curls.	Take care with tools, avoid pulling on the hair and work with the curls wherever possible. Use diffusers to style the hair.	As the hair is fragile, avoid wherever possible the use of heated styling equipment.

Head and face shapes

Head and face shape	Effect on the style
Oval 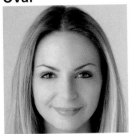	Oval is known as the ideal face shape. Be creative with your style confidently knowing you are working with this face shape.
Round 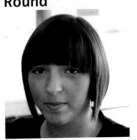	Suggest a style that gives an illusion of an oval face shape. Avoid width at the sides and too much height.
Square 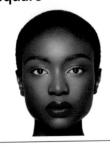	Suggest a style that gives an illusion of an oval face shape. Aim for styles that soften the jawline and are swept on the face slightly.
Oblong 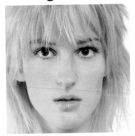	Suggest a style that gives an illusion of an oval face shape. Avoid height but add width. Avoid hair length finishing just below the jaw. Fringes can visually help reduce the length of the face.
Heart 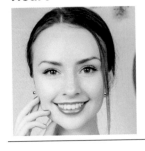	Suggest a style that gives an illusion of an oval face shape. Avoid width at the temple area, which exaggerates the heart shape. Add balance near the jawline. If the client has pointed features, such as nose or chin, avoid a centre parting which brings unwanted attention to the areas – opt for side partings instead.

It is not just hair and skin colour that varies across ethnicities; facial characteristics vary enormously too:

- face and skull shapes
- width of the cheeks
- nose shapes – nasal openings and the bridge of the nose
- eye shape
- lip shape and fullness/thickness.

Activity

Search for images of people of different ethnicities and compare their varying characteristics. Discuss how these variants may affect the styling and finishing service.

WHY DON'T YOU...
Practise identifying face shapes on your colleagues.

Tools, equipment and products

You must confirm the finished look your client requires so that you can choose the most suitable products, tools and equipment to achieve the best result.

Tools and equipment

When styling and finishing the hair you will use a variety of tools and equipment, such as brushes and combs, hand-held hairdryers, straightening irons or curling tongs. To achieve the best results for the style and to maintain the condition of the hair, always follow the MFIs.

The table below shows the tools and equipment available for use.

Tools and equipment	Use
Wide-toothed comb 	To detangle the hair before styling
Cutting comb 	To cleanly section the hair
Dressing-out comb 	For backcombing, teasing and dressing out the finished result
Section clips 	To secure hair in place

Tools and equipment	Use
Denman brush (flat)	To create a smooth, straight finish – such as a 'bob' style
Vent brush (flat)	To create a textured straight finish
Dressing-out brush (flat)	To dress and finish a blow dry
Small radial brush (round)	To create root lift, volume and small curls in layered hair
Medium radial brush (round)	To create root lift and medium curls in short to medium layered hair, and waves in longer hair
Large radial brush (round)	To smooth and straighten, and create soft waves in longer hair
Rake attachment	To blow dry African type/very curly hair
Hand-held hairdryer	To dry the hair during blow drying
Diffuser	To aid finger drying and encourage curls and lift in curly or wavy hair
Nozzle	To direct the airflow and heat from the hairdryer

Tools and equipment	Use
Straightening irons	To smooth and straighten dried hair
Tongs	To create curls and body
Wands	To create soft curls on long hair

Activity

Write down the tools and equipment you would need to:

- blow dry long hair smooth and straight
- finger dry short, curly hair
- blow dry loose, medium-length curly/frizzy hair smooth but with body.

Which products would you use for these styles?

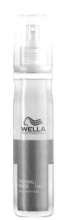

Heat protector spray

Before using heated appliances, always protect the hair with a heat protector to prevent damaging the hair and to prolong the style. You must take into consideration the texture and density of the hair, as fine, sparse hair will need considerably lower temperature settings to prevent damaging the cuticle scales and cortex. Always avoid contact with the skin when sectioning the hair and using the appliance. Check all appliances for safety before using.

Products

You are likely to use different products for styling and finishing the hair. Some products are designed to be used on wet, some on dry and some are suitable for both wet and dry hair.

Styling products

Styling products are designed to aid the styling of wet hair.

The table below shows which styling products should be used to achieve the most effective result.

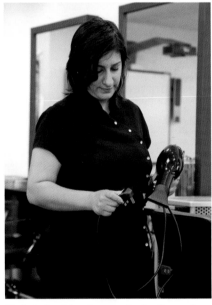

Stylist checking for cracks in the main body of the hairdryer

Styling product	How to use	Effect achieved and benefit to the client
Mousse/activators	Apply a golf-ball-sized amount to towel-dried hair and comb through evenly.	Enhances curls and offers support and hold to hair blow dried with a radial brush.
Blow dry lotion	Spray or sprinkle near the root area and work through to the ends.	Longer-lasting volume, lift and support for fine hair of any length. Can strengthen the structure when blow drying.
Anti-frizz lotion/moisturiser	Distribute evenly through damp hair, dry and style with a brush and hairdryer.	Achieves a smoother, straighter appearance by taming frizz and curls. It coats the hair and forms a barrier to prevent moisture from humidity affecting the finished look. Ideal for any hair length.
Serum	After shampooing, rub two to three drops of serum into your palms and apply to wet hair, distributing evenly.	Ultra-shine finish for all styles and hair types, enhances coloured hair and provides an anti-frizz effect by coating the hair with a smoothing liquid which forms a barrier to moisture.
Heat protector	Spray evenly through towel-dried hair.	Protects the hair from the drying effects and heat of the hairdryer, prevents frizz and gives an even finish.
Gel	Use on damp hair and distribute evenly through the hair before blow drying or finger drying.	Provides volume and texture for all hair lengths and hair types.
Cream	Rub a liberal amount between your palms and distribute evenly throughout the hair.	Provides flexible body and pliable style support. Adds texture to shorter hair lengths, eliminates frizz and maintains moisture.

Finishing products

Finishing products are applied to dried hair and are designed to support the finished look and give the style longevity.

The following table shows which finishing products are recommended to achieve longer-lasting effects.

Finishing product	How to use	Effect achieved and benefit to the client
Serum	Rub two to five drops of serum into your palms and apply to dry hair, distributing evenly before straightening.	To calm frizzy hair and flyaway ends, and protect from heated appliances by coating the hair and forming a protective barrier.
Cream/paste	Apply using your fingertips, moving from root to point to create texture and movement.	Adds texture to shorter hair lengths and supports, lifts and adds shine and body to medium-length or longer hair.
Gloss	After drying, lightly mist the hair or apply cream gloss with your fingertips, avoiding the root area.	Optimal shine, texture and condition – ideal for medium to longer hair lengths.
Gel	Massage a small amount into your palms and work evenly into the hair, shaping and moulding it into shape with your fingers.	For stronger-hold looks. Gel can provide an elastic effect, causing the hair to bounce back into style.
Hairspray	Shake well and spray on the hair from about 20cm away.	Finishes the style with a shine and long-lasting shape, leaving the hair touchable and without stiffness. The spray forms a barrier to prevent absorption of moisture. Ideal for medium to longer hair lengths.

Finishing product	How to use	Effect achieved and benefit to the client
Wax	Apply with your hands and fingertips through the hair, avoiding the root area. For funky, messy looks, apply using your palms and target the ends of the hair.	For soft, supple hold and great shine. Ideal for short hair.
Heat protector	Spray onto clean, dry hair prior to using heated appliances.	Provides a protective film over the outside of the cuticle scales and protects the hair from the heat of the appliance. Ideal for all hair lengths.

Activity

In pairs, identify your salon's product range for styling and finishing and list their benefits to the client. Choose one styling product and one finishing product that a client may purchase and calculate the costs. What would your 10% commission be?

Activity

Look at your fellow stylists and identify what products you would use on their current hairstyles.

Commercially viable times

To enable you to work to commercially viable times, you need to be prepared for the service and use your time effectively. Ensure you have set up your workstation and trolley with the tools you need, and that all products and equipment are at hand. It is essential you work to schedule to prevent lateness for following appointments. Test all your equipment before the service to ensure that no interruptions occur during the service. Your salon would have judged the prices charged to the clients to include salon costs and your time. Working to salon time guidelines helps the salon to maintain profit and increase its revenue. If you work on a commission basis, time is money!

VALUES & BEHAVIOURS

Refer to the values and behaviours chapter for more information on the importance of completing services in commercially viable times.

Science and techniques

The basic science

Hair is mostly composed of a hardened fibrous protein called keratin. Keratin is made up of amino acids and peptide bonds which originate in the hair follicle. These many amino acids and peptide bonds form the **polypeptide** chains (coils). The polypeptide chains are held together by permanent and temporary bonds inside the cortex layer of the hair.

The bonds in the hair

Hair can be naturally curly, wavy or straight. It is held in its natural state by the permanent and temporary bonds. The permanent bonds are broken by chemicals, such as perm solution, and can be changed from naturally straight to chemically curly. Styling the hair softens the weak temporary bonds and temporarily changes the natural state, such as changing from straight to curly, or wavy to straight. The flow chart below shows what makes up the hair.

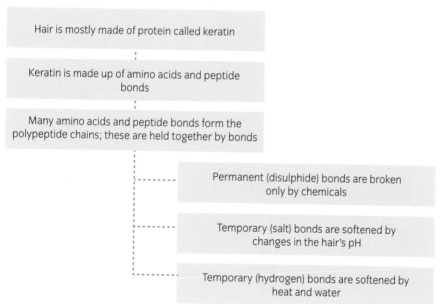

Hair is mostly made of protein called keratin

Keratin is made up of amino acids and peptide bonds

Many amino acids and peptide bonds form the polypeptide chains; these are held together by bonds

Permanent (disulphide) bonds are broken only by chemicals

Temporary (salt) bonds are softened by changes in the hair's pH

Temporary (hydrogen) bonds are softened by heat and water

Polypeptide

This word is derived from poly (many) and peptos (broken down).

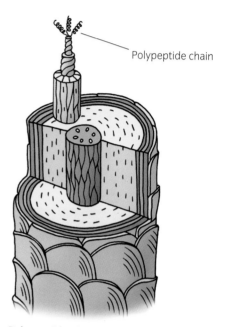

Polypeptide chain

Polypeptide chains inside the cortex of the hair

Salt bonds

The salt bonds are weak bonds that are temporarily softened by changes in pH, by the use of weak acids or alkalis. They are reformed by normalising the pH.

Hydrogen bonds

The main bonds that are broken when styling the hair are hydrogen bonds. These are broken by heat or water and hardened by drying or cooling the hair. Hydrogen bonds give the hair its strength and its flexibility to move freely; it is what makes the hair elastic. Well-conditioned hair with a strong cortex can stretch up to a further half of its original length when wet; this is due to the temporary breaking of the hydrogen bonds.

Alpha and beta keratin

Hair in its natural state of curly, wavy or straight is described as being in an alpha keratin state. When hair has been wetted, stretched and dried into a new shape it is described as being in a beta keratin state.

Heat from styling equipment, such as tongs and straightening irons, can also change the state from alpha keratin to beta keratin when the hair has cooled into its new shape. The temporary bonds that are changed during the heat styling process are hydrogen bonds (shown as H–O) and salt bonds (shown as – and +).

The permanent bonds that are changed during a perming or relaxing process are called disulphide bonds and are shown in the diagram as S–S; you will learn about these in chapters CH5 and AH2.

This diagram shows the polypeptide chains and how the permanent and weak temporary bonds hold the hair together. When styling the hair, the hydrogen (H–O) bonds are broken and reformed.

> **HANDY HINT**
>
> The weak temporary hydrogen bonds are softened by water and heat, and hardened by drying and cooling of the hair.

> **HANDY HINT**
>
> Hair in its natural state is in an alpha keratin state; when wetted, stretched and dried, its new state is beta keratin.

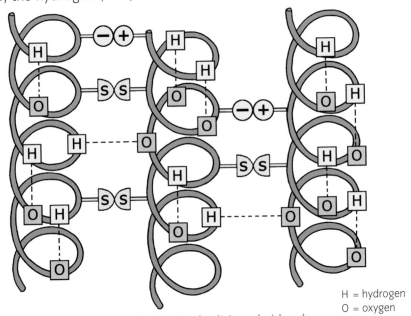

Hydrogen (H–O), disulphide (S–S) and salt (+ and –) bonds

H = hydrogen
O = oxygen
S = sulphur

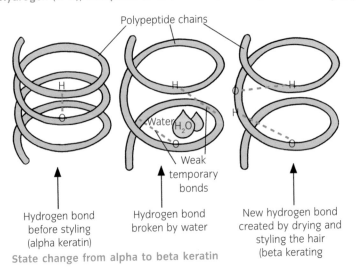

Polypeptide chains

Water H_2O

Weak temporary bonds

Hydrogen bond before styling (alpha keratin)

Hydrogen bond broken by water

New hydrogen bond created by drying and styling the hair (beta kerating

State change from alpha to beta keratin

THE CITY & GUILDS TEXTBOOK

Humidity

Hair is hygroscopic, which means it can absorb moisture from the atmosphere. The hairstyle is therefore affected by the humidity and moisture present in the air. The hair absorbs the moisture from the air and the beta keratin state changes back to alpha keratin, because the moisture softens the temporary hydrogen bonds and the hair reverts back to its original state.

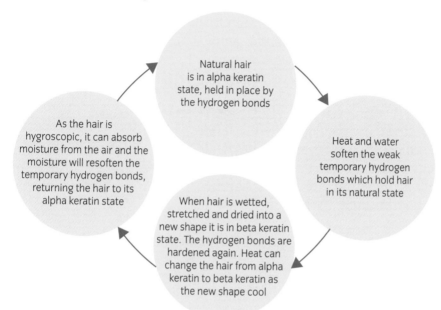

Natural hair is in alpha keratin state, held in place by the hydrogen bonds

Heat and water soften the weak temporary hydrogen bonds which hold hair in its natural state

When hair is wetted, stretched and dried into a new shape it is in beta keratin state. The hydrogen bonds are hardened again. Heat can change the hair from alpha keratin to beta keratin as the new shape cool

As the hair is hygroscopic, it can absorb moisture from the air and the moisture will resoften the temporary hydrogen bonds, returning the hair to its alpha keratin state

The alpha to beta keratin process

> **HANDY HINT**
>
> Keeping the hair misted and with even moisture balance helps you to produce a smooth even effect when blow drying the hair.

> **HANDY HINT**
>
> Humidity returns the hair to the alpha keratin state by adding moisture from the air.

Effects of the styling and drying process

Each client's hair will dry out at a different rate, and, as wet hair stretches allowing a new shape to form, an even moisture balance is required. If areas of the hair have started to dry during the styling process, then hair will lose its elasticity and the ability to stretch sufficiently, so the result may be uneven. You must mist the hair sections lightly with a water spray if you notice an uneven elasticity when drying the hair, to allow the bonds to be reformed evenly into their new position.

After blow drying or when using heated appliances, always allow the hair to cool, or use the cool setting button on the hairdryer for a minute or so at the end. This enables the hydrogen bonds to harden in their new shape and the result will be longer-lasting.

> **HANDY HINT**
>
> Always allow the hair to cool, which allows the hydrogen bonds to harden in their new shape and prolong the style.

> **HANDY HINT**
>
> When styling the hair with heated appliances, you must always use a heat protector. These products create a protective barrier around the cuticle scales, preventing moisture in the air from penetrating.

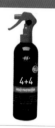

Techniques

Your clients may have their hair styled for a special occasion or at the end of a hairdressing service to complete the look. You will need to be able to smooth and straighten the hair, create volume, movement and curls, support the style with the aid of backcombing and backbrushing, and create looks on a variety of hair types and lengths. This includes: very curly, curly, wavy and straight hair; above- and below-shoulder lengths, and layered or one-length looks.

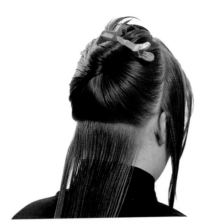

Sectioned hair

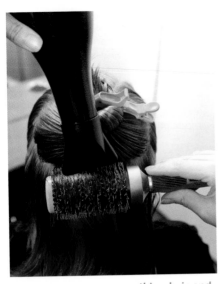

Brush at root area, smoothing hair and achieving volume

Blow drying the hair

Whether you are blow drying short or long hair you must have control. Curly hair can be challenging to even the most able stylist, but using suitable products and tools helps control the hair. A methodical working pattern with clean sections is also very important.

Sectioning the hair

When you are working on medium to long hair you must section it cleanly, and secure the hair you are not currently working on out of the way. This will prevent it from drying too quickly and disturbing the areas that you are working on.

Take manageable sections to enable you to dry each part thoroughly and obtain the required amount of root lift. Part the hair and section it from ear to ear, crown to nape, and finally from the crown to the front hairline. Clip and secure the front two sections out of the way, and, starting from the bottom of the nape section, take a 2cm thick section, securing the rest.

Styling – airflow, brushes, tension and angles
Airflow

You must always ensure you direct the airflow away from the client's scalp to prevent burning the client and causing discomfort. Always keep the airflow moving, as keeping it in one area could cause damage to the hair and scalp.

You should direct the airflow in the direction of the style to ensure root lift where required. Follow the cuticle direction, aiming downwards from root to point to follow and smooth the cuticle scales, avoiding disturbing the hair you have already dried.

Brushes

Your brush choice and size will vary, depending on the desired look, degree of curl, and the movement and volume required.

Tension

Pulling the hair with tension as you dry it will make the style last longer. Curly hair being blow dried straight will need a lot more tension than straight or wavy hair. A large radial brush will help you to smooth and straighten curls, but still create volume and movement. Ensure the tension is firm but without causing discomfort to your client.

Angles

The angle in which you direct the brush and airflow through the hair will aid you in achieving root lift and volume where required.

You should keep the brush on the base of the section if you require lift (on base) and drag the hair back away from the section (off base) if you require a flatter look.

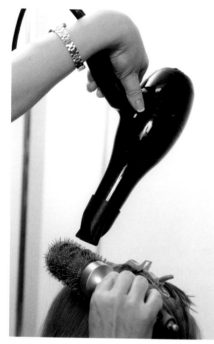

Airflow directed away from scalp, following direction of cuticle scales root to point

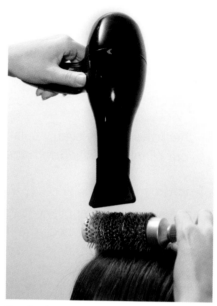

Brush sitting on base at the root area for lift and volume

HANDY HINT

Make sure the dampness of the hair is consistent throughout the service to ensure an even curl result and to enable you to control the curl and movement. If you find some areas are drying more quickly than others, re-dampen them.

HANDY HINT

Always allow the hair to cool before removing the hair meche from the brush or the curl will not hold and the style may drop.

Finger drying

When finger drying the hair, you must ensure you achieve the required amount of volume, movement and/or curl. You should massage the root area in the direction in which the lift and volume are required. Applying products at the root area will support the style.

Short hair can be styled using a hand-held hairdryer and using your hands and fingers as the tools. This works particularly well for hair with movement and texture, requiring a finished look that is modern and funky. Your choice of styling products will influence the end result, as support from the product is required.

Diffuser drying

Hair with movement, curl or body can be finger dried with a diffuser attachment. This technique works particularly well with medium to longer hair lengths. You should use curl-activating products to enhance curls and movement, and to support the style.

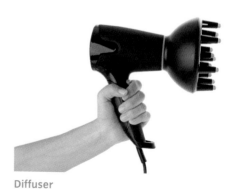

Diffuser

Natural drying

Hair that is naturally curly or has been permed can be left to dry naturally with an accelerator. To do this you should:

- apply your suitable chosen products
- position the hair into the desired style, considering the natural partings rather than manipulating the hair into a direction it does not naturally want to fall into
- sit your client comfortably at a workstation with an accelerator correctly positioned above the hair
- set the timer on your accelerator to dry the hair, taking into consideration the hair length, density and texture
- check throughout the drying process that the temperature is suitable and that your client is comfortable (and offer them a drink)
- check the style is evenly balanced when the hair is dry and that your client is satisfied with the finished look.

Finishing hair

When using heated appliances to finish the hair, you must always use a heat protector and check that the temperature setting is suitable for the hair condition, type and density. You should use a bristle brush to smooth and detangle the hair before straightening, and cleanly section the hair into manageable sections. Allow the hair to cool in its new state prior to finishing the style.

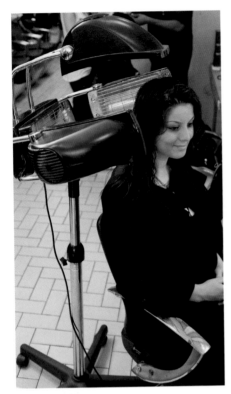

Accelerator

Providing advice and recommendations

During and after the service you should recommend aftercare and give your client advice on maintaining the style and condition of the hair. During your consultation you would have identified what the client does on a day-to-day basis and how much time they have to spend on styling and finishing the hair.

You should provide advice on how to maintain their look, products and their use, and when to return for future or additional services:

- advise your client on how to maintain their look
- advise on present and future products and services
- advise on the time interval between services.

Creating and maintaining the style

Together with advising on the best products and equipment for maintaining the style at home, you should give advice on which tools to use. Recommend brushes that will help the client to recreate the look, explain how to use them and show them how to follow the direction of the cuticle. You should explain how to section the hair and demonstrate how to clip hair out of the way to help them control their hair and methodically style it, enhancing the end result and using their time effectively.

Products and their use

Your advice should include which products are best suited for styling the hair and supporting the finished look. You must clearly advise which products you recommend for styling the hair while it is wet, and those that will aid longevity on dry hair.

You should consider the following.

- Condition of the hair – recommend shampoo and conditioning products to maintain condition and improve porosity and elasticity. You should advise the client on how to remove the products from the hair in order to prevent a build-up.

- Density and texture – recommend products that will protect, support and give root lift if required for fine/sparse hair, and smooth and give shine to coarse/abundant hair. Advise on how much product is required and how to apply it.

- Required result – suggest products that provide strong or light control to the hair, movement, root lift or curl enhancers where required.

Equipment and its use

If you are recommending the use of hairdryers, straightening irons or tongs, ensure you offer advice on using them safely. Explain that using heated appliances repeatedly, too close to the scalp and concentrating on one area for too long can cause damage to the hair and scalp, increase porosity, decrease elasticity and cause colour to fade. You must recommend the use of heat-protecting products.

When to return

Advise your client when to return to the salon for either a weekly style and finish service, or a haircut when the style becomes difficult to manage themselves. You may also have discussed any additional services that your client may benefit from, such as colour, body perms or treatments. Suggest to your client a date and time when these services could be carried out.

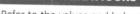

VALUES & BEHAVIOURS

Refer to the values and behaviours chapter for more information on:

- selecting appropriate ways to communicate with your client
- checking with the client that you have understood their expectations
- responding promptly and positively to the client's questions and comments
- allowing the client time to consider their response and give further explanation when appropriate
- quickly locating information they need about the services or products offered by the salon
- recognising information that the client may find complicated and checking they fully understand.

Provide hair styling and finishing services

Prepare for styling and finishing services

Prepare your client for the service ahead – gown and protect them, discuss their requirements, shampoo and condition their hair and comb the hair through so it is tangle-free.

Work safely and hygienically

You should always follow safe and hygenic methods of working. Remember to:

- maintain your responsibilities for health and safety
- protect your client throughout the service
- consider your posture and your client's body position for health and safety and comfort
- minimise risks of injury and damage to tools and test the temperature of heated styling equipment throughout the service
- use clean resources and minimise the risk of cross-infection
- promote environmental and sustainable working practices and minimise waste
- ensure your personal hygiene, protection and appearance are up to salon standard
- minimise risk of injury to self and others and follow MFIs
- use your time effectively and complete the service in a commerically acceptable time.

Consult with clients

When you consult with clients, remember to:

- identify any factors that may prevent or affect the service
- identify client requirements
- confirm and carry out client requirements.

Select products, tools and equipment

After the consultation choose your tools, equipment and products to use. Set up your trolley with the final items and work effectively. Always follow the instructions of the manufacturer, suppliers and your salon when working with tools, equipment and products. Apply products to your client's hair to suit the style requirements, hair length and density, so as not to overload the hair.

Carry out styling and finishing services – review

To style the hair:

- control your styling tools to minimise the risk of damage to the hair length, client discomfort and to achieve the desired look

- take sections of hair that suit the size of the styling tools

- maintain an even tension throughout the blow drying process

- keep the hair damp throughout the blow drying process

- test the temperature of heated styling equipment throughout the service

- control the hair length during the blow drying/styling process taking account of factors influencing the service

- use tools and equipment in a way that achieves the desired blow dry finish.

- ensure that blow drying/finger drying achieves the direction, volume and balance for the desired look.

To finish the hair:

- use heated styling equipment, when necessary, that is at the correct temperature for your client's hair and the desired look

- control your use of heated styling equipment, when used, to minimise the risk of damage to the hair and scalp, client discomfort and to achieve the desired look

- take sections of hair that suit the size of the heated styling equipment, when used

- use back-combing and back-brushing techniques, when required, to achieve the desired look

- apply and use suitable products, when required, to meet manufacturers' instructions

- ensure the finished look takes into account relevant styling factors influencing the service

- ensure the finished look meets the intended shape, direction, balance and volume agreed with your client.

WHY DON'T YOU...
Practise blow drying a short hairstyle in 30–40 minutes and longer hair within 45 minutes.

Step by steps

Chelsea blow dry

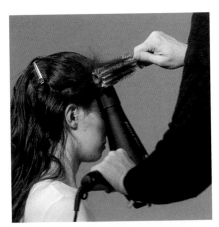

STEP 1 – Starting with the right-hand side, work a diagonal section from the front hairline using a round medium brush. Ensure that the heat from the dryer is facing down the cuticle to smooth and seal.

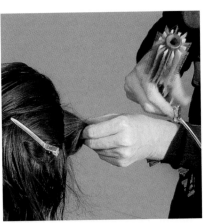

STEP 2 – Once you have dried this section, roll the hair and secure with a long silver clip, then leave to cool.

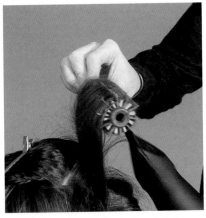

STEP 3 – Next work a subsequent section on top of the previous one with the same process. Repeat these two sections on the opposite side and add a third. Return to the original side and complete the third section, directing the hair onto the opposite side and slightly back giving direction to the parting.

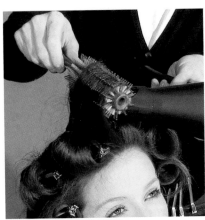

STEP 4 – Finish the front hairline with the very top section which you direct onto the second side. Work the top section behind the fringe area and direct the hair back and down. Repeat this process, working with a brickwork pattern until you complete all sections. Throughout this drying process, apply a suitable product.

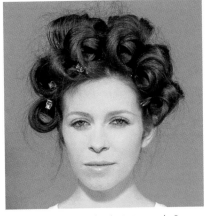

STEP 5 – Leave the hair to cool. Once cooled, let down the hair and apply a suitable product, and style visually with a dramatic, bold look.

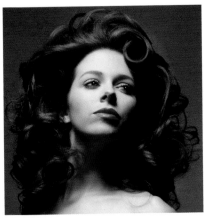

STEP 6 – Final look.

Mid-length layer shape above shoulders

A medium layered, mid-length shape above the shoulders employing slight root lift and control of bevel with a variety of brushes.

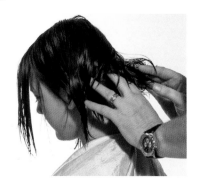

STEP 1 – Add a suitable product to ensure a medium hold.

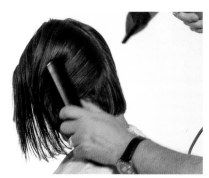

STEP 2 – Begin by wrap drying. Wrap dry by directing the airflow along the lengths of the hair whilst brushing it in multiple directions, wrapping it around the head in order to utilise the natural curves of the head. This process reduces the amount of water through the regrowth, roots and mid-lengths and ensures that the root areas move in a natural way.

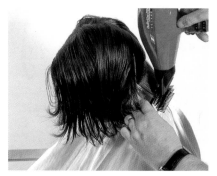

STEP 3 – Once the moisture has been reduced, change brush to a small curved brush to allow you to work in smaller sections. Start in the nape area, picking up the hair with the first two rows of the brush, then turn to brush over in an anticlockwise direction and direct the air flow downwards.

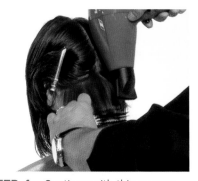

STEP 4 – Continue with this process throughout the nape area.

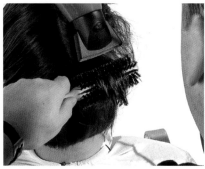

STEP 5 – Continue with this process working horizontal sections up the head using a medium diameter pure bristle radial brush.

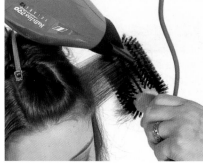

STEP 6 – Work two sections on one side, then two sections on the other side up to the back of the ear. Then revert back to the seven row ceramic brush to take away moisture from the side root area using a wrap dry technique. This also avoids any harsh partings.

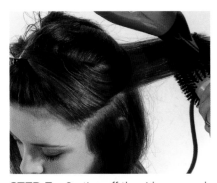

STEP 7 – Section off the side area and use a large diameter pure bristle radial brush. Continue with the process – picking up the hair with your fingers, laying over the brush and once again directing air flow down the cuticle.

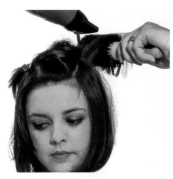

STEP 8 – Work with parallel sections up the head to where the head rounds on the first side.

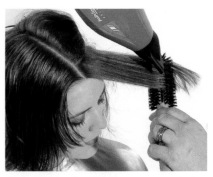

STEP 9 – Release the top area, which is the heavier side from the parting. Use diagonal sections from the parting in the front and dry from regrowth/roots to ends with the same process with the medium brush. Dry the hair turning the ends in a backward direction to get a kick in the front – enabling the hair to move naturally away from the face.

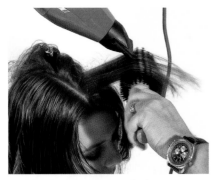

STEP 10 – Continue with this process working back towards the crown using the larger brush on the longer lengths.

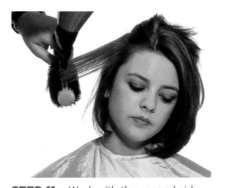

STEP 11 – Work with the second side area ensuring correct tension.

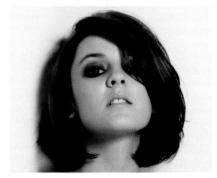

STEP 12 – Final look.

Diffuser drying curly long hair

Hair with movement, curl or body can be scrunch-dried with a diffuser attachment. This technique works particularly well with medium to longer hair lengths. You should use curl-activating products to enhance curls and movement, and to support the style. However, use minimal handling of the hair.

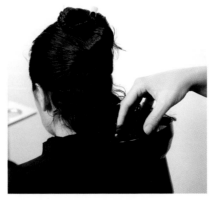

STEP 1 – Apply the styling product and section the hair; place the hair into the diffuser.

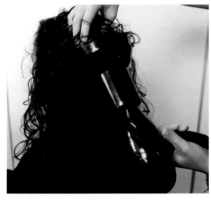

STEP 2 – Continue the finger dry, gently manipulating the hair at the root area for lift.

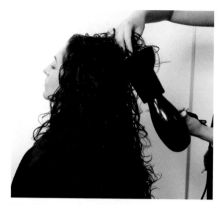

STEP 3 – Avoid 'overplaying' with the curls: let the diffuser curl the hair where possible.

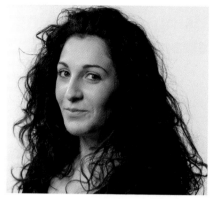

STEP 4 – Check the balance and ensure that the client is happy with the end result.

Finger drying short hair

Finger dry short hair to create movement and texture.

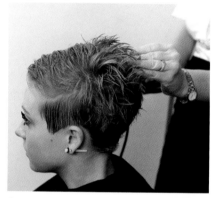

STEP 1 – Apply the product, removing any excess moisture by 'rough' drying.

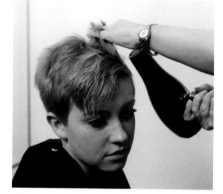

STEP 2 – Manipulate the root area to create body and movement.

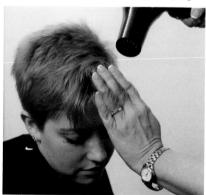

STEP 3 – Ensure the airflow follows the direction of the hairstyle.

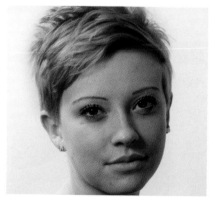

STEP 4 – Check the balance and ensure that the client is happy with the end result.

Using straightening irons to smooth and straighten the hair

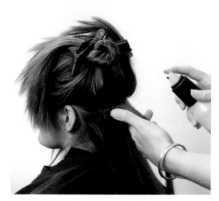

STEP 1 – Section the hair and apply a heat protector.

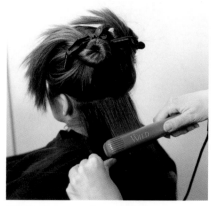

STEP 2 – Heat the straightening irons to the desired temperature and slowly move them from root to point.

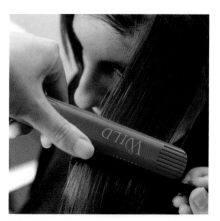

STEP 3 – Continue around to the side section, taking small sections at a time.

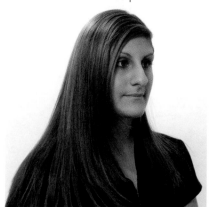

STEP 4 – Check the balance and ensure that the client is happy with the end result.

Using a wand to create volume, curls and movement

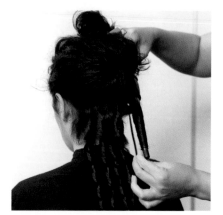

STEP 1 – Taking small clean sections, wrap the hair around the wand and wind down from root to point.

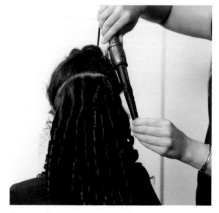

STEP 2 – Continue with your sections and curl the hair from root to point.

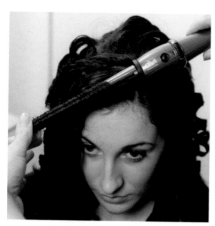

STEP 3 – Direct the hair sections to suit the chosen style.

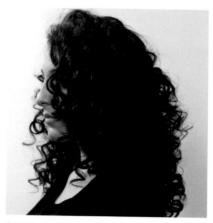

STEP 4 – Tease the curls if required, check the balance and ensure that the client is happy with the end result.

Using tongs to curl hair

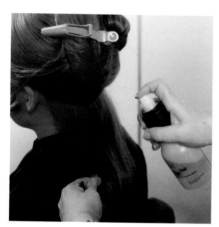

STEP 1 – Section the hair and apply a heat protective lotion.

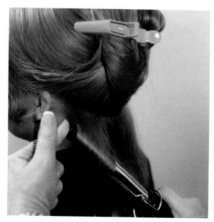

STEP 2 – Clasp the hair in the end of the tongs and wind from tip to root.

Answers in the back of the book.

1 Which one of the following is a risk associated with styling wet hair?

  a Electric shock

  b Chemical burns

  c Trips and falls

  d Cuts and abrasions

2 Which one of the following is the best way of avoiding contact dermatitis?

  a Washing hands after each client

  b Visiting the doctor for regular checks

  c Wearing gloves when applying products

  d Using moisturiser before applying products

3 Which one of the following is used to obtain detailed information during consultation?

  a Closed questions

  b Open questions

  c Listening techniques

  d Body language

4 Hair with a coarse texture will need which one of the following products to give it shine?

  a Gel

  b Serum

  c Spray

  d Mousse

5 Which one of the following should be avoided when styling very porous hair?

  a Bristle brushes

  b Heat protector

  c Wide-toothed combs

  d Finger drying

6 Which one of the following describes the effect of using a hairdryer nozzle?

  a Smooth cuticle

  b Root lift

  c Wave movement

  d Natural curls

7 Which one of the following describes the effect of using a vent brush when drying hair?

  a Textured straight finish

  b Volume and root lift

  c Waves in longer hair

  d Curls in shorter hair

8 Which one of the following describes the changes to the hair structure during wet styling?

  a Disulphide binds are weakened by water and rebuilt by acids

  b Salt bonds are permanently broken and reformed by mild alkalis

  c Hydrogen bonds are broken and alpha keratin changes to beta keratin

  d Polypeptide chains in keratin are reformed by the addition of hydrogen

9 What is the meaning of the term hygroscopic?

  a The ability to absorb water from the atmosphere

  b The ability to repel water vapour in the air

  c The bonds in hair are broken by acids

  d The bonds in hair and broken by alkalis

10 Why is it important to section long hair when blow drying?

  a To maintain client care

  b To look professional when working

  c To direct the airflow from root to point

  d To avoid disturbing areas that have been worked on

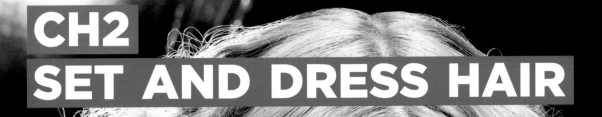

CH2
SET AND DRESS HAIR

Setting and dressing hair can be very exciting and rewarding. It gives you the chance to be creative and produce a variety of different looks. Long gone are the days when setting was all about short hair sets on older clients – modern setting is at the forefront of fashion. Of course, traditional setting skills are still required but long hair-setting can create soft curls and catwalk styles, giving you the chance to have fun, show off your creative flair and your dressing skills!

After reading this chapter you will:

- know how health and safety affects setting and dressing services
- understand the factors that influence setting and dressing services
- know the tools, equipment, products and techniques used to set and dress hair
- be able to provide setting and dressing services.

Health and safety

When setting and dressing the hair you must ensure you gown and protect your clients, and position them comfortably. Always stand with your body weight evenly distributed to prevent fatigue and back problems, and maintain your personal health and hygiene.

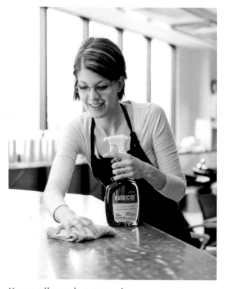

Keep all work areas clean

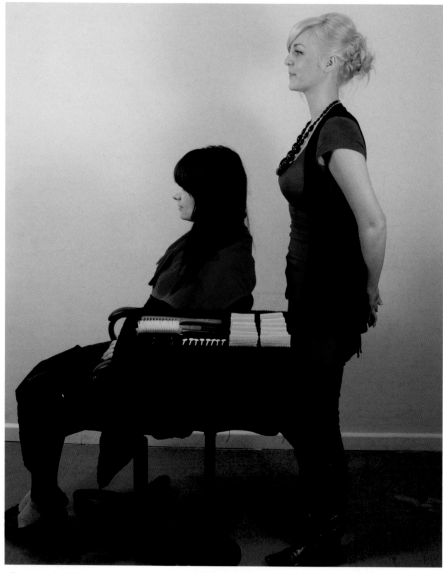

Client and stylist positioning

HEALTH & SAFETY

Refer to the health and safety and salon policies chapter for a recap on the health and safety Acts you must follow when setting and dressing hair.

HEALTH & SAFETY

Refer to the health and safety chapter to recap on protecting the environment and maintaining sustainable working practices, such as:

• reducing waste and disposing of it safely

• using disposable items

• reducing energy usage

• preventing pollution.

Always ensure you follow the salon's, suppliers' and manufacturers' instructions (MFIs) for the products and electrical appliances you will use. You should wear personal protective equipment (PPE) when applying products to protect your hands and clothes.

You must ensure that you and your work area are prepared for the service, and your tools and equipment are at hand and sterilised, to promote a professional image and prevent cross-contamination. This will also help you to work methodically, and keep the salon running to time.

Maintain an effective working environment and carry out safe working practices

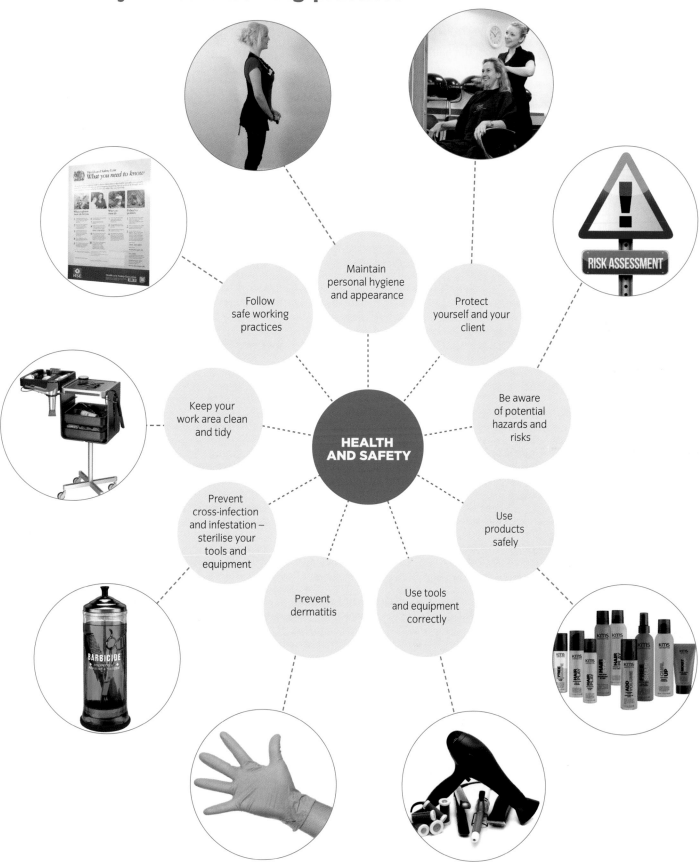

HEALTH AND SAFETY

- Maintain personal hygiene and appearance
- Follow safe working practices
- Protect yourself and your client
- Be aware of potential hazards and risks
- Keep your work area clean and tidy
- Use products safely
- Prevent cross-infection and infestation – sterilise your tools and equipment
- Prevent dermatitis
- Use tools and equipment correctly

Factors that influence setting and dressing services

The following factors need to be considered when setting and dressing hair:

- hair characteristics
- hair classifications
- head and face shape
- hair cut and length
- the occasion for which the style is required.

Hair characteristics

The table shows the types of hair characteristics that can affect the style, causing you to have to adapt your choice of products and their quantities, and your choice of tools and equipment.

VALUES & BEHAVIOURS

Refer to the values and behaviours chapter for a recap on effective, hygienic and safe working methods.

VALUES & BEHAVIOURS

Refer to the values and behaviours chapter for more specific information on how to clean, sterilise and disinfect setting and dressing equipment.

HANDY HINT

Carry out a porosity test to identify whether the hair is porous, and an elasticity test to check the strength of the cortex.

Factors	Effect on the style	Effect on product choices	Effect on tool choices	Effect on equipment choices
Density Abundant hair Chignon	Carefully consider the style for abundant hair, as it may make the style look too big. Abundant hair will also take longer to dry. If styling hair into a **chignon**, avoid too much backcombing or backbrushing as this will promote more volume. Sparse hair will dry more quickly and backcombing may be required to aid support within some styles.	Abundant hair will need more product. Choose products that do not provide any volume or lift, but help smooth the hair. For sparse hair less product is required and take care not to overload it. **Chignon** Roll of hair, worn at the back of the head.	Avoid root movement that promotes volume and makes hair look thicker. Rollers with pins may help you to control the hair. Extra pins and grips may be required when putting hair up. Take care with pins on sparse hair and avoid causing your client any discomfort.	Abundant hair should be rough dried first to reduce any excess moisture and then set and dried to decrease the drying time, making effective use of your time. Use straightening irons to help flatten thick hair if a smooth style is required. Avoid excessive heat on sparse hair.

Factors	Effect on the style	Effect on product choices	Effect on tool choices	Effect on equipment choices
Texture Long thick hair	You need to consider the length of fine hair, as longer lengths can look thinner and may require gentle backcombing for more support. Coarse hair may need taming and controlling to ensure the style looks its best.	Use less product on fine hair to support the style and give the hair body and volume. Coarse hair may need smoothing products such as serum.	Fine hair will need rollers to give root lift and support the style.	For fine hair use more rollers and smaller sections to give the illusion of thicker hair. When using heated appliances, lower the heat settings on fine hair and increase heat for coarse hair to help smooth and tame it.
Elasticity Dry hair	Take extra care when stretching dry hair if there is poor elasticity.	For hair with poor elasticity, avoid 'sticky' products that offer strong hold, as the hair will tangle easily. You should suggest smoothing products, such as serums. Use heat protectors with heat appliances.	You should avoid non-bristle brushes and velcro rollers on hair with poor elasticity, as these may cause the hair to snag and break. Use smoothing brushes and wide-toothed combs.	You should suggest minimal use of heated appliances as these will cause further deterioration of condition.
Porosity Porous hair	If the hair is porous it may have a 'fluffy' appearance on the ends and will tangle easily; take care not to catch the hair in the equipment.	Avoid 'sticky' products that offer strong hold as porous hair will tangle easily. You should suggest smoothing products, such as serums. Use heat protectors with heat appliances.	You should avoid non-bristle brushes and velcro rollers on porous hair as these may cause the hair to snag and break. Use smoothing brushes and wide-toothed combs.	You should suggest minimal use of heated appliances, as these will cause further deterioration of condition.

Factors	Effect on the style	Effect on product choices	Effect on tool choices	Effect on equipment choices
Hair condition 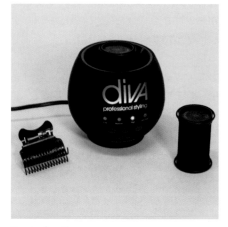 Hair in poor condition	Hair in poor condition may have weak elasticity and poor porosity – the style may look lacklustre in appearance and be hard to manage. Backcombing or backbrushing may need to be avoided.	For hair in poor condition, products will be needed to help the hair look shiny in appearance – such as oils or serums. Be careful not to use 'sticky' products such as gel that may make the hair feel even worse. Use heat protectors if using heated styling equipment.	Use wide-toothed combs to comb through hair in poor condition to avoid it tangling and causing discomfort to your client. Use bristle brushes to brush tangles through on dry hair. Avoid fine-toothed combs and plastic firm bristle brushes.	Avoid excessive heat on the hair and small rollers that may get tangled in damaged hair. Velcro rollers may catch on damaged cuticles, so use rollers with minimal grip.

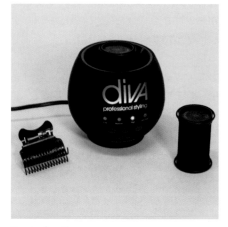

Heated rollers

Hair growth patterns

Consider nape whorls and double crowns on shorter hair. When styling fringes, identify potential problems with cowlicks and widow's peaks. Consider winding techniques to overcome some hair growth patterns.

Adjust the roller size if need be on the double crown. Use off-base rolling where needed to avoid additional lift.

Consider winding techniques to overcome some hair growth patterns with heated rollers. When rolling tip to root, avoid too much curl near the root area of double crowns and cowlicks.

Use finishing products to hold fringes in place and strong styling products on double crowns.

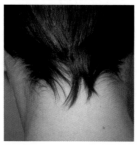

Nape whorl

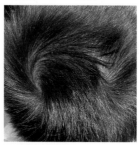

Double crown

Hair classifications

For hair classifications, the main information can be found in the table in chapter CH1. Coarse and curly hair will benefit from wet setting prior to dresssing the hair. Wet setting will help produce a more even curl that will be smoother in appearance than if you used heated rollers. If curling, tongs may help even out the curls. As curly hair can be frizzy it will tangle easier. Take care with combs and hard brushes. Take care with all tools, avoid pulling on the hair and work with the curls wherever possible. As very curly hair is fragile, avoid wherever possible the use of heated styling equipment.

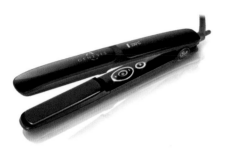
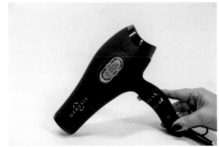

Heated styling equipment with heat settings for fragile/African type hair

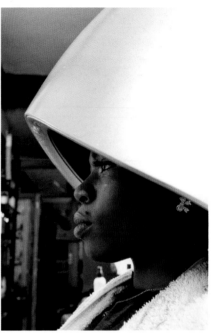

Wet set

Head and face shapes

Always try to enhance the face shape and create an oval look finish. Avoid additional width and height on round faces. For square face shapes soften the jawlines. Consider features – faces with sharp noses should not be styled with centre partings; if ears protrude you should avoid styles that expose the entire ear. For more information, see Chapter CH1.

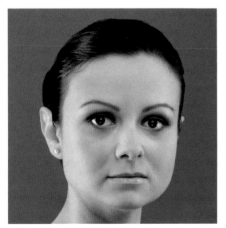

Square face

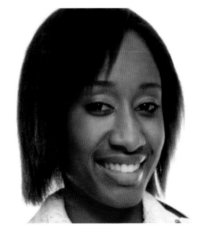

Prominent nose

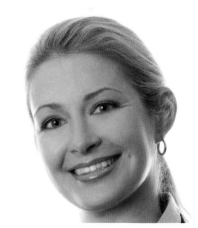

Protruding ears

Activity

As shapes of the skull, face, nose and eyes vary so much, discuss in pairs how techniques and styles may need to be adapted to ensure the desired chosen style would suit diverse people (think about ethnicity, age, etc.).

At the end of your discussion present your findings to the group and compare shared ideas.

Length, cut and intended occasion

Factors	Effect on the style	Effect on product choices	Effect on tool choices	Effect on equipment choices
Hair length	Longer hair requires more maintenance and can make setting difficult. Longer layers will need to be supported with suitable products and styling tools. Ensure the hair is long enough to be put up and meet the client requirements.	More supporting products, such as hairsprays and root lift products may be required. You must use heat protectors with any heated appliance. Use serums on the ends of the hair. Use less product for shorter hair lengths.	Larger rollers will help to obtain lift and smooth the hair. Small rollers may get caught in long hair.	Straightening irons/tongs or heated rollers can be used, but wet setting techniques will have a longer-lasting effect on the style.
Haircut	This is very important, as this is how the hair has been cut for the style; you must work with it not against it. If you're setting the hair for a special occasion, check the layer lengths are long enough for the setting roller chosen and the desired look.	You should suggest and use products to support the style. Identify whether you need root lift, curls and/or volume. Use products to suit the length of the cut (as well as the condition of hair).	Identify whether you'll need lift and volume to help decide on roller size if setting.	If using heated appliances, again decide on the most suitable appliance – tongs or heated rollers for curls and lift, straightening irons for straight looks and flat curls.

Factors	Effect on the style	Effect on product choices	Effect on tool choices	Effect on equipment choices
The occasion for which the style is required	The longevity of the style needs to be considered – does the client want a style for day wear, evening wear or a special occasion? A special hair up-do may last only for a day or evening; a curly set may last a few days.	Depending on the style, choose products to support and enhance the style.	Depending on the style, choose tools that help create the style.	Depending on the style, choose equipment that helps to create the look.

Physical effects of setting

Hair is composed of amino acids that form polypeptide chains; these are held together by the chemical bonds in the cortex. The weak temporary hydrogen bonds are softened by water and heat, and hardened by drying and cooling the hair.

Here is a reminder of the alpha to beta keratin change process.

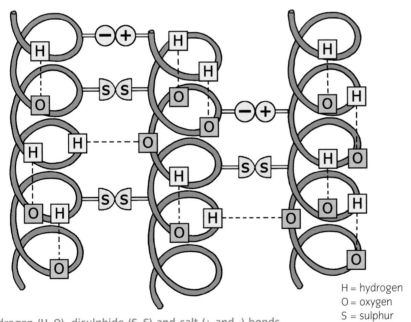

H = hydrogen
O = oxygen
S = sulphur

Hydrogen (H–O), disulphide (S–S) and salt (+ and -) bonds

Refer to CH1 for a full recap on the basic science when setting and dressing the hair.

Humidity

Hair in its natural state, curly, wavy or straight, is in an alpha keratin state. When hair has been wetted, stretched and dried into a new shape, it is in a beta keratin state.

Hair is hygroscopic, which means it can absorb moisture, for example from the atmosphere. Hair absorbs moisture from the air and the beta keratin style reverts back to an alpha keratin state. This is because the moisture softens the temporary hydrogen bonds and the hair changes back to its original state.

Keeping hair damp during the setting process

When setting hair, ensure the elasticity is even throughout and keep the hair damp when sectioning and winding the hair.

Sectioning and securing hair out of the way prevents the hair from drying too quickly and disturbing the areas that you are working on.

Using heat

Heat alone can also change the keratin state, for example using heated styling equipment, such as heated rollers, tongs and straightening irons. After dry setting or dressing, and once the hair has cooled, the hair will be in its new state of beta keratin.

Avoid using too much heat on African type hair, as this will dry out the moisture from the hair. African type hair is naturally low in moisture (1% moisture, 99% protein) due to the natural curl pattern and slightly open cuticle. Excessive use of heat will make the hair, which already lacks moisture, feel and appear drier. As with all hair types, African type hair is moisturised from the sebaceous gland. However, due to the curl pattern it takes longer for the sebum produced by the sebaceous gland to wind its way down the length of the hair. This is why we have to add moisture using products to constantly rebalance the moisture level in the hair.

HANDY HINT

Keeping the hair misted with water maintains a consistent moisture balance to produce a smooth, even effect.

HANDY HINT

The incorrect application of heat can cause damage to the hair and the scalp. If the cuticles are damaged then the hair will increase in porosity and the hair may lose some of its elasticity. The hair may also be discoloured if damaged by heat.

HANDY HINT

Use heat protectors before setting and dressing; these products coat the cuticles in a protective layer to shield the hair from direct heat.

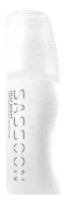

Heat styling protector

Avoid using too much heat when straightening hair

Tools, equipment and products

Preparing for setting and dressing services

You must always complete a thorough consultation with your client to identify their needs, decide on the most suitable tools and equipment to use, and ensure you achieve the desired result. You will need to demonstrate different styles for a variety of occasions. In the section 'Be able to set and dress hair' and the step by steps towards the end of this chapter, you will have the opportunity to set and dress hair for clients going to a ball, a wedding, the races, nightclubbing and, of course, for everyday styles, suitable for work or a day at the beach.

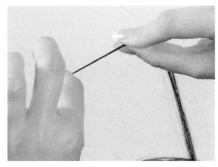

Carrying out an elasticity test

Confirming the style required

You must always thoroughly analyse your client's hair and scalp, completing visual checks and relevant hair tests. Feel the hair to identify whether the hair is porous or has good/weak elasticity. Ask open and closed questions to identify your client's requirements.

You'll need to ask your clients the following types of question:

- What is their vision of the finished look?
- What is the occasion for which the style is required?
- What will they be wearing? If you are setting the hair for a night out, can they fit their clothes over the hairstyle?
- Would they like any accessories in their hair?
- How long does the style need to last for the occasion?
- Do they want to be able to recreate the style themselves?
- What products do they have at home to recreate the style?
- Are there any lifestyle factors that could affect recreating the style at home?
- Do they have any allergies?

You'll need to visually check and feel the hair to identify:

- the condition of the hair and scalp
- the length, style, type, texture and density of the hair
- any growth patterns
- the head and face shape
- any scalp problems
- how long the service will take
- the necessary tools and equipment needed to achieve the particular style.

> **HANDY HINT**
>
> Open questions require the client to give a more in-depth answer and may start with 'what', 'why', 'how' and 'when'. Closed questions help to confirm and define details as they are answered with 'yes' or 'no' or one-word responses.

> **HANDY HINT**
>
> You must always record on a record card the outcome of any tests and your client's verbal responses to any questions asked in case you need to refer back to the information in the future, or if there are any problems and you need evidence of the client's comments.
>
> Always write clearly, checking your spellings and accuracy.

> **VALUES & BEHAVIOURS**
>
> Refer to the values and behaviours chapter for more information on:
> - maintaining customer care
> - greeting clients respectfully and in a friendly manner
> - identifying and confirming the client's expectations
> - treating the client courteously at all times
> - giving the client the information they need about the services or products offered by the salon
> - recognising information that the client may find complicated and checking they fully understand.

Activity

List the types of question you would ask your client if they wanted their hair put up for a day at the races.

Highlight which of your questions are open and which ones are closed.

Tools and equipment

When setting and dressing the hair you will use a variety of tools and equipment, such as rollers, pins, grips, combs, heated rollers, straightening irons and tongs.

This chart shows the tools and equipment available for use.

Tools and equipment	Use
Wide-toothed comb	To detangle wet hair prior to setting
Cutting comb	To cleanly section the hair and allow it to be secured out of the way
Tail/pintail comb	To cleanly section the hair when setting
Dressing-out comb	For backcombing, teasing and dressing the finished result
Section clips	To secure the hair in place
Flat brush	To detangle dry hair, or to smooth hair when brushing it for an up-do
Dressing-out brush (flat)	To remove roller marks from setting and to dress the hair

Tools and equipment	Use
Velcro rollers	Ideal for dry hair setting; hair is dampened with setting lotion and dried under a dryer
Setting rollers	To set wet hair
Pin curl clips	To hold pin curls in place
Hood dryer	To dry wet sets
Grips and pins	To secure and hold chignons, rolls and up-dos
Backcombing brush	To backbrush the hair for volume and support
Heated rollers	To set dry hair

Tools and equipment	Use
Straightening irons	To smooth and straighten dry hair
Tongs	To create curls and body on dry hair
Wand	To create soft varied curls on long dry hair

Activity

Prepare a trolley and work area with all the tools you would need for a hair-up style on long hair to be set using heated rollers. What products could you use to set and dress this style?

Calculate how long it will take for you to set up the trolley, set the hair, allow for it to cool and then dress it out. What is your estimation? How would this time vary between clients with long or short hair?

HANDY HINT

You should explain to your client how to use heated appliances at home safely, as these can cause damage to the hair, increase porosity and decrease elasticity, as well as fade hair colour.

Heated styling equipment

When using electrical equipment, be aware of potential hazards and follow the Electricity at Work Regulations. Always ensure your equipment is in good working order and fit for use to prevent harm to you and others. Use equipment correctly, following the MFIs.

To use heat styling equipment correctly:

- never use electrical appliances with wet hands
- know how to use the appliance
- visually check the body and plug of the appliance
- check the wires and remove the kinks and knots
- follow the Electricity at Work regulations
- follow MFIs to ensure you use the appliance correctly and achieve the best results
- use it for the correct purpose.

Heated appliances can damage the hair and burn you and the client, so it is essential that you use the equipment correctly and safely.

Using and maintaining heated styling equipment

Equipment	How to use	Safety considerations and maintenance
Heated rollers	1 Heat the appliance. 2 Use a flat brush to detangle the hair. 3 Section the hair cleanly – no bigger than the rollers' width or depth. 4 Take a heated roller carefully in your fingers. 5 Protect the ends of the hair with an end paper. 6 Roll the hair section from point to root either on base or off base depending on the style, and secure with the pin. 7 Complete the full head using the chosen winding technique. 8 Leave to cool and then remove the rollers. 9 Dress the finished result.	1 Check the appliance is safe to use. 2 Check the appliance is fit for purpose. 3 Visually check the body and plugs for cracks. 4 Check the wires for kinks and knots. 5 Check the temperature before use. 6 Avoid contact of heated rollers with the skin. 7 Ensure pins are not touching the skin and scalp. 8 Use heat-protecting products. 9 Clean and sterilise rollers after use.
Straighteners	1 Heat the appliance. 2 Use a flat brush to detangle the hair. 3 Section the hair cleanly. 4 Comb the section of hair to be straightened. 5 Run straighteners down the hair section from root to point. 6 Complete the whole head in a methodical manner. 7 Leave to cool. 8 Dress the finished result.	1 Check the appliance is safe to use. 2 Check the appliance is fit for purpose. 3 Visually check the body and plugs for cracks. 4 Check the wires for kinks and knots. 5 Check the temperature before use. 6 Avoid contact of straighteners with the skin and scalp. 7 Use heat-protecting products. 8 Clean the heating plates once cooled and ensure they are free of products.
Tongs and wands	1 Heat the appliance. 2 Use a flat brush to detangle the hair. 3 Cleanly section the hair. 4 Comb the section of hair to be curled. 5 Curl the hair section from root to point (wand) or point to root (tongs). 6 Complete the whole head in a methodical manner. 7 Leave to cool. 8 Dress the finished result.	1 Check the appliance is safe to use. 2 Check the appliance is fit for purpose. 3 Visually check the body and plugs for cracks. 4 Check the wires for kinks and knots. 5 Check the temperature before use. 6 Avoid contact of tongs/wand with the skin and scalp. 7 Use heat-protecting products. 8 Clean the body of the tongs or wand once cooled and ensure they are free of products.

Equipment	How to use	Safety considerations and maintenance
Hood dryers	1 Place the client comfortably under the dryer. 2 Set the timer for the suitable time considering the density and length of the hair. 3 Check that the hair is dry. 4 Allow to cool once dried.	1 Check the appliance is fit for use and safe. 2 Check the temperature setting with your client. 3 Ensure the metal pins are not touching the skin or scalp. 4 After styling, wipe over the hood of the dryer with a sterile wipe or disinfecting spray and cloth.

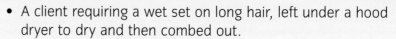

Activity

How long will the following services take?

- A client requiring a wet set on long hair, left under a hood dryer to dry and then combed out.
- A client requiring a dry set, cool down and hair up.
- A client requiring a wet set and pin curls, dried and dressed out.

HANDY HINT

Maintain the condition of your tools by ensuring they are cleaned effectively and free from oil, product build-up and hair.

Ineffectively maintaining your tools and equipment can lead to poor health, safety and hygiene, risk of cross-infection and infestation, and a negative salon image.

Range of products

Make sure you use suitable styling products for wet or dry setting. When you're using heated appliances you must use products that protect the hair from heat and prevent damage.

To use products effectively:

- always follow MFIs
- follow COSHH regulations
- wash your hands after application and ideally wear gloves to apply products
- take precautions to prevent dermatitis
- use the correct quantity of product – avoid overloading the hair
- avoid product waste
- choose the correct product to achieve the best result possible

The following table shows which products should be used to achieve the most effective result.

WHY DON'T YOU...
Ask a stylist in your salon what finishing products they are using when dressing and finishing the hair and why they have chosen these products.

Products and their benefits

Product	How to use	Effect achieved and benefit to the client
Mousse	Use on wet hair. Apply a golf-ball-sized blob to towel-dried hair and comb through evenly.	Enhances curls and offers support and hold to sets and pin curls.
Setting lotion	Use on wet hair. Spray or sprinkle near to the root area and work through to the ends.	Longer-lasting volume, lift and support for fine hair of any length.
Wax	Usually applied on dry hair. Apply with your fingertips through the hair, avoiding the root area. For funky, messy looks, apply using your palms and target the ends of the hair.	For soft supple hold and great shine. Ideal for short hair and smoothing flyaway ends on longer hair or up-dos.
Serum	Can be used on wet or dry hair. Rub two to five drops of serum into your palms and apply to the hair, distributing evenly prior to setting and when using heated appliances.	To calm frizzy hair and flyaway ends, and protect from heated appliances.

Product	How to use	Effect achieved and benefit to the client
Cream/paste	Usually applied to dry hair. Apply using your fingertips, moving from root to point to create texture and movement.	Adds texture to shorter hair lengths, supports and lifts, adds shine and body to medium/longer hair lengths.
Heat protectors	Can be sprayed on wet or dry hair prior to use of heated appliances.	Covers the hair with a protective film, protecting it from heat damage.
Gel	Can be used on wet or dry hair. Massage a small amount into your palms and work evenly into the hair. Shape and mould with your fingers.	For stronger-hold looks, gel can provide an elastic effect, allowing the hair to bounce back into style. Can be used to tame or enhance curls.
Hairspray	Used on dry hair. Shake well and spray onto the hair from about 20cm (7¾ in) away.	Finishes style with a shine and long-lasting shape memory, which is touchable but without stiffness. Ideal for any hair length.

Activity

In pairs, identify your salon's product range for setting and dressing hair and list the benefits to the client. Describe how each product should be used.

Activity

Make up and design your own products and then create a poster marketing them. List their features and benefits, making sure your spelling, punctuation and grammar are correct.

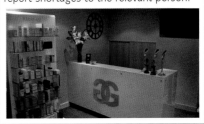

Setting techniques

When setting the hair you will need to consider whether volume, lift and curl are required. Hair can be rolled to sit on base or off base, and the wind can be directed to suit the style, or a brick wind can be used to avoid roller and section marks.

Rollering and winding techniques

The wide choice of winding techniques helps you to create lift and curl, with varied root movement and direction. Changing your roller size enables you to achieve tighter or looser curls.

Setting the hair in the direction in which it is to be styled ensures the root movement falls in line with the desired style result. This method enables you to work with partings – style the hair to one side, creating the look of the style, in the same way you would blow dry.

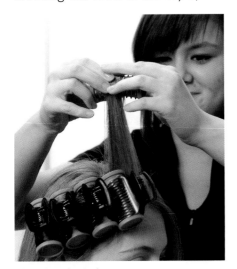

Directional wind

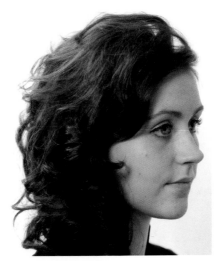

Directional wind result – final look

If the style requires a more blended look that is free from partings and section patterns, then the ideal technique is brick winding. This involves setting the hair in horizontal rows across the head, ensuring that the following row is offset, so that it looks like brickwork.

Activity

Adapting the size of your rollers and estimating size of sections and number of rollers required is about using your maths skills. The angles in which you roll the hair will also involve you using and applying maths.

Estimate how many rollers you would use to create a brick wind set and a spiral set. Carry out these services on a training head and compare your estimates to actual requirements.

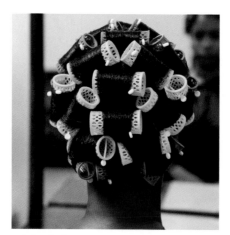

Brick wind

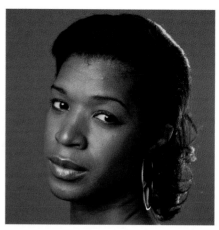

Brick wind – final look

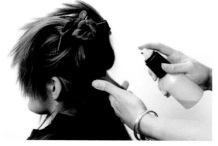

Long hair sectioned while setting

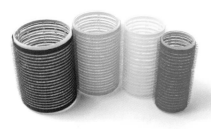

Various size rollers

Sectioning the hair

You must always section the hair cleanly using a pintail or tail comb, depending on your personal preference. When you are working on long hair, always secure the hair you are not working on out of the way.

You must always ensure you take manageable size sections (meches), which are no larger or wider than your roller choice. Small rollers give tighter curls, and medium to large rollers give looser curls, so choose your roller size to suit the required style, taking into consideration the hair's length and density.

Ensure your section meche is combed directly upwards for on-base winds (90°) and combed slightly backwards for off-base winds (45°). For more details, see 'Angle of winding' below.

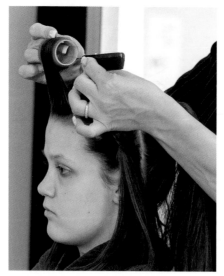

On-base winding – comb the hair directly upwards to create lift and volume

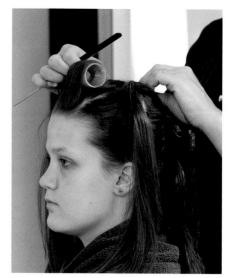

Off-base winding – comb the hair at a 45° angle with root dragged to create flatter curls

Tension and controlling the hair

Pulling the hair with tension as you wind will make the set last longer and the hair stretch into its new position. Long hair can tangle easily and get caught in a roller, so take care when winding the hair around the roller: control the wind; make sure you have all the required sectioned hair neatly wrapped around the roller. When you are happy that the roller has been wound effectively, secure it in place with a hairpin.

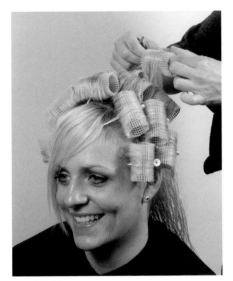

Neatly winding the hair

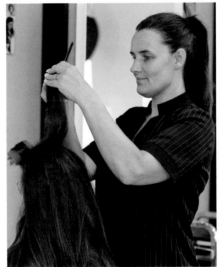

Badly rolled hair – hair not sectioned cleanly and not held with tension

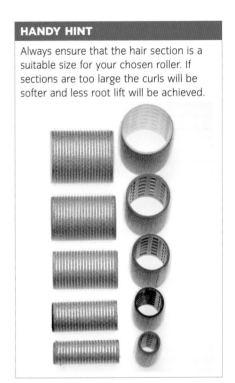

HANDY HINT

Always ensure that the hair section is a suitable size for your chosen roller. If sections are too large the curls will be softer and less root lift will be achieved.

Make sure that you keep the hair damp throughout the winding process to maintain an even elasticity and to allow the hydrogen bonds to set in their new stretched position, setting the hair in a beta keratin state.

Angle of winding

The more volume that is required, the more root lift needed; this requires on-base winding.

When winding the hair to sit on base you must:

- take the section of hair to be rolled and comb it upwards, straight from the head
- hold the section at 90° from the head
- wind the hair downwards from point to root around the roller, ensuring that the completed roll sits on the base of its own section, at the root area.

Ensure that you wind the hair considering the root direction required, to give maximum support to the style.

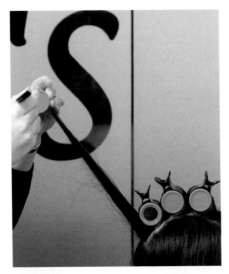

On base

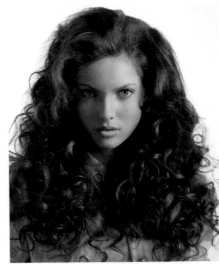

On-base winding – curls with volume and lift

If the style you are creating needs less root lift and a flatter look, you should direct your wind off base. This involves dragging the root back, slightly away from the roller base and section. Use a 45° angle and complete the wind with the roller almost sitting on the root of the section below. The roots then dry or cool without creating lift.

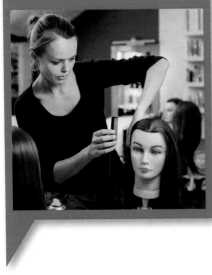

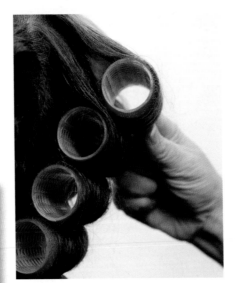

Off base

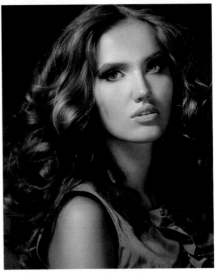

Off-base winding – flat curls

Spiral curls

You can achieve spiral curls with tongs, rollers or 'bendy rods'. The technique used is the same as with conventional setting or tonging, except the hair is wound along the length of the roller or tong (instead of the hair being wound back over itself). Starting from the points and working towards the roots, wind the hair along the tong or roller, in a spiral wind allowing for the direction of the root movement required. This technique gives soft or tight curls, depending on roller size, which fall in a similar way to natural curls.

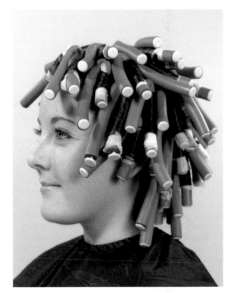

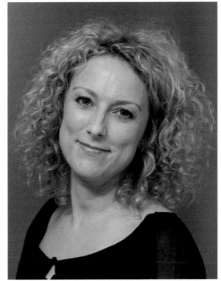

Bendy rods

Bendy rods – spiral curls

How to wrap set hair

Wrap setting is where you section, comb and then wrap the wet hair around the head in a clockwise or anticlockwise direction. This wrapping of the hair around the head means that the contours of the head form the finished shape of the hair. The hair is dried under a hood dryer for up to 90 minutes and then dressed out into a straight smooth style. This setting method is popular on African type hair and very curly hair, and the use of styling products such as Africare foam wrap setting lotion are very important in order to achieve the end result.

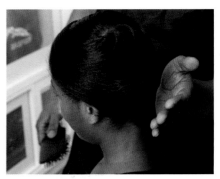

Wrap set

Pin curling

Pin curling involves a setting technique of winding without the aid of a roller. Great skill and hand **dexterity** are required, and once this craft is mastered it is a skill in its own right! You may not need to set without the aid of rollers often, but imagine going to a photoshoot or visiting a bride's home to style their hair, only to find you do not have enough rollers, or worse, you have forgotten them! The ability to pin curl gives great curl results and the hair dries much faster than when it is tightly wrapped around a roller.

These curls are created by a wet setting technique. The section patterns and winding techniques can be the same as for winding with a roller, and the hair is wound from point to root.

Pin curls can be used on very straight African type hair or on woven hairstyles, for example, with hair additions. Hair that is texturised or curly may not be suitable for this hairstyle, as the hair may be too frizzy when dry and the finished curl will not be structured enough.

Dexterity

Precise and flexible handling.

WHY DON'T YOU...
Practise these setting techniques and time yourself.

Pin curls for volume

To create curls with root lift and volume, you can use 'stand-up' pin curls, sometimes called barrel curls. Use a suitable product and comb the wet hair upwards, at about 90° to the head. Roll the hair downwards from point to root, without a roller. Secure the hair on base with a pin curl clip. This technique produces soft curls or waves and volume.

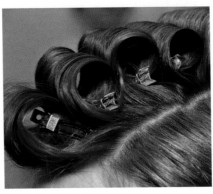
Pin curls for volume

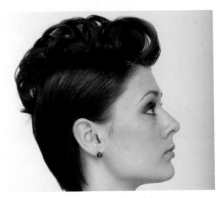
Pin curls for volume – final look

Pin curls for flat movement

To create movement through the hair but without root lift and volume, you can use 'lie-down' pin curls, sometimes called a flat barrel curl. After you have applied a suitable styling product, comb the wet hair downwards at about 45° and feed the hair through your fingers to create a flat, open-coiled curl. Secure the hair off base with a pin curl clip. This technique produces flat movement and waves throughout the hair.

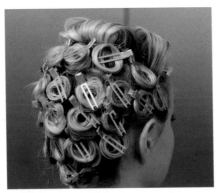
Pin curls for flat movement

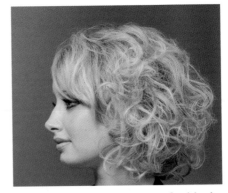
Pin curls for flat movement – final look

Clock-spring pin curls for flat movement

For 'clock-spring' pin curls follow the technique described above for pin curls for flat movement, but feed the hair through your fingers and create a closed-in coiled curl that is smaller in the centre and gradually gets larger towards the outside of the coil. Clock-spring pin curls create flat movement that has tighter curls and body at the ends of the hair, where the coil was at its tightest, and gradually loosens towards the root.

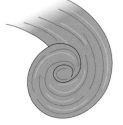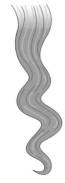
Clock-spring pin curl

Dressing techniques

Now that you have learnt the art of setting the hair, it is time to have fun dressing it out and putting it up. By setting the hair first, you have a solid foundation to build on. Most hair-up styles require some body or curl to be added to support the up-do. For chignons and bouffant styles, the hair may need to be straightened to obtain a smooth finish.

The dressing techniques you may use are curls, rolls, smoothing and backbrushing and backcombing. You can see these in detail in the step by steps at the end of the chapter.

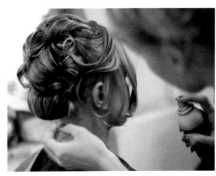

Hairspray for special occasion style

Providing advice and recommendations

It is important that you have thorough and up-to-date knowledge on tools, equipment, products and techniques so that you can carry out the services your clients require and so that you can make recommendations and provide your clients with advice.

Maintaining the look

Providing your client with advice for maintaining an everyday style will be a little more straightforward than the aftercare required for hair-up styles and dressed looks. For all options you should advise your client on which products, tools and equipment work best and how to maintain the look. You could offer some tips for recreating the style themselves, but it is fair to say that the look they will achieve is unlikely to be of a professional standard. After all, the client came to you, the expert, to obtain the required look.

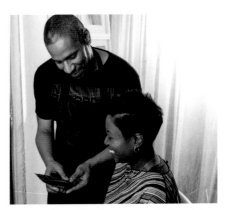

Suggest new products to suit the style

Taking down the hairstyle

If your client has had their hair put up, you will need to advise them on how to remove the grips and pins and take the hair down. At the end of the service advise your client of where the last pins were inserted, so they know roughly where to start when taking them out. Advise the client on how to remove them so they don't cause themselves any discomfort and once all of the pins are out explain how to brush the hair through. Advise them on what brush to use when removing backcombing or backbrushing from the hair to avoid damaging the hair and discomfort being caused.

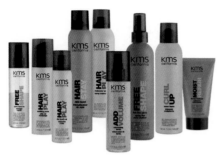

Products that may benefit the style

Present and future products and services

You should advise your clients on the products you used to create their initial style, asking them about the products they already have, and suggesting which new products they would benefit from purchasing and using. Always advise your client on how to use the products and how to remove them from the hair to prevent build-up. If you are recommending backcombing or backbrushing techniques, they would also benefit from conditioning treatments.

Time interval between services

You should explain to your client how long the style is likely to last. If it's hair-up, then the client is likely to take the style down at the end of the evening, but a set to create curls may last for a few days. Advise your client when to return for the same service and book any appointments for future services you have suggested to your client, such as cuts, colours, treatments, etc.

Be able to set and dress hair – review

Prepare for setting and dressing services

Before you carry out the service, ensure your client is gowned and protected and the hair prepared. This may include a shampoo and conditioning service prior to a wet set, or checking the hair is clean and ready for a dry setting service.

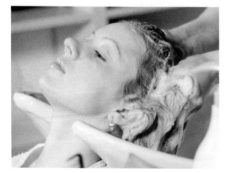

Shampoo and conditioning prior to service

Work safely and hygienically

When carrying out hair setting, you must always remember to work safely and hygienically:

- maintain your responsibilities for health and safety
- protect yourclient throughout the service
- consider your posture and your client's body position for health and safety, and comfort
- minimise risks of injury and damage to tools and test the temperature of heated styling equipment throughout the service
- keep area clean and tidy, use clean resources and minimise the risk of cross-infection
- promote environmental and sustainable working practices and minimise waste

- ensure your personal hygiene, protection and appearance are up to salon standard
- minimise risk of injury to self and others and follow MFIs
- use your time effectively and complete the service in a commerically acceptable time.

Consult with clients

Client consultation:

- identify client requirements
- identify any factors that may prevent or affect the service
- confirm and carry out client requirements.

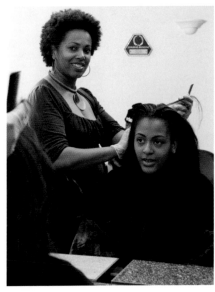

Client consultation

Carry out setting and dressing services

Set hair

When setting hair:

- control your tools and equipment to minimise the risk of damage to the hair, client discomfort and to achieve the desired look
- apply suitable products following manufacturers' instructions
- control your client's hair throughout the setting process taking account of factors influencing the service
- take sections of hair that suit the size of the tools and equipment
- keep the hair damp throughout the setting process, when necessary
- section and wind the hair cleanly and evenly to achieve the desired look
- ensure all wound rollers, when used, are secure and sit on or off base to meet the style requirements
- maintain the correct tension throughout the setting process
- remove any items used for setting, avoiding discomfort to your client
- ensure your setting techniques achieve the desired look.

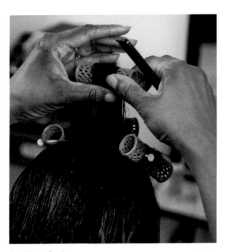

Setting hair

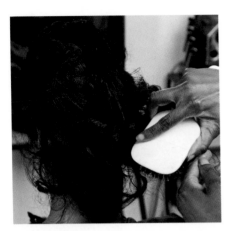

Dressing out

Dress hair

When dressing hair:

- leave your client's hair free of all section marks (from the setting technique)
- use heated equipment, if required, at the correct temperature for your client's hair and the desired look
- control your tools and equipment to minimise the risk of damage to the hair and scalp, client discomfort and to achieve the desired look
- apply and use suitable products following the manufacturers' instructions
- ensure the finished look takes into account relevant factors influencing the service
- ensure your dressing techniques and effects achieve the intended shape, direction and volume agreed with your client
- confirm your client's satisfaction with the finished look
- give your client advice and recommendations on the service provided
- complete the service within a commercially viable time.

Provide advice and recommendations

When providing setting and dressing services, you should provide your client with advice:

- advise on the time interval between services
- advise on present and future products and services
- advise your client on how to take down the style
- advise your client on how to maintain their look.

Step by steps

Set and dress hair to create curls

Traditional wet set wound in a brick wind pattern

WHY DON'T YOU...
Practise these wind settings and time yourself.

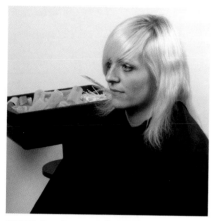

STEP 1 – Gown and prepare your client for the service.

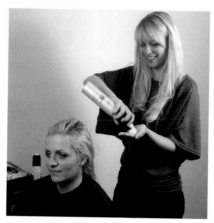

STEP 2 – Shampoo the hair and apply styling products.

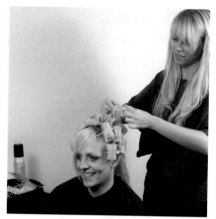

STEP 3 – Wind the rollers from point to root in a brick wind formation.

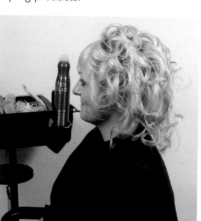

STEP 4 – Complete the whole head wind and dry the hair with a hood dryer or similar.

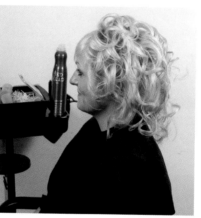

STEP 5 – Allow to cool and remove the rollers.

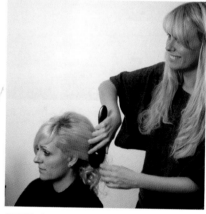

STEP 6 – Using a dressing-out brush, remove the roller marks.

HANDY HINT

When dressing out a wet set, brush the hair thoroughly to ensure you break up all the roller marks and remove all partings to blend the hair. This will also help to reduce the stiffness of the dried setting product and create a softer appearance.

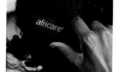

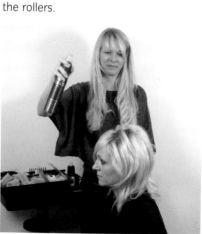

STEP 7 – Dress the hair into the desired style and apply your finishing products.

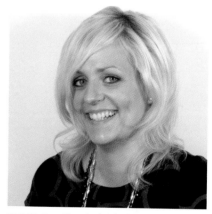

STEP 8 – Check the balance and ensure that the client is happy with the end result.

Dry setting directional wind technique using heated rollers

Long hair is dry set with heated rollers wound in a directional style to produce volume and root lift.

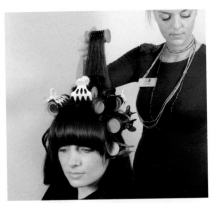

STEP 1 – Wind the hair from points to roots in a directional manner.

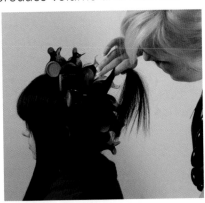

STEP 2 – Roll the hair on base to maintain root lift and volume.

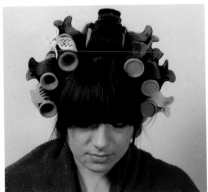

STEP 3 – Allow the rollers to cool before you remove them.

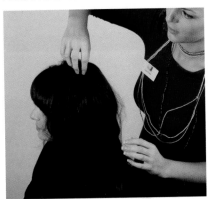

STEP 4 – Use your hands or a brush to remove roller marks.

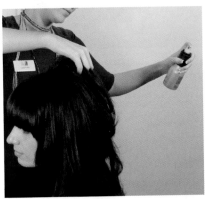

STEP 5 – Dress and backcomb the hair into the desired style. Apply your chosen finishing products.

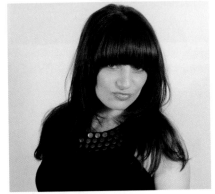

STEP 6 – Check the balance and ensure that the client is happy with the end result.

Dry setting directional-wind technique using velcro rollers

Long, layered hair is dry set on larger velcro rollers and combed out to produce a curly style with body and root lift.

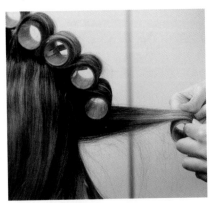

STEP 1 – Apply your products to your client's dry hair and wind from point to root.

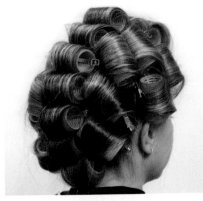

STEP 2 – Wind all the hair into your chosen wind.

THE CITY & GUILDS TEXTBOOK

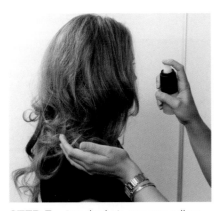

STEP 3 – Dry the hair, remove rollers and run your fingers through the hair or brush through to remove roller marks; then apply finishing products.

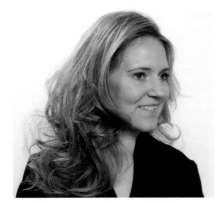

STEP 4 – Check the balance and ensure that the client is happy with the end result.

Pin curls to create volume

Stand-up pin curls (barrel curls) styled on wet hair that is medium to long in length.

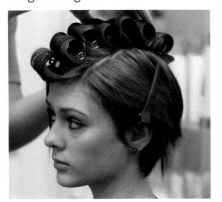

STEP 1 – After gowning and preparing your client, apply styling product and section the hair. Roll the hair from point to root around your fingers into the direction of the style. Secure the curl with a pin curl clip.

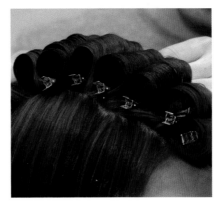

STEP 2 – Repeat as required.

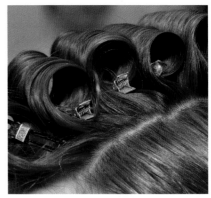

STEP 3 – Ensure the pin curl sits on base for maximum root lift.

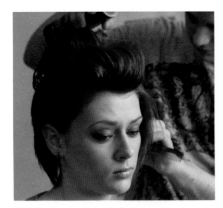

STEP 4 – Dry the hair, leave it to cool, remove the pin curl clips, dress and tease it into the desired style, and apply finishing products.

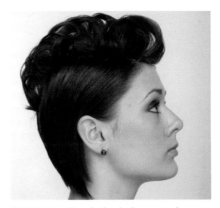

STEP 5 – Check the balance and ensure that the client is happy with the end result.

Pin curls to create flat movement

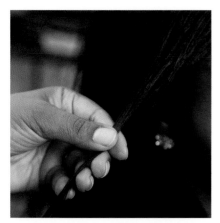

STEP 1 – Create a side parting and take a small section of hair. Comb the section of the hair from ends to roots. The section should be 6–12mm in width.

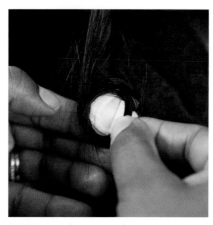

STEP 2 – Place an end paper on the ends. Curl the hair in a flat circle between your fingers in an anticlockwise direction.

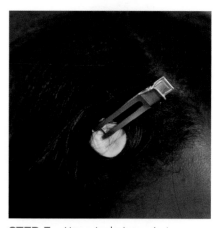

STEP 3 – Use a Lady Jane pin to secure the hair, following the root direction of the hair.

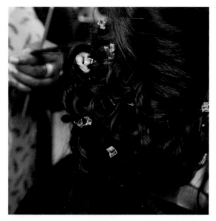

STEP 4 – Using a brick wind, place clockwise pin curls from the right side of the head around to the left of the head.

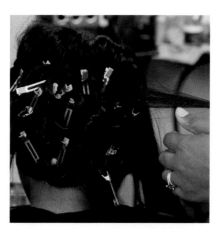

STEP 5 – In the following row place the pin curls in the reverse order using a row of anticlockwise pin curls, working left to right.

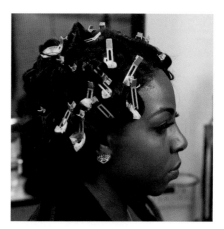

STEP 6 – Continue using this reverse pin curling technique of anticlockwise and clockwise pin curls until you have completed the whole head. Leave the hair to dry for 45 minutes to one hour (depending on the length).

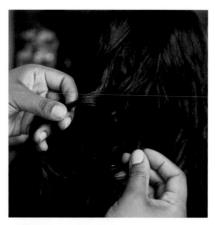

STEP 7 – Comb the hair out into ringlets and soft curls. Apply serum, oil sheen spray and holding spray if required.

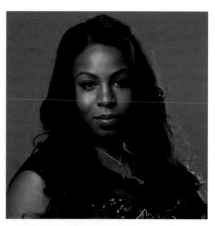

STEP 8 – Check the balance and ensure that the client is happy with the end result.

Set and dress hair to smooth

Wrap setting

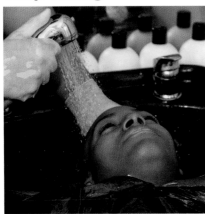

STEP 1 – Shampoo and condition the hair and apply plenty of smoothing cream.

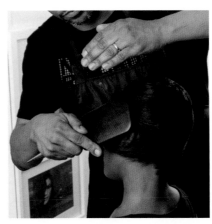

STEP 2 – Section the hair and comb it smooth, wrapping it around the contours of the head.

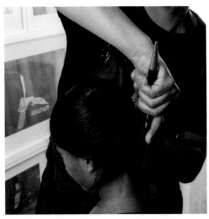

STEP 3 – Continue this process around the head, smoothing the hair and adding more product if required. Secure the hair in place with either hair clips or a hair scarf/wrap.

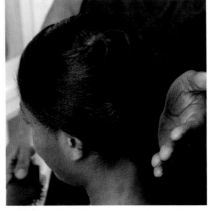

STEP 4 – Dry the hair under a hood dryer for up to 90 minutes and check it is dry before dressing out. Dress the hair into style and add finishing products to add shine and hold.

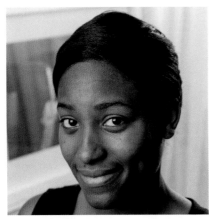

STEP 5 – Final look

Set and dress hair to create a roll

Creating a bouffant roll

Bouffant style using a 'beehive' attachment for extra root lift.

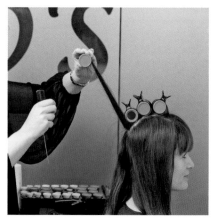

STEP 1 – Gown and prepare your client and set the hair with heated rollers.

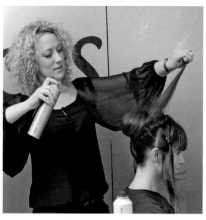

STEP 2 – After removing the rollers, apply hairspray to the sections of hair and secure the back section into a bun.

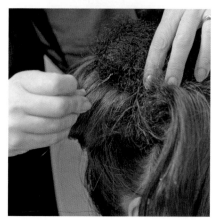

STEP 3 – Attach and secure the hair padding on top of the bun.

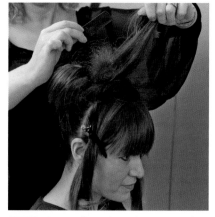

STEP 4 – Backcomb each section of hair.

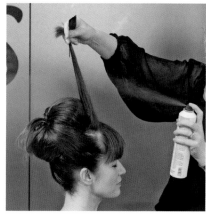

STEP 5 – Dress the hair over the hair padding into a bouffant, and secure with grips and pins. Tease the hair into place and apply finishing products.

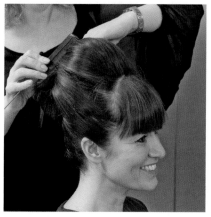

STEP 6 – Smooth any stray hairs with a comb or dressing-out brush and add more spray.

HANDY HINT

Always ensure you handle and control the hair effectively when dressing it, setting the hair first. Using backcombing or backbrushing helps you to manipulate the hair into place. To help secure the hair, use grips, pins and hairspray.

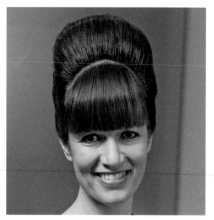

STEP 7 – Check the balance.

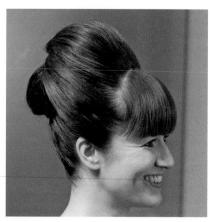

STEP 8 – Ensure that your client is happy with the end result.

Creating a vertical roll

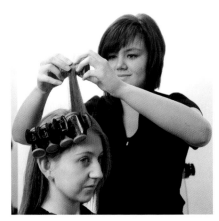

STEP 1 – Gown and prepare your client, and set the hair.

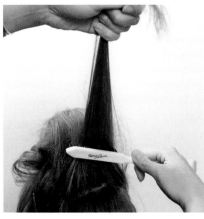

STEP 2 – Apply styling products to dry hair and backcomb the roots.

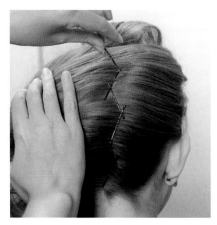

STEP 3 – Grip the hair down the centre, criss-crossing the grips.

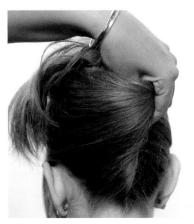

STEP 4 – Fold the hair, and slightly twist it over the grips, securing the hair with pins.

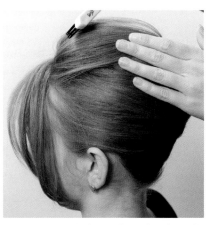

STEP 5 – Tuck the ends under the roll, smooth over the top section and apply finishing products.

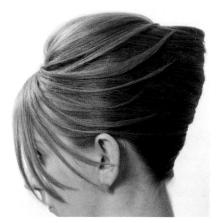

STEP 6 – Check the balance and ensure that your client is happy with the finished result.

HANDY HINT

To remove backcombing/backbrushing from the hair, advise your client to take small sections and, using a soft bristle brush, gently brush through the hair starting at the points and working down towards the roots.

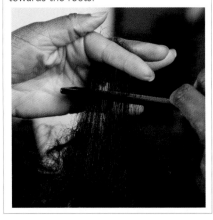

Answers in the back of the book.

1 **Statement one**

Standing with feet hip width apart will minimise the risk of fatigue when working.

Statement two

To avoid contact dermatitis, personal protective equipment should be worn when applying products before setting.

Which one of the following is correct for the above statements?

a True   True

b True   False

c False   True

d False   False

2 Which one of the following is best used to achieve a chignon on fine hair?

a Back-combing

b Mousse

c Heat protector

d Serum

3 What is the best advice to be given to a client with split ends?

a To always use clarifying shampoo

b To hide them by using grips

c To shampoo the hair regularly

d To minimise the use of heated appliances

4 Off-base rollering can minimise the look of

a An oval face shape

b Very coarse hair

c Thick, full hair

d Very fine hair

5 Which one of the following is considered the ideal face shape?

a Rectangular

b Square

c Round

d Oval

6 How does alpha keratin change to beta keratin?

a By breaking and re-forming the disulphide bonds

b By breaking and re-forming the hydrogen bonds

c By changing the pH from alkali to acid

d By removing oxygen in the amino acids

7 Why is it important to keep the hair evenly damp throughout the setting process?

a Because it is more elastic and workable when wet

b Because it is easily damaged when dry

c Because it absorbs atmospheric moisture

d Because it will take less time under the dryer

8 African Caribbean hair lacks moisture and is

a Elastic and delicate

b Coarse and dense

c Fine and brittle

d Dry and fragile

9 Which one of the following is the best tool to use to section hair cleanly?

a Cutting comb

b Pin tail comb

c Dressing-out comb

d Wide-toothed comb

10 **Statement one**

Setting lotion should be used on dry hair only.

Statement two

Mousse should be used on wet hair.

Which one of the following is correct for the above statements?

a True   True

b True   False

c False   True

d False   False

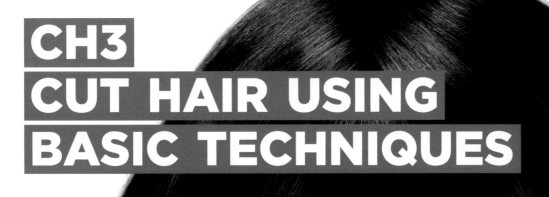

CH3
CUT HAIR USING BASIC TECHNIQUES

Cutting hair is the foundation of all styles and combined with the other services it makes you a stylist. Having learnt the art of a good consultation, you can now style and cut the hair. The cut and shape of every style is paramount to the end result and learning these basic techniques will be the foundation for the rest of your styling and cutting career. So what are you waiting for? Get your scissors and let's get started.

After reading this chapter you will:

- know how health and safety affects cutting services

- understand the factors that influence haircutting services

- know the tools, equipment, products and techniques used to cut hair

- be able to provide haircutting services.

HEALTH & SAFETY

Refer to the health and safety and salon policies chapter for more information on the health and safety Acts you need to follow when cutting hair.

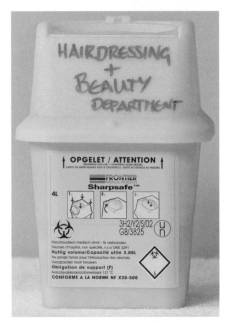

Sharps bin

HANDY HINT

You must ensure that you remove hair cuttings during and at the end of the service. Wet and dry hair can be slippery and cause accidents. Sweep up the hair and place it in the salon's designated hair bin.

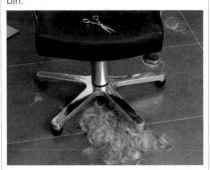

HANDY HINT

Protect clients from hair clippings to ensure they are comfortable at all times and to prevent any stray hairs from entering the skin or eyes.

Health and safety

Your responsibilities for health and safety

Your responsibilities for health and safety include:

- following your salon procedures and all of the health and safety Acts
- preparing a clean working environment
- maintaining your personal hygiene and presentation
- carrying out a consultation with your client
- gowning and protecting your client for the cutting service
- behaving in a suitable manner that does not cause risk of injury to you and those around you.

Hazards and risks

Throughout the cutting hair service you're surrounded by sharp objects such as scissors and possibly razors. Care must be taken when using and transporting these tools to avoid the risk of injury. Sharps must be disposed of in a sharps bin.

Other potential hazards and risks include:

- infected clients or staff – could result in cross-contamination
- unsupervised children – if unruly they may run into stylists or clients whilst scissors or razors are being used – risk of injury
- electrical appliances – clippers – there is risk of electric shock if, for example, your clippers are faulty or used incorrectly
- hair on the floor – risk of slipping over/injury
- spillages – there is a risk of slipping over/injury.

Safe working practices

To maintain a safe and effective working relationship, remember:

- complete a thorough consultation
- gown and protect your client from hair cuttings
- position your client comfortably – support their back at all times, keeping legs uncrossed
- maintain a good posture – stand with body weight evenly distributed
- maintain good personal hygiene
- prepare your tools, equipment and work area in advance

- clean and sterilise tools and equipment prior to and after the service
- take care with sharp tools and use them for the correct purpose
- remove waste and hair cuttings throughout the service.

Safe use of equipment, materials and products

You must always use your tools correctly. Scissors are extremely sharp and accidents can occur. Always carry your scissors with the blades closed and keep them safe by storing them in a cutting case. Your scissors are likely to be the most expensive item in your tool collection and dropping them with the blades open or pointing downwards can affect the position of the blades and be very costly.

Instructions for the care of scissors include:

- using them only for their intended purpose – cutting hair
- not carrying them in the pockets of your clothes
- carrying them in a safe manner and storing them after use
- ensuring they are fit for purpose
- using the correct type of scissors for specific styles
- cleaning and sterilising them after use
- removing all hair cuttings and oiling them regularly
- having them professionally sharpened when required.

Care of razors should include:

- using them only for their intended purpose
- carrying them in a safe manner and storing them after use
- ensuring they are fit for purpose and using a new blade when required
- cleaning and sterilising them after use
- removing all hair cuttings and oiling them regularly
- disposing of used razor blades in a sharps bin.

You might, on occasions, use clippers. These must be maintained by removing all excess hair from the blades and oiling the blades. Adjusting the blade settings while oiling helps lubricate the entire blade area.

HEALTH & SAFETY

Refer to the health and safety and salon policies chapter to recap your knowledge on using environmental and sustainable practices when cutting hair.

HANDY HINT

Take care with scissors so as not to cut yourself or your client. If you do cut yourself or your client, cover any open wounds and take care not to cause any cross-contamination. Remember to record the details in the salon's accident book.

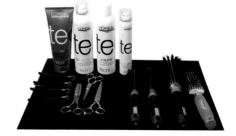

Hygienic, well-maintained tools and products

Activity

Discuss with a colleague how you think a client would feel if you used combs, scissors or clippers with the previous client's hair still on them!

Working safely and hygienically

Working safely with cutting tools is very important: you must ensure that your tools and equipment are well maintained and fit for use. Always protect your client's clothes from hair cuttings by gowning them and using a clean towel or cutting collar to ensure client comfort throughout the service. As we saw in previous chapters, your own personal hygiene must be maintained and you must correctly clean and prepare your workstation in advance of your client's arrival.

Preventing cross-infection and infestation

The tools you are likely to use during the cutting service are:

- scissors
- thinning scissors
- razors
- combs
- sectioning clips
- clippers/trimmers.

You must disinfect or sterilise your cutting tools after every service, to maintain a good reputation, ensure a professional image and to prevent cross-infection and infestation. You must ensure that you protect yourself and your client from the risk of cross-contamination.

Make sure all your towels and gowns are contamination-free, and that scissors and combs are sterile. If you encounter any infections or infestations, you must boil wash all towels and gowns. Use heat such as boiling water or an autoclave for scissors and combs and remember that a UV light will only *maintain* sterilisation but is not an effective method of removing micro-organisms from your tools.

Methods of cleaning, disinfecting and sterilising

The table below shows the most appropriate methods of sterilising or disinfecting your tools.

Cutting tools	Appropriate method of disinfecting/ sterilisation
Scissors and thinning scissors	Autoclave – moist heat
	UV light cabinet
	Chemical solutions, e.g. Barbicide (oil the blades after disinfecting)
Razors	Autoclave – moist heat
	UV light cabinet

Cutting tools	Appropriate method of disinfecting/ sterilisation
Combs	UV light cabinet Chemical solutions, e.g. Barbicide
Sectioning clips	UV light cabinet Chemical solutions, e.g. Barbicide
Clippers and trimmers	Chemical wipes or sprays (oil the blades after disinfecting)

HANDY HINT

Always clean your non-electrical tools prior to disinfecting or sterilising, using detergent with warm water. Toothbrushes or nail brushes work particularly well for removing hair cuttings and scalp debris from between the teeth of combs and clipper blades.

Positioning

The positioning of you and your client is most important when cutting the hair, as the result and balance of the finished look can be affected.

Your client's positioning

Once gowned and protected, you must ensure that your client sits comfortably with their back supported in the chair, in an upright position with their legs uncrossed and evenly balanced.

Your body position

Stand with your body weight evenly distributed throughout the entire cutting process. This will not only prevent fatigue and back problems but also ensure the hairstyle is balanced. Sit on a cutting stool while cutting hair short or for working on the back of the client's head. This will prevent you from bending and overstretching, and help to maintain your comfort, which is essential during the cutting service.

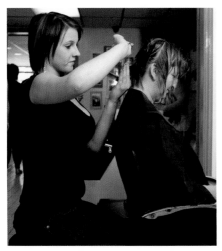

Stylist sitting on a cutting stool to cut a short graduation into the nape of the neck

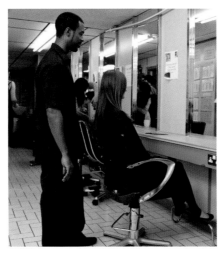

Good client positioning

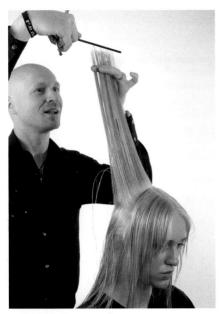

Agree and check with your client how much length to remove

WHY DON'T YOU...
Ask a colleague to pretend to be your client. Ask them to visualise a style and then ask the relevant questions to identify the image and look they require.

VALUES & BEHAVIOURS
Refer to the values and behaviours chapter for more information on client care and effective communication.

HANDY HINT
Revisit chapter CHB9 for more in-depth information on consulting with your client.

Importance of questioning clients

You must always carry out a thorough consultation with your client, to identify their needs and to be able to carry out their wishes. During the consultation you should tell them how long the service should take and how the client can maintain the look between salon visits. The consultation process should continue throughout the cutting service, as you should update them on the progress of the haircut and check you are cutting to the agreed lengths.

The consultation process

It is advisable to begin the initial consultation before you gown your client, to see their style of dress and overall image. You should ask your client about their day-to-day lifestyle and available time to commit to styling their hair. Always listen to what your client is asking of you, and be honest yet tactful with the advice you give them. You should use open questions to obtain as much information as possible and finish with closed questions to confirm what has been agreed.

During the consultation you should ask questions about how much hair they would like taken off the length and the layers. You must be specific with your questions to achieve an accurate account of their needs. Show them in the mirror how much hair you are going to remove to confirm what you assume to be the agreed lengths and amounts. Use visual aids such as magazines to agree on styles and shapes. Always give your clients the option to try something different from their current style and give them the opportunity to express what their vision of the finished look should be.

When you have decided on a style together, ask your client which products they currently use to style their hair to identify whether you need to recommend any alternative products for their new image.

Reasons why clients leave their hairstylist:

- The hairstylist didn't recommend anything new and interesting.
- The hairstylist didn't listen to the client request.
- The hairstylist created a style that was not suitable for the client.
- The hairstylist cut the hair too short, even after consultation and agreeing the lengths.

Factors that may affect services

You need to consider factors that might affect the outcome of the service required. Always ensure that you check the hair and scalp for any lumps and bumps that could cause discomfort to the client when you are combing or cutting the hair. Some scalp disorders may require consideration in the style recommended, as the client might want them covered up. Always ask about scalp disorders during your consultation and check for infections and infestations which would prevent the service from being carried out. Check the eyebrows and ears for piercings that could cause an injury if you were accidentally to catch them with the comb.

You must consider the following different factors prior to and during cutting and understand how these may impact on the cutting service:

- hair classifications
- hair characteristics
- head and face shape.

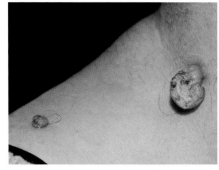

A skin tag – something that a client may want their hair to cover up

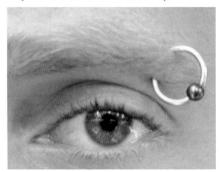

Take care with your scissors and combs, and check for piercings

How hair classifications might affect the service

Hair classification	Description	Impact on service
Straight hair – type 1 Fine/thin hair	Fine/thin – hair tends to be very soft, shiny and oily, and it can be difficult to hold a curl.	Fine/thin straight hair might not achieve the desired result. Avoid using deep texturising techniques that will make the hair thinner. Instead use club cutting techniques and choose styles to suit the hair type.
Medium hair	Medium – hair has lots of volume and body.	When cutting fine and medium straight hair, every 'scissor cut' can show in the hair; accuracy is very important and subtle texturised cuts, such as point cutting, can help to prevent the cutting lines from being so apparent.

Hair classification	Description	Impact on service
 Coarse hair	Coarse – hair is normally extremely straight and difficult to curl.	Coarse straight hair may benefit from deeper texturising and thinning out techniques to remove some bulk, and improve the end result and style.
Wavy hair – type 2 Fine/thin hair	Fine/thin – hair has a definite 'S' pattern. Normally can accomplish various styles.	Wavy hair can be great to work with. It's easy to mould it straighter or enhance the body. Most techniques work well with this hair type. Fine/thin wavy hair – you may need to leave some length to aid body within the cut.
 Medium hair	Medium – hair tends to be frizzy and a little resistant to styling.	Medium and coarse wavy hair can be frizzy so avoid texturising techniques that will enhance a fluffy appearance such as razor cutting. Club cutting can help, by keeping all hair lengths the same.
 Coarse hair	Coarse – normally very frizzy; tends to have thicker waves.	Coarse wavy hair can be resistant to styling, so it may benefit from being texturised or thinned out but avoid using a razor on the hair.

VALUES & BEHAVIOURS

Equality and diversity – you will work on many different hair types to cover the range required. Some of the hair types you may cut could be European hair, Asian hair or African type hair. Clients will come from different ethnic groups, have different cultures and have different religions (or no religion). Make sure you respect other people's cultures and religions, even if they differ from your own personal views. See the values and behaviours chapter for more information on personal ethics.

Hair classification	Description	Impact on service
Curly hair – type 3 Loose curls	Loose curls – the hair can be thick and full with lots of body, with a definite 'S' pattern. It also tends to be frizzy.	Soft loose curly hair can have a combination of textures to consider; it may be frizzy in appearance and have lots of body. Avoid using razors or heavily texturising the hair if the hair tends to be frizzy.
 Tight curls	Tight curls – with a medium amount of curl.	Tight curly hair can also have combined textures and will spring up after the hair has been cut when it is dried – particularly fine curly hair. Consider the amount of tension you place on the hair during the cutting service and use a wide-toothed comb.
Very curly hair – type 4 Soft	Soft – tightly coiled and has a more defined curly pattern.	Soft very curly hair is often fragile, so be careful if using razors or clippers. Comb the hair gently using a wide-toothed comb and use a conditioning spray to prevent client discomfort. Choose a style to suit and work with the curls, rather than try to fight them.
 Wiry	Wiry – tightly coiled but with a less defined curly pattern. The hair has more of a 'Z' pattern shape.	Wiry curly hair is also very fragile but can have less of a defined curly pattern. Avoid techniques that texturise the hair and use mostly club cutting and freehand techniques. Take care with tools if using razors or clippers. Comb the hair gently using a wide-toothed comb and use a conditioning spray to prevent client discomfort and damage to the fragile hair.

HANDY HINT

Curly hair will spring up when dry – use less tension when cutting curly hair.

How hair characteristics might affect the service

Factor	Impact on service
Density 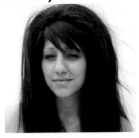 Abundant hair 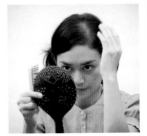 Sparse hair	Density can affect the choice of style and cutting technique. Abundant hair may need to be thinned out to create the desired look. Consider whether abundant hair will complement the look; if not, suggest alternatives. Sparse hair will need to be blunt cut/club cut to maintain as much thickness as possible. Avoid cutting the hair too short, but equally avoid suggesting keeping fine hair long.
Texture 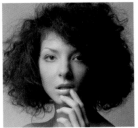 Coarse hair 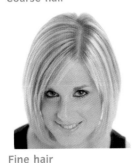 Fine hair	Texture can affect the choice of style and cutting technique. Coarse-textured hair may not suit the desired look; you will need to recommend smoothing products to help achieve the result. Texturising techniques may help to remove some of the coarseness, but razor cutting the hair can make the hair look coarser and more frizzy. Fine hair may also need supporting hair products and style recommendations to enhance the finish.
Elasticity 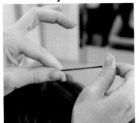 Elasticity test	Elasticity can affect the cutting technique. If the hair is weak avoid using razor blades and fine-tooth combs to detangle the hair. Wet hair has more elasticity than dry hair. If the hair is weak avoid overstretching the hair. Spray the hair with water throughout the cut to maintain an even moisture balance which helps avoid the hair tangling and snagging.

Factor	Impact on service
Porosity and hair condition 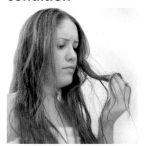 Porous hair	Hair that is damaged is likely to be porous. This can affect the cutting technique and client comfort. If the hair is porous and the cuticles are open, then the hair is more likely to tangle during the cut, and this may cause client discomfort. You should use a wider-toothed comb and spray the hair with leave-in conditioner to aid the combing process. Avoid using a razor on porous hair and take care if using clipper grades, as they may get caught in the dry porous hair.

Hair growth patterns

Hair growth patterns can affect the choice of style and cutting technique. For cowlicks avoid full fringes; instead, suggest a side half fringe that works with the cowlick. Cut this area of the hairline once dry to clearly see the jump and length of hair remaining. For widow's peaks avoid fringes completely and suggest styles that are created with the top area of hair going over to one side or straight back. For double crowns suggest maintaining a little length around the crown area and ideally work the natural fall into the style. For nape whorls suggest maintaining the length at the nape area, or at least a little weight. Avoid cutting into the hairline. For more detail on these hair growth patterns, see the hair characteristics table in chapter CHB9.

HANDY HINT

Always check the hair for growth patterns prior to shampooing the hair – when the hair is wet some growth patterns are not as easy to detect.

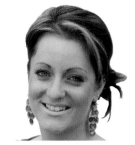

Cowlick

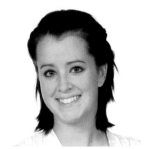

Widow's peak

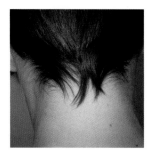

Nape whorl

How head and face shapes might affect the service

The head and face shape can affect the choice of style. Always aim to achieve a style which makes the face look oval-shaped.

Head and face shape

For round face shapes, avoid styles that add more roundness, such as too much width or height. Try to suggest styles that come onto the face. For oblong face shapes, avoid styles that come onto the

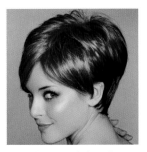

Question mark head shape

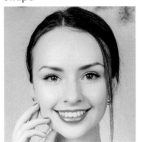

Heart shaped face

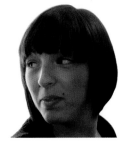

Round face

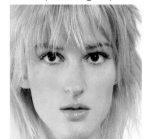

Oblong face

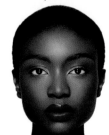

Square face

face; encourage width, avoid height and suggest a fringe to shorten the impression of a long face shape. For square face shapes, suggest softer styles that soften the jawline.

For heart face shapes, avoid width at the temple area and add width near the jawline area; try to avoid the finished length being at jawline level. The head shape should be considered within the overall shape of the style. The ideal head shape will look a little like a question mark from the side view. The head should be rounded from the crown to the occipital bone and then dip in slightly towards the nape.

Prominent features

Facial features can also affect the choice of style. For clients with **protruding** ears, suggest styles that cover the entire ear. For strong nose features or jawlines, avoid centre partings that encourage the eye to follow down from the parting to the nose and chin.

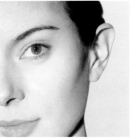

Protruding ears

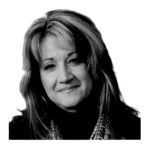

Strong nose and jaw features

Factors when cutting hair wet and dry

Along with the above factors, whether you cut the hair wet or dry will affect the technique used and the end result. Hair should be checked while dry and rechecked after shampooing.

Dry haircutting

You must check the hair while it is dry to see how the client is currently wearing their hairstyle, to identify any natural hair growth patterns and to feel the density and texture of the hair. Always carry out a porosity test on dry hair prior to the service and an elasticity test on wet hair.

Freehand and scissors-over-comb cutting techniques are best carried out on dry hair. Thinning scissors and clippers must only be used on dry hair.

Protruding

Sticking out.

Activity

To aid your development in maths it is important you understand and recognise different shapes.

Draw and label the different face shapes, and then add sketches of hairstyles that will complement each one to give the illusion of an oval face.

HANDY HINT

When checking dry hair before the service, you are looking at a styled head of hair which may have products on it or have been styled to change the natural fall and make the hair feel thicker. Always recheck the hair type and the natural movement and fall of the hair when it has been shampooed.

Wet haircutting

Once the hair has been shampooed and prepared for the service, check through the hair to identify the natural parting. On wet hair you will be able to see the hair type in its natural state, such as curly or straight, and recheck the movement of the hair.

The elasticity in the hair allows wet hair to be stretched up to 50% of its original length, and you must consider this when you are cutting the hair wet, as the dried result could be much shorter than you or your client anticipated. Always carry out an elasticity test on wet hair. Razors and any slice cutting techniques should only be used on wet hair.

Tools, equipment and products

Choosing suitable cutting tools

For most basic cutting techniques, you will use scissors with an average blade length of 5 inches (or 12.5cm), depending on the size of your hands. Choosing the right scissors for you to work with comfortably is important. As you become more experienced you are likely to want a selection of scissors for a variety of techniques, and you'll probably buy more expensive scissors as your skill level increases.

Activity

Convert the following imperial size scissors to centimetres:

- 4.5 inch scissors
- 5.5 inch scissors
- 6 inch scissors.

Scissors

Although, at a glance, all scissors look the same, they are indeed very different. They can vary in size and weight due to the metals they are made from, and the type of cutting blade may also vary. At varying costs, you can purchase scissors that have a movable thumb area, which can make it more comfortable for you to cut baselines and achieve exaggerated angles. Scissors are available with serrated or straight blades.

Serrated scissors are most suitable when you first start cutting hair, as they aid control and grip the hair as you cut. However, if you wish to use texturising techniques and slide or slice cut the hair, these will not be suitable as they pull the hair, affecting the cut, and may cause discomfort to your client.

HANDY HINT

Shorter-length scissors are good for chipping into the hair; 5 inch (12.5cm) scissors are good for most techniques; and longer-length scissors are ideal for scissors-over-comb techniques used by many barbers.

Straight scissors, or non-serrated blades, are the sharpest for cutting, slicing and chipping. You can use these for most techniques and can buy them from £30 up to a few hundred pounds.

Thinning scissors are used to remove bulk at the end of the haircut and have 'teeth' or 'notches' all the way up one or both blades. Thinning scissors with notches on both blades remove less bulk than those with only one notched blade.

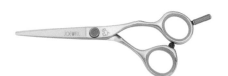

Straight edge blades

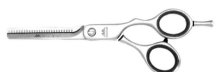

Thinning scissors – one blade with notches

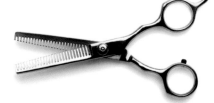

Thinning scissors – two blades with notches

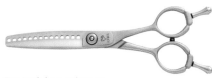

Texturising scissors

Texturising scissors can be used to add texture to a finished haircut. These have wider notches along the blades and remove weight from the hair section as you cut.

What size scissors should I buy?

To help you choose the correct size scissors, rest the scissors in the palm of your hand, starting with a 5 inch (12.5cm) blade length. If they are slightly shorter than the length of your hand, from middle finger to wrist, then these should be suitable. For smaller hands try a 4–4½ inch (10–11cm) length and for longer hands try a 5½–6 inch (14–15cm) length.

The thumb and finger holes vary in size too; try them for size before buying, and ensure they are comfortable but not so loose that you could lose control over the cut.

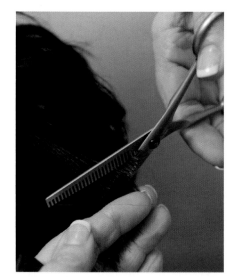

Texturising

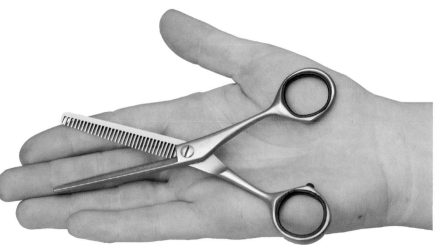

These scissors are the correct size for this hand

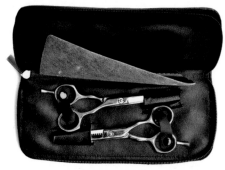

Store your scissors in a cutting pouch

Activity

Use the internet to research the types of scissors available. Decide which ones would be most suitable for you and consider the following:

- How much can I afford to spend?
- What size do I need?
- What size is most suitable?
- What type of blade would I like?
- What cutting techniques do I need my scissors for?
- How am I going to store them when they are not in use?

Look at colours and styles that are available too!

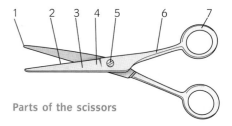

> **WHY DON'T YOU…**
> Practise holding your scissors correctly, moving only your thumb.

The parts of your scissors

1 The points of the scissors – used for point cutting or chipping techniques and freehand.

2 The cutting blade edges – used for all club cutting techniques, scissors over comb and some freehand angles.

3 The blades – outside of blade edges.

4 The heel – the strength of the scissors.

5 The pivot – an adjustable screw to loosen or tighten the movement of the blades.

6 The shanks – give the length from the blades to the handles.

7 The handle – thumb and finger holes.

Parts of the scissors

Activity

To help you to decide on how tight or loose your blades should be, try this simple exercise. Do not have your thumb in the hole during this exercise. Place your ring finger in the finger hole and support your scissors with your other fingers; lift and open the thumb blade and let the thumb blade drop towards the finger blade. Ideally, the thumb blade, when dropped, should stop just short of the finger blade. If the blades touch, they may be too loose; if there is a large gap between the blades, they are too tight. This can be adjusted by loosening or tightening the pivot screw.

Razors

Razors can be used once you are confident with your cutting techniques. They are used to add texture or definition to your style and to taper and remove bulk from the hair.

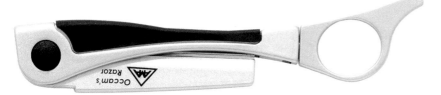

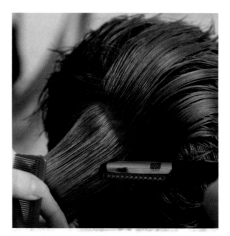

Razor being used on wet hair

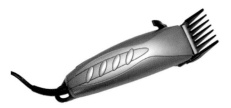

Clippers – using mains electricity

Clippers

Clippers can be used to blend in hair on the back of the neck, create outlines and definition, or for clipper-over-comb techniques. Trimmers can also be used to blend or remove neck hair. These are mostly used for cutting men's hair. They can be mains electrical or rechargeable battery-operated clippers.

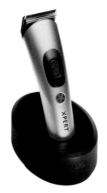

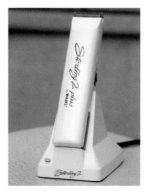

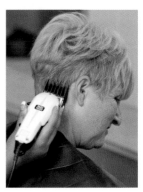

Clippers – rechargeable

Trimmers

Clippers being used on female client

Techniques

The looks that you will create may involve a number of techniques, including club cutting, freehand, texturising and scissors-over-comb cutting techniques to achieve one-length, uniform layers, short-graduation and long-graduated-layer looks.

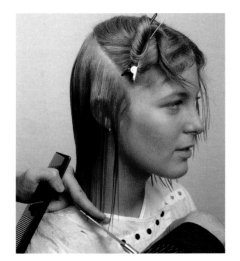

Holding the hair for club cutting

Club cutting technique

Club cutting is also know as blunt cutting and involves cutting the hair straight across while holding the hair with tension between your fingers. This technique will reduce the length of the hair and layers but will retain the thickness of the hair.

Freehand technique

When using the freehand technique, you must not hold the hair with any tension, but instead comb the hair into position and cut. This technique can be used when tension is not required, such as when cutting fringes, or allowing for the natural fall of the hair over the ears when cutting hair one length.

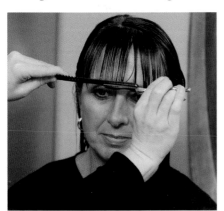

Use freehand for fringes and one-length cuts to allow for natural fall

Texturising

Texturising the hair reduces the bulk at the ends of the hair, it helps to soften styles, adds personalisation and encourages movement throughout the style.

To texturise hair:

1 take a larger section of the hair
2 leave 5–7cm (2–2¾ in) above your fingers

3 carefully cut inwards and slightly vertically towards your fingers. removing bulk and maintaining length (unlike club cutting where the hair is taken to the ends of your fingers and then cut straight across horizontally).

Scissor-over-comb technique

When using the scissor-over-comb technique, run the comb up the hair, and use it to lift and support the hair to be cut. The hair is cut with the scissors over the comb. This technique gives a graduated effect to the cut and blends short hair into the neck.

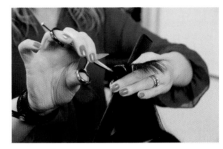
Texturising

Considerations when cutting hair

Establishing and following guidelines

The guideline is the most important part of the haircut. If you are cutting and lose your guideline – STOP! The guideline determines the finished length of the cut and the overall shape and balance. Without a guideline you cannot work methodically through the haircut or maintain accuracy. Even the most experienced stylists will follow a guideline.

Guidelines are the first cuts of the hairstyle. You first cut in a baseline length; once the length has been agreed with your client, this becomes your guideline for the length of the haircut.

Once the baseline length has been agreed and cut, you are ready to begin the guideline for the internal layers of the hair. This internal guideline will help you achieve the shape of the style. Again, agree the desired length of the layers with your client and then cut in your internal guideline to suit the angle at which the hair will be cut. You can either cut in your internal guideline from front to back and ear to ear, or work in stages, cutting the back first from crown to nape, and then working towards a front guideline.

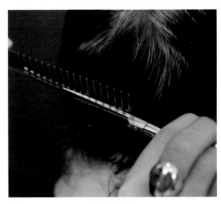
Scissor-over-comb technique

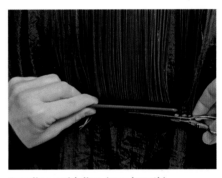
Baseline guideline (one length)

HANDY HINT

If you can't see your guideline, stop cutting, go back a few sections and find it. Or you can section the hair the opposite way to work out where you have cut up to.

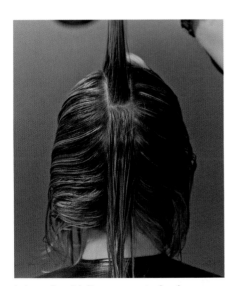
Internal guideline crown to back

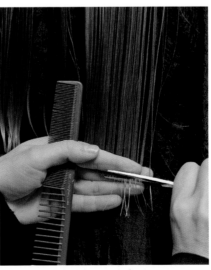
Stylist following guideline when cutting

HANDY HINT

With any cutting technique you must always work with the natural fall of the hair, taking account of the weight distribution to ensure the expected shape can be achieved.

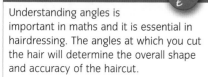

HANDY HINT

Understanding angles is important in maths and it is essential in hairdressing. The angles at which you cut the hair will determine the overall shape and accuracy of the haircut.

Once you have cut your guideline, every section you cut afterwards will follow this guideline to the same length and hold the hair at the same angle. Always ensure that your cutting sections are clean and that you take manageably sized sections.

Cutting hair with tension

When you are cutting hair with tension, you must remember that wet hair stretches more than dry hair. So make sure that the end result is not shorter than you expected. You must always keep the same tension to ensure an even result. This includes keeping an even moisture balance during the cutting service so that the hair is not of mixed porosity or elasticity, which could cause tangles, damage to the hair or uneven cutting results.

Angles and weight distribution

The weight distribution and angles that the hair is held at will vary for every haircut and style. It is the angles that the hair is cut at that give the weight distribution.

The diagram shows the most common angles that you hold the hair at whilst cutting, for creating one-length, uniform layers, short-graduation and long-graduation looks.

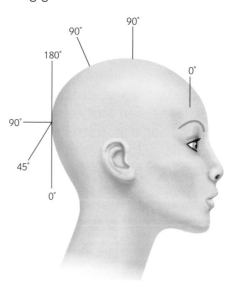

WHY DON'T YOU...
Practise sectioning and pulling the hair out at the angles described in the diagram.

- One length – the hair is pulled directly down at a 0° angle.

- Uniform layer – use 0° for the baseline, and for the layers the hair is pulled out at a 90° angle throughout the entire haircut.

- Short graduation – the inner layers of the hair lengths are longer than the outline shape and generally pulled out at 45°.

- Long graduation – use 0° for the baseline, and between 90° and 180° for creating the longer layer effects.

- Fringes – often cut freehand to allow for the natural movement and fall of the hair growth patterns, but fringes can be cut under tension and pulled down to 0°.

The following table shows the angles at which the hair is cut and where the weight distribution falls.

Look	Angle of graduation	Weight distribution	Balance of style
One length 	The hair is pulled down at 0°. 	The weight of this hairstyle sits at the perimeter.	The balance of this style is even all around the **perimeter**. **Perimeter** Length or baseline of the cut.
Uniform layers 	The whole haircut is pulled out at 90°. 	The weight distribution of this haircut is even throughout the style.	The balance of this style is even throughout.
Short graduation 	The hair on top may be cut at 90°. The back and sides are tapered in and cut at 45°. 	The weight distribution of this style would be where the shape changes from 90° to 45° – around eye level at the sides and the **occipital** bone at the back. **Occipital** The bone between the crown and the nape area that normally sticks out a little bit.	The balance of this style is even on both sides.
Long graduation 	The layers are cut between 90° and 180°. 	The weight distribution for this style would be at the back and sides, where the length is mostly around the neck and below.	The balance of this style is even on both sides and around the head.

Asymmetric

Unequal – not symmetrical.

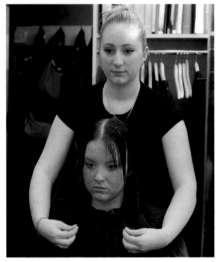

Cross-checking in the mirror

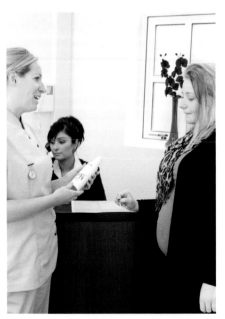

Recommend aftercare to your clients

Cross-checking your cut

Cross-checking the haircut during the service and at the end ensures an accurate finish. You can cross-check the haircut at any point during the service to check for balance and even cutting lengths. Using a mirror will help you to check for balance.

If the one-length look, short graduation or long layers have been cut with a side parting, then the balance of the look may be **asymmetric** and the weight distribution could be heavier on one side, with an uneven balance.

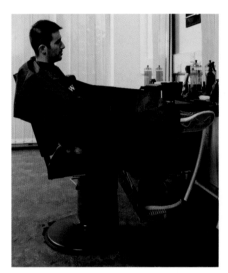

Poor sitting position could cause a poor end result

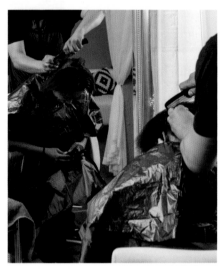

Ensure that your client is sitting straight

For layered haircuts you can cross-check the evenness of the whole cut by sectioning the hair in the opposite direction to which you cut the layers. If you cut the layers in vertical sections, then cross-check horizontally and vice versa.

The final and most commonly used method of cross-checking is used as you progress through the haircut. Pull out sections of cut hair on both sides to feel if the lengths are the same. For longer hair you can pull sections forward and see if they meet evenly under the chin.

Providing advice and recommendations

Recommending retail products

If your client has had a full cut and blow dry service, you should have discussed the products that you used during the styling service and explained why you used them. If the service was a wet cut, then a discussion should take place on how the client should finish the look themselves.

Advise your client on which styling and finishing products would enhance and support their finished look. Explain how particular styling products will aid the drying and styling process, help control the hair and provide longevity to the finished result. You should advise them on how much product to use and how to apply it. If the product could cause a build-up on the hair, ensure that you advise them on how to remove the product effectively.

Recommending tools and equipment

Throughout the styling service you should advise your client on which tools to use at home to recreate their look, and during the blow dry service demonstrate what you are doing and why. This gives the client a thorough understanding of what they will need to do when styling their hair at home. Talk to them about how to create root lift if required or how to prevent it. Discuss which brushes are needed and the correct sizes to use. Remember to discuss the health and safety side of styling and the use of electrically heated styling equipment on the hair and the damage it could cause.

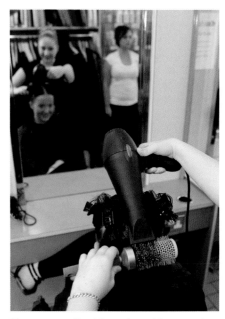

Show your client how to achieve root lift

Recommending further services

During the cutting and styling service is a good time to recommend colouring services to your clients to enhance the image created. Adding colour and highlights to a haircut helps to add texture and definition to the shape. A modern block colour can add a striking finish to any cut. Without doubt, colour enhances and complements every look you create.

Recommending when to return

You should advise your client on when to book their cutting service. To help guide them, explain that it depends on how quickly their hair grows, but four to six weeks is commonly suggested. You should suggest that they return to the salon when the style grows out of shape and when they have trouble maintaining the style, as this may mean it is ready for a cut.

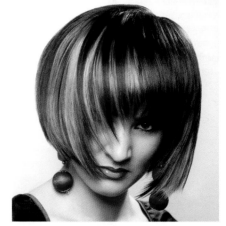

You could recommend enhancing a haircut with subtle colours to add depth, tone and shine

Provide cutting services

In this part of the chapter you will look at the assessment criteria and how to provide the cutting services. The final section shows you how to create the following looks:

- one length
- uniform layers
- short graduation
- long graduation.

Prepare for cutting services

As your client arrives you must follow your salon requirements for gowning and protecting your client to ensure they are protected from hair cuttings. You will also need to prepare the hair for the service.

Work safely and hygienically

Throughout the whole service you must maintain your responsibilities for health and safety and ensure that you, your client and others are not at risk of injury. Use your time effectively to ensure you work to commercially viable times and prepare most of your tools in advance. Take care when handling your tools and use them for the correct purpose, following your workplace and the suppliers and manufacturers' instructions for use.

To prevent cross-contamination, work safely and hygienically, cleaning and sterilising your workstations, tools and equipment. Sweep the floor during and after the service and correctly dispose of any waste in an environmentally friendly manner.

During the service check your client's positioning and that they are comfortable and well balanced for the cutting service. Check that they remain protected by the gown and their skin is free of excess hair. Make sure your own posture is balanced throughout the service.

Consult with clients

Always carry out an in-depth consultation with your client to ascertain what the client would like. Establish any factors that may affect the service – check the hair classifications, hair characteristics, the head and face shape, and any hair growth patterns. Before you commence the cut confirm with your client, in client-friendly language, the look you have both agreed.

Select products, tools and equipment

From the outcome of the consultation select the appropriate products, tools and equipment you will need for the service and complete the preparation of your work area.

When using the products, tools and equipment always follow the instructions and ensure that you use, handle and store them correctly and safely.

HANDY HINT

If your client's posture is unbalanced or they are sitting with their legs crossed, your resulting haircut may also be unbalanced as your client may have a tendency to lean to one side. Always ensure your client is sitting upright with their legs uncrossed.

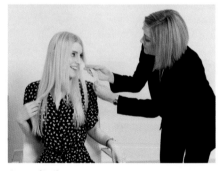

Consultation process

HANDY HINT

When using your consultation skills you are also developing and maintaining your English speaking and listening skills. These skills are vital in hairdressing.

Carry out cutting services

Continue to consult with your client during the cutting process to confirm the desired look and to reassure your client that you are following the agreed style.

Throughout the service, control your tools to minimise the risk of damage to hair and scalp, client discomfort and to achieve the desired look.

Use cutting techniques suitable for your client's hair type and to achieve the desired look, such as club cutting, freehand, texturising and scissor-over-comb, adapting these cutting techniques to take into account the factors that influence the service.

When cutting hair to one length, uniform layers, short graduation or long graduation, create and follow the cutting guideline to achieve the required look.

Change and adapt your own position and that of your client to help you ensure the accuracy of the cut, and cross-check and balance the cut to establish accurate distribution of weight, balance and shape.

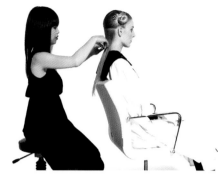

Stylist using tools correctly

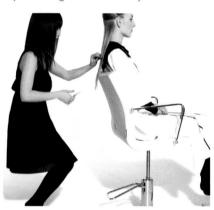

Try to ensure that your back is straight, although not rigid, and your shoulders are relaxed

Activity

- If a client had her hair cut every three months, how much would her hair have grown between cuts?
- How much does your hair grow on average over a six-month period?
- How much does your hair grow on average over a year?

At the end of the haircut, make a final visual check of the hair to ensure the finished cut is accurate, remove any unwanted hair outside the desired outline shape and confirm your client's satisfaction with the finished cut.

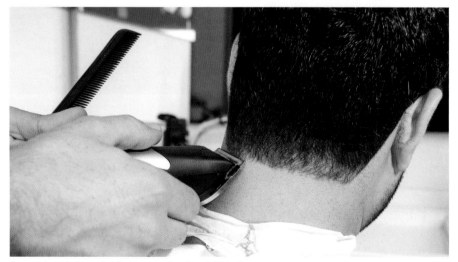

Removing hair outside the desired outline shape

HANDY HINT

As hair only grows about 1.25cm (½ inch) each month, it is important that you do not cut the hair too short.

HANDY HINT

To enable you to complete the service in the commercially viable time, you'll need to know your salon's expected service times for different cutting looks.

Provide advice and recommendations

You have just created a fabulous haircut for the client – when they leave, they are an advert for you and your salon. Not only does your client want the new style to look great every day until their next visit, so do you! Every compliment the client receives about their hairstyle could be a potential new client for you or the salon. Therefore it is essential that you provide suitable aftercare for your client on maintaining the look you've created.

During and at the end of the haircut give your client advice and recommendations on the service provided. These should include additional products and services that would benefit them, now and in the future, and advice on how to maintain the look and the time intervals between services.

Step by steps

Creating a one-length look

When cutting the hair to create a one-length look, you need to take very thin sections to enable you to follow your guideline, and take into consideration the natural fall of the hair. The hair is pulled straight down at 0°.

One length above shoulders

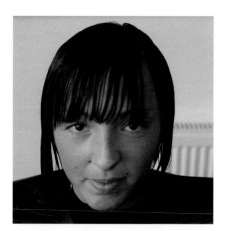

STEP 1 – Gown the client and position the head.

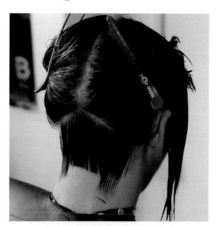

STEP 2 – Use a horizontal section at the back for the guideline.

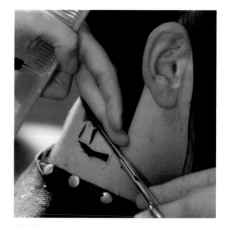

STEP 3 – Make the horizontal cut following the guideline, using a club cutting technique.

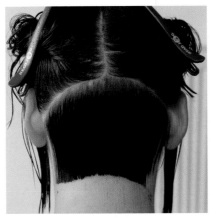

STEP 4 – The next horizontal section.

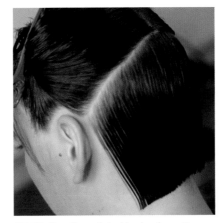

STEP 5 – Complete the back sections.

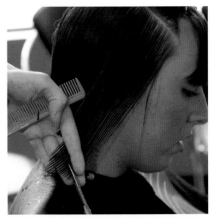

STEP 6 – Take a section from the sides to blend into the back.

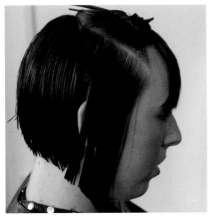

STEP 7 – Blend in the side section and take a guideline.

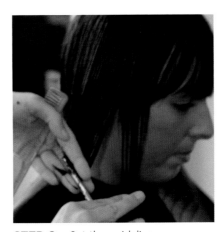

STEP 8 – Cut the guideline.

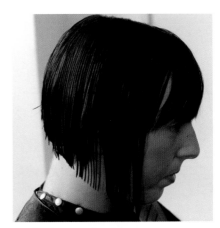

STEP 9 – Cut the sides.

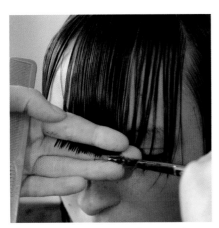

STEP 10 – Cut a fringe if required.

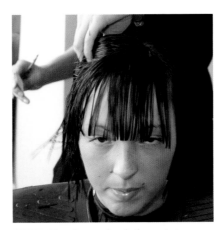

STEP 11 – Cross-check the cut, to ensure it is evenly balanced.

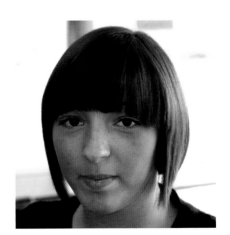

STEP 12 – The completed look.

One length below shoulders

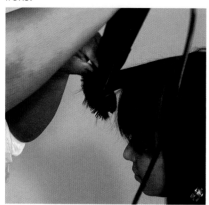

STEP 1 – Start in the fringe area which is prepared with a sleek finish using appropriate product, hair dryer and flat irons.

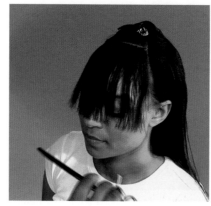

STEP 2 – Section the fringe from temple to crown on both sides with a slight curve towards the crown.

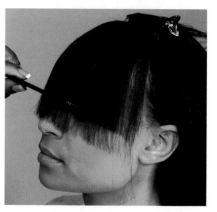

STEP 3 – Continue with parallel sections using the previous section as a guide and ensuring that the hair falls naturally into position.

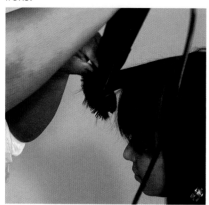

STEP 4 – Next, re-dry the hair, checking proportion and balance.

WHY DON'T YOU...
Create a mood board of varying one-length looks and write up how to achieve one of the images.

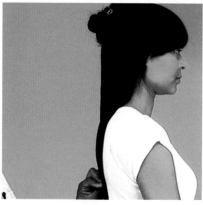

STEP 5 – Then determine the perimeter outline in the back and sides. Cut the guidelines. Using a club-cutting technique, cut the back and sides. Remember to cross-check the cut to ensure it is evenly balanced.

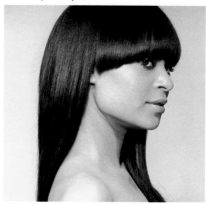

STEP 6 – The final result is a sleek, elegant one-length natural look with an impactful deep wide fringe – a perfect aesthetic match.

Creating a uniform layer look

When cutting the hair to create a uniform layer look, you will need to make a guideline section for the length of the hair and one for the internal layers of the hair. The hair is cut at 90° all over.

Uniform layers

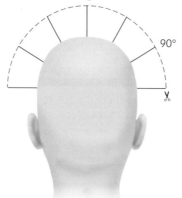

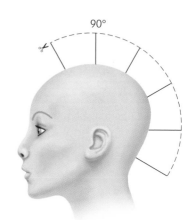

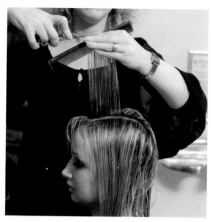

STEP 1 – Take clean vertical sections of hair and pull the hair up at 90°.

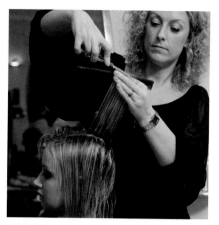

STEP 2 – Cut the hair in sections from the top to the back, following the head shape.

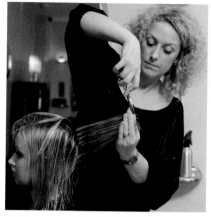

STEP 3 – Ensure you pull the hair directly away from the head, maintaining a 90° angle.

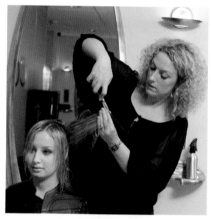

STEP 4 – Blend the length into the base guideline.

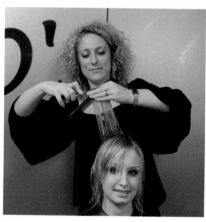

STEP 5 – Cut the internal guideline – using club cutting techniques.

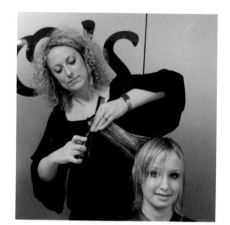

STEP 6 – Work around the back sections taking hair at 90°.

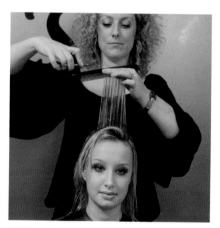

STEP 7 – Cross-check the hair using a horizontal section.

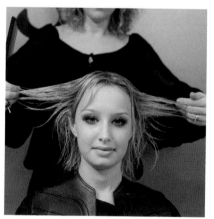

STEP 8 – Cross-check the cut, pulling sections out evenly to the sides.

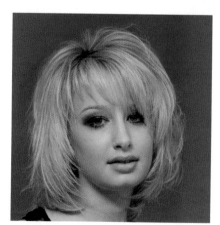

STEP 9 – The completed look.

WHY DON'T YOU...
Create a mood board of varying uniform-layer looks and write up how to achieve one of the images.

Creating a precision cut

Precision cuts with clear sharp edges work well on long or short styles. On a long look, it may be the sides or fringe that are not connected to the rest of the style. On shorter hair the disconnection could be an undercut or as part of an asymmetric look, or a creative style designed by you.

Short graduation

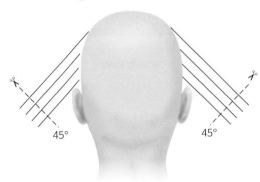

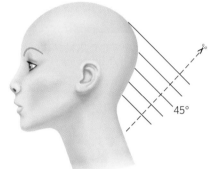

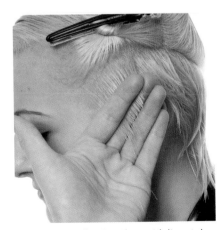

STEP 1 – Before haircut.

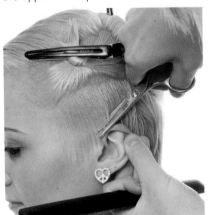

STEP 2 – Take a section from the front temple off-centre through the back nape area, then from the diagonal point to the opposite temple.

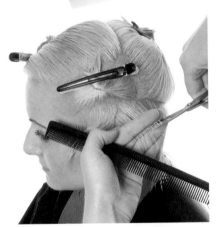

STEP 3 – Take a vertical section at the top of the ear, and cut it holding it out at a 45° angle.

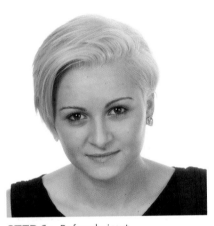

STEP 4 – Following the guideline, take a further vertical section at a 45° angle and work towards the front section.

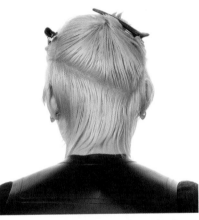

STEP 5 – Holding the ear back, use a freehand technique to cut and shape around the ear.

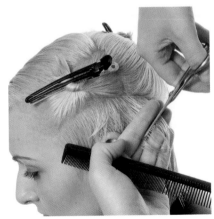

STEP 6 – Continue with the sectioning pattern behind the ear, following the guideline and taking the hair shorter through the nape section.

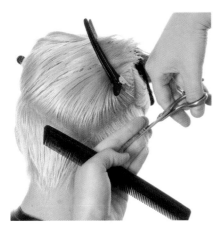

STEP 7 – Continue through the opposite side at the nape area on the off-centre diagonal, graduating the shorter disconnected area.

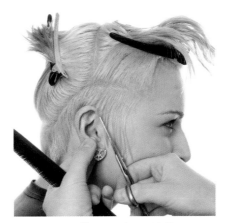

STEP 8 – Following the guideline around the ear area, build the weight and length in front of the ear using a freehand technique.

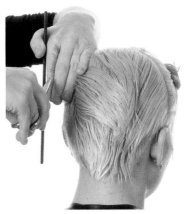

STEP 9 – Working through the top section at the back of the head, hold the section at a 90° angle. Working vertically, take radial sections and blend into the underneath section using a point cutting technique.

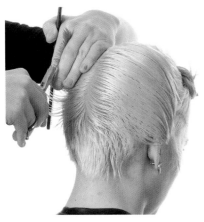

STEP 10 – Over-direct the hair to the original section, point cutting the hair to maintain the length.

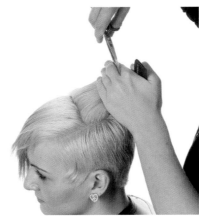

STEP 11 – Working through the top section, take a guideline on the crown area, holding the hair out at a 90° angle. Use a point cutting technique.

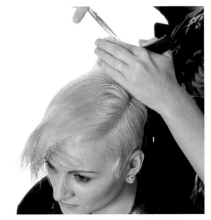

STEP 12 – When working through the top section, over-direct the hair back to the guideline on the crown to maintain length.

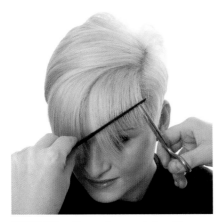

STEP 13 – Use a deep point cutting technique to personalise the fringe.

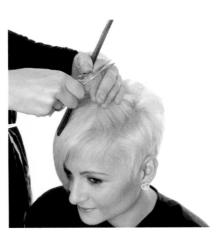

STEP 14 – Use a slicing technique to give texture through the top of the haircut.

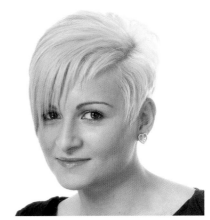

STEP 15 – The finished look.

Creating a long graduated layer look

When you create a long graduated layer look, the hair must gradually get longer as you move up the head towards the crown. This style maintains the length of the hair. The layers are held out between 90° like the uniform layer and up to 135° or 180°, depending on the length of the hair and the layers.

Long graduation

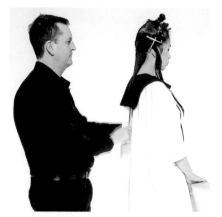

STEP 1 – Before commencing, assess the hairline and growth patterns. Apply the appropriate protective clothing. Comb the natural parting into position to assess full movement in this area.

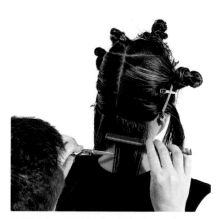

STEP 2 – Divide the hair down the centre back, finding the natural centre using the top of the spine as a guide. Then divide the section to behind the ear to separate the back section.

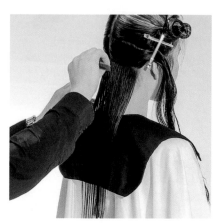

STEP 3 – Start by taking a curved horizontal line in the nape area. Note that the size of this section will depend on the texture and density of the hair. Comb this section as close as possible to the shoulders or the back with very little tension and cut the hair using the comb as a guide.

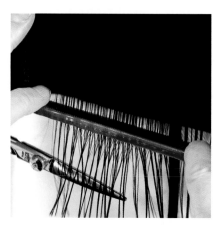

STEP 4 – Take a section from the centre down to the back of the ear on a diagonal line. This mirrors the outline shape. Assess the outline before cutting.

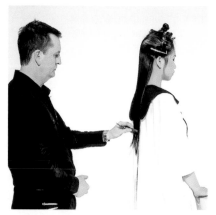

STEP 5 – Now repeat this on the second side.

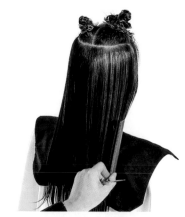

STEP 6 – Then take subsequent sections parallel to the first, moving back toward the crown, again mirroring the outline.

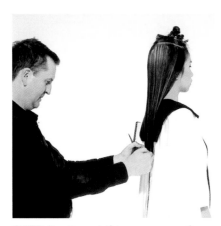

STEP 7 – Repeat this process on the other side.

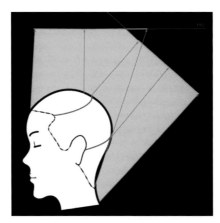

STEP 8 – Next divide the hair from the front hairline vertically to the nape in 2cm (¾ in) sections.

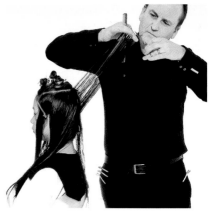

STEP 9 – Elevate the hair vertically, straight out from the head and cut a straight line from short to long (graduation) using the previously cut fringe section as a guide. Ensure enough weight is established through the outline.

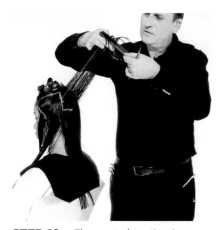

STEP 10 – The central section is a guide for the internal layering. Take a pivoted section from the crown down to the front hairline incorporating a part of the central section already cut. The hair is elevated, over-directed and cut using the previous section as a guide.

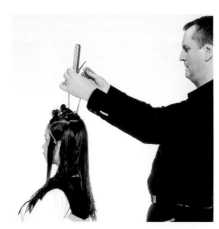

STEP 11 – Take subsequent parallel sections. Over-direct using the previous section as a guide. Again these sections are elevated and cut short to long (graduation). Repeat this process on the second side and cross-check.

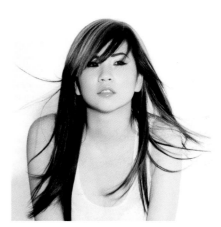

STEP 12 – The final look.

Thinning to create a textured look

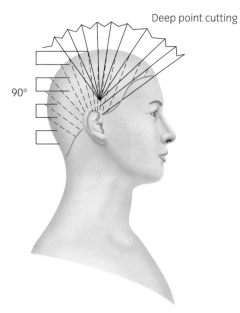

Deep point cutting

90°

90° 90°

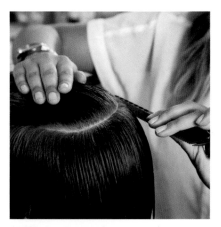

STEP 1 – Section hair using the recession and upper occipital bone as guidelines, to create horseshoe sections.

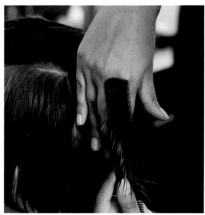

STEP 2 – Take a vertical section from the centre of the occipital bone at a 90° angle to create the first guideline.

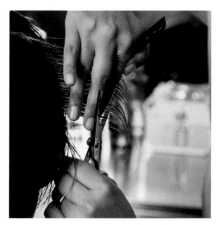

STEP 3 – Using the initial guideline, take radial sections throughout the back of the head.

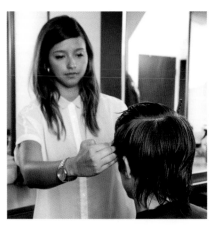

STEP 4 – Cross-check your cut and check the weight and balance of the hair.

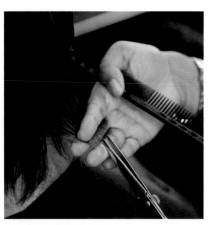

STEP 5 – Cross-check, taking horizontal sections.

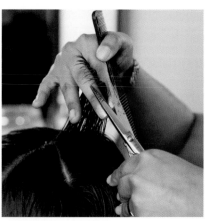

STEP 6 – Using your initial guideline section, cut a guideline for the crown.

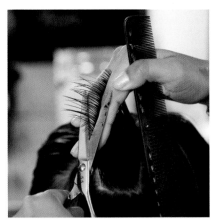

STEP 7 – Follow the crown guideline and cut your profile line through the top of the head.

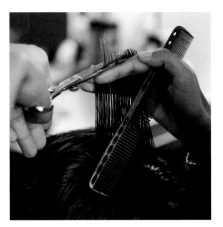

STEP 8 – Use the profile guideline to cut square layers through the top sections.

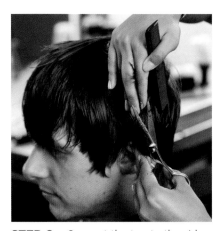

STEP 9 – Connect the top to the sides, removing the corners, connecting both guidelines.

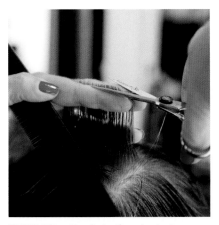

STEP 10 – Dry hair, then texturise following your initial cutting pattern, using a deep point cutting technique.

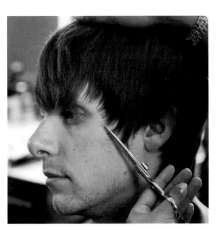

STEP 11 – Refine the perimeter using a freehand technique.

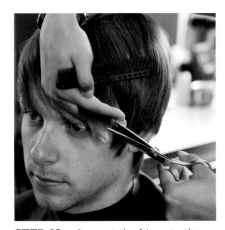

STEP 12 – Connect the fringe to the rest of the hair, removing any corners.

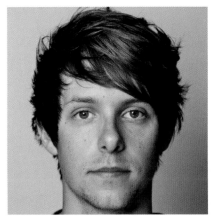

STEP 13 – The finished look.

Answers in the back of the book.

1 Which one of the following best describes a sharps bin?

a A covered black bin for disposal of razors

b A waste bin kept safely in the staff room

c A yellow bin emptied by specialists

d A lined bin for disposal of needles

2 Which one of the following is the main reason to remove hair cuttings immediately?

a Because it presents a slipping hazard

b Because it will put clients off

c Because it presents a tripping hazard

d Because it looks unprofessional

3 Which one of the following is the best way to maintain hairdressing scissors?

a Remove and store securely

b Oil and sharpen regularly

c Wash in hot soapy water

d Sterilise every evening

4 Which one of the following is recommended to remove hair clippings and debris from combs?

a Sponge

b Toothbrush

c Cotton wool

d Pintail comb

5 A cutting stool is used to

a Enable the stylist to reach very long hair

b Ensure that the client can talk to the stylist

c Present a professional image of the stylist and salon

d Prevent the stylist having to bend or stretch too far

6 Why is it important to begin the consultation before gowning the client?

a To avoid client complaints

b To avoid the client feeling too hot

c To see the style of dress and image of the client

d To see the size of the client's head in relation to their body

7 Straight hair is classified as

a Type 4

b Type 3

c Type 2

d Type 1

8 **Statement one**

Fine hair should be kept long to avoid it looking too sparse.

Statement two

Fine hair should be texturised with a razor to give it support.

Which one of the following is correct for the above statements?

a True   True

b True   False

c False   True

d False   False

9 Which of the following tools and techniques should only be used on dry hair?

a Freehand, club cutting, razors and clippers

b Texturising, club cutting, razors and thinning scissors

c Freehand, scissor-over-comb, thinning scissors and clippers

d Texturising, slicing, scissor-over-comb and thinning scissors

10 Which one of the following should be tightened if scissors become too loose?

a The pivot

b The shank

c The heel

d The handle

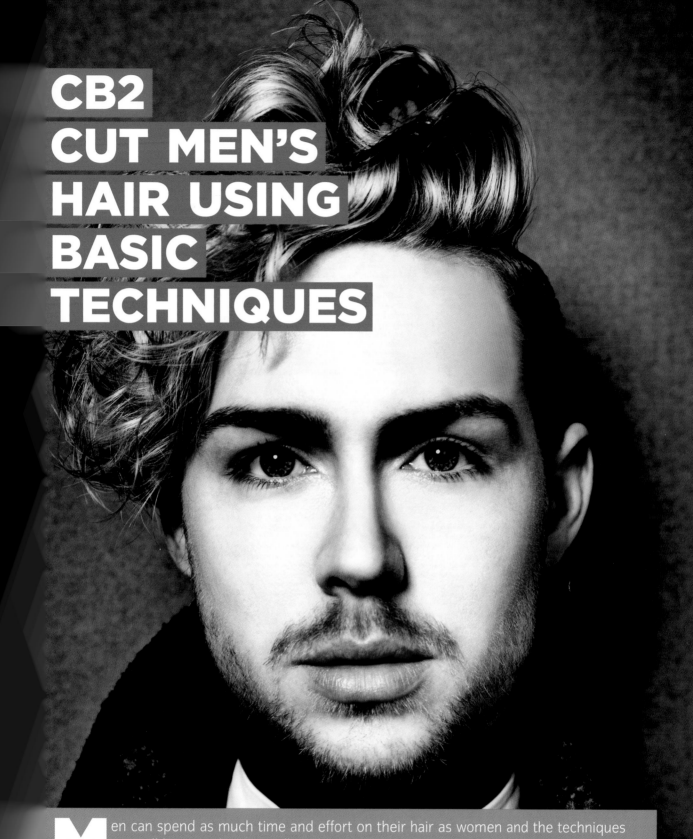

CB2
CUT MEN'S HAIR USING BASIC TECHNIQUES

Men can spend as much time and effort on their hair as women and the techniques you will learn in this unit will enable you to create a variety of looks from one haircut. Learning the basic techniques will give you the knowledge, skills and confidence to generate a clientele that you can build on. Enhancing your skills will give you the opportunity to produce a variety of different styles.

After reading this chapter you will:

- know how health and safety affects cutting services
- understand the factors that influence cutting services
- know the tools, equipment, products and techniques used for basic barbering services
- be able to provide cutting services using basic barbering techniques.

Your responsibilities for health and safety

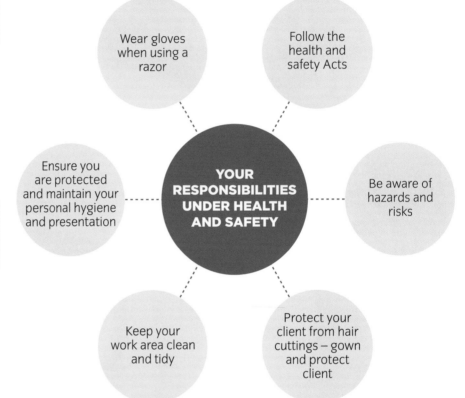

- Wear gloves when using a razor
- Follow the health and safety Acts
- Ensure you are protected and maintain your personal hygiene and presentation
- **YOUR RESPONSIBILITIES UNDER HEALTH AND SAFETY**
- Be aware of hazards and risks
- Keep your work area clean and tidy
- Protect your client from hair cuttings – gown and protect client

As with all services, you must follow the health and safety Acts when cutting men's hair and minimise the risk of harm to you and others.

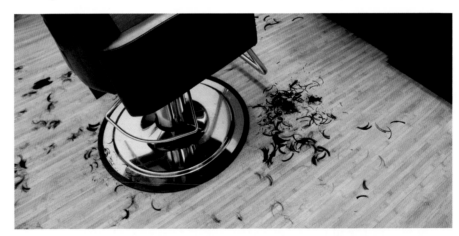

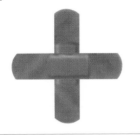

Activity

List all the potential hazards and risks that you and your client may encounter during the service. How could you prevent each hazard becoming a risk?

Safe working practices

The safe working practices that must be followed are:

- working safely and hygienically, including avoiding cross-contamination
- client preparation, protection and positioning
- barber positioning and posture, including ensuring that you can easily reach your tools.

Working safely and hygienically

When preparing for your client's arrival, you must ensure that all work surfaces are cleaned and sterilised with chemical disinfectant spray/wipes. Use your time effectively and prepare all tools and equipment in readiness for the service, checking that your workstation is ready for your client's service, with clean sterile tools and equipment. Make sure the floors are hazard-free – that there are no hair cuttings/wet floors that your client could slip on and no trip hazards from trailing wires, etc.

To minimise the risk of cross-infection always ensure that the salon has a plentiful supply of clean, washed gowns and towels, and check whether any need to be washed or dried. You should change your Barbicide solution regularly, so that it can be used between every client for disinfecting your cutting tools.

Once your client arrives, complete a thorough consultation, gown and protect your client, position them comfortably, and maintain a good posture yourself.

Throughout the service ensure that you take care when using tools and equipment to minimise the risk of damage and that you use sustainable working practices. When using a razor you must wear gloves to prevent any cross-contamination.

At the end of the service remove any waste, ensuring you protect the environment and recycle where possible. Turn off all electrical items and prepare your tools and work area for the next service.

Activity

Discuss how you can protect the environment when cutting men's hair.

Activity

In pairs, discuss the safety considerations that are relevant to cutting men's hair. Refer to the health and safety chapter if you need further guidance.

Activity

Discuss with a colleague how you think a client would feel if you used combs, scissors or clippers with the previous client's hair still on them!

HEALTH & SAFETY

Refer to the health and safety and salon policies chapter for more information on best practices for working safely and hygienically.

VALUES & BEHAVIOURS

Always turn off taps after you have shampooed the hair, switch off electrical appliances when not in use and use products sparingly to prevent wastage and overloading the hair. Always dispose of used razor blades in a sharps box and take care when removing blades.

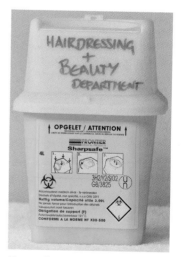

Sharps bin

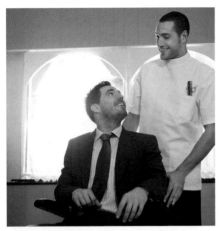

Always listen to your client and be honest yet tactful with advice

HANDY HINT

Keep your client free of hair cuttings to protect his clothes and ensure he is comfortable throughout the service.

HANDY HINT

If your client's posture is unbalanced or he is sitting with his legs crossed, your resulting haircut could be unbalanced, as your client might have a tendency to lean to one side. Always ensure your client is sitting upright with his legs uncrossed.

HANDY HINT

During the service you will need to adapt and change your body position, and that of the client, to ensure you maintain a balanced, even and accurate haircut throughout.

VALUES & BEHAVIOURS

Refer to the values and behaviours chapter for more information on maintaining effective, hygienic and safe working methods.

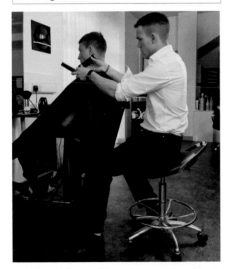

Comfortable working on a cutting stool

Client preparation, protection and positioning

It is advisable to begin the initial consultation before you gown your client, to ascertain his style of dress and overall image. You should ask him about his day-to-day lifestyle, work patterns and available time to commit to styling his hair. Always listen to what your client is asking of you and be honest yet tactful with the advice you give him. You should use open questions to obtain as much information as possible and finish with closed questions to confirm what has been agreed.

Activity

List the protective clothing available for clients during barbering services.

The positioning of you and your client are most important when cutting the hair, as the result and balance of the finished look can be affected.

When he is gowned and protected, you must ensure that your client sits comfortably with his back supported by the chair, in an upright position with his legs uncrossed and evenly balanced.

Barber positioning and posture

You must stand with your body weight evenly distributed throughout the entire cutting process. This will not only prevent fatigue and back problems but also ensure the haircut is balanced. Sit on a cutting stool while cutting hair short or for working on the back of your client's head and adjust the height of the barber's chair to ensure you work comfortably. This will prevent you from bending and over-stretching and help to maintain your comfort, which is essential during the cutting service.

Importance of questioning clients

You must always carry out a thorough consultation with your client to identify the service objective, your client's needs and whether you are able to carry out his request. During the consultation you should tell him how long the service should take and how he can maintain the look between salon visits. The consultation process should continue throughout the cutting service, as you should update him on the progress of the haircut and check you are cutting to the agreed lengths.

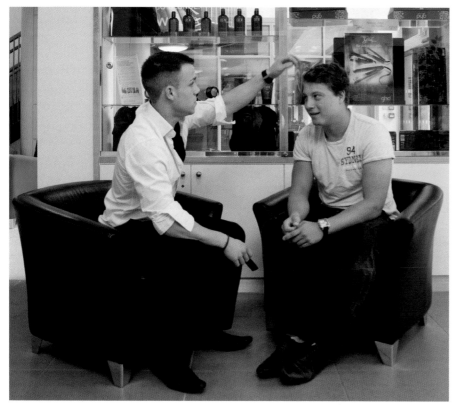

Client consultation

WHY DON'T YOU...
Use a smart phone or tablet to search for men's styling images online?

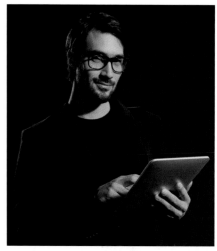

The internet is a great source of ideas for men's styles

Carry out a consultation with your client

During the consultation you should ask questions about how much hair he would like taken off the length and the layers. You must be specific with your questions to achieve an accurate account of his needs. Show him in the mirror how much hair you are going to remove to confirm what you assume to be the agreed lengths and amounts. Use visual aids, such as barbering images/magazines, to agree on styles and shapes. Always give your client the option to try something different from his current style, and give him the opportunity to express his thoughts about the finished look.

When you have decided on a style together, ask him which products he currently uses to style his hair, to identify whether you need to recommend any alternative products for his new image.

Confirm client satisfaction

Now you have carried out a consultation and discussed the client requirements, you will need to consider the relevant factors to confirm with your client whether it will be achievable. If a style is not suited to the hair type, you should politely explain why and offer your professional opinion, suggesting alternative options.

At the end of the service you must ask your client whether he is satisfied with the end result to ensure that he leaves the salon happy and pleased with his haircut.

HANDY HINT

You may use different communication skills with male clients which involve more banter and mockery, and your topics of conversation may also be very different from those you have with female clients. You will, however, still need to remain professional throughout the service and ensure your communication skills are effective and clear.

HANDY HINT

Always give clear instructions and repeat back what your client has asked of you; this will help you to gain the client's confidence in the service.

HANDY HINT

Reasons why clients leave their barber/hairstylist:

- The barber did not recommend anything new or interesting.
- The barber did not listen to the client's request.
- The barber created a style that was not suitable for the client.
- The barber cut the hair too short/left it too long, even after consultation and agreeing the lengths.
- The service took too long.

HANDY HINT

Revisit chapter CHB9 for more in-depth information on consulting with your client.

Activity

Ask a male colleague to pretend to be your client. Ask him to visualise a style and then ask the relevant questions to identify the image and look he requires. Use at least three open and two closed questions to obtain as much information as possible about his requirements. (Refer to chapter CHB9 for more information on open and closed questions.)

Factors that may influence services

HANDY HINT

Ask your client where he wears his parting, but always check visually for the natural fall of the hair.

You need to consider factors that might affect the outcome of the service required.

There are many factors that could affect how you cut the hair, the tools that you use and the styles that you recommend. You must consider these factors prior to and during the service. The first factor that you must take into consideration is what your client wants. His requirements are what your whole consultation is all about, and now you must determine whether there are any factors that might affect your achieving the desired result.

You should discuss your client's lifestyle to ensure that he does not have any barriers that could prevent him achieving the desired result. Is the chosen style easy to maintain and does it fit around work requirements?

As some men have a more manual job, they can be prone to bumps on the head; as they tend to wear their hair shorter than women the head is not as well protected. Always check the hair and scalp for any lumps and bumps that could cause discomfort to your client when you are combing through the hair.

HANDY HINT

For more information on hair characteristics and classification, see chapter CHB9.

Hair characteristcs

Characteristic	Impact on service
Elasticity 	Elasticity can affect the cutting technique. For medium to longer hair with poor elasticity you should avoid pulling with too much tension during the cutting process. Ensure the hair has an even moisture balance when you cut it – either all wet or all dry – to ensure the effects of poor elasticity are not worsened.

Characteristic	Impact on service
Porosity and hair condition 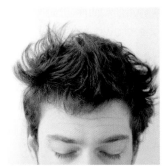 Porous hair	Hair that is damaged is likely to be porous – this can affect the cutting technique and client comfort. If the hair is porous and the cuticles are open, then hair is more likely to tangle during the cut and this may cause client discomfort. You should use a wider-toothed comb and spray the hair with leave-in conditioner to aid the combing process. Avoid using a razor on porous hair and take care when using clipper grades as they may get caught in the dry porous hair.
Density 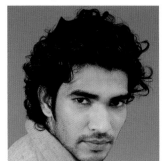 Abundant hair 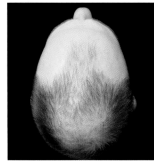 Sparse hair	Density can affect the choice of style and cutting technique. Abundant hair might need to be thinned out to create the desired look. Consider whether abundant hair will enhance the look; if not, suggest alternatives. Sparse hair will need to be blunt cut/club cut to maintain as much thickness as possible. Avoid cutting the hair too short.
Texture 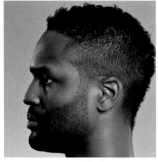 Coarse-textured hair 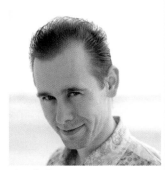 Fine hair	Texture can affect the choice of style and cutting technique. Coarse-textured hair might not suit the desired look; you will need to recommend styling products to help achieve a smoother result. Clipper cuts or very short cuts might not suit fine hair; you might also need to use supporting hair products.
Hair growth patterns 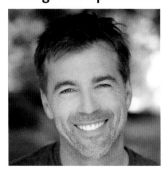 Cowlick 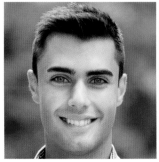 Widow's peak	Hair growth patterns can affect the choice of style and cutting technique. For cowlicks avoid fringes; instead suggest a side half fringe that works with the cowlick. For widow's peaks avoid fringes completely and suggest styles that are constructed with the top area going over to one side or straight back.

Characteristic	Impact on service
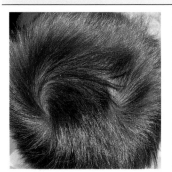 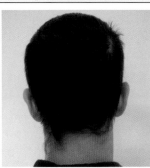 Double crown Nape whorls	For double crowns suggest maintaining a little length around the crown area and ideally work with the natural fall into the style. Alternatively, very short haircuts around the crown area will prevent the hair from sticking up. For nape whorls suggest maintaining the length at the nape area, or at least a little weight, and avoid cutting into the hairline unless you are using the clippers or cutting the nape area very short. This growth pattern can affect many men's hairstyles, as they generally like to wear their hair shorter than women.

Hair classifications

Hair classifications can affect the choice of style and cutting techniques.

You will need to consider whether you should cut the hair wet or dry, when looking at the hair classifications.

Classification	How it can affect the service
Straight hair 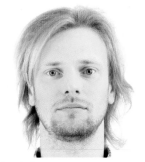 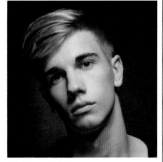 Fine hair Medium hair 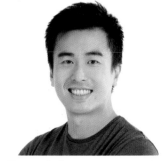 Coarse hair	When cutting fine and medium straight hair every 'scissor cut' can show in the hair. Accuracy is very important and subtle texturised cuts can help to prevent the cutting line's from being so apparent. Fine/thin straight hair might not achieve the desired result. Avoid using texturising techniques that will make the hair thinner; instead use club-cutting techniques and choose styles to suit the hair type. Medium straight hair can have lots of volume and body and suits most techniques Coarse straight hair can be difficult to curl or add movement. It may benefit from texturising and thinning out techniques to remove some bulk and improve the end result and style.

Classification	How it can affect the service
Wavy hair 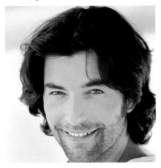 Fine hair 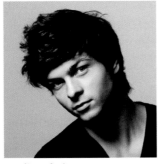 Medium hair 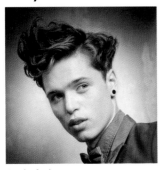 Coarse hair	Wavy hair can be great to work with. It is easy to mould straighter or to create enhanced body. Most techniques work well with this hair type. Fine/thin wavy hair – you may need to leave some length to aid body and use club-cutting techniques to give the appearance of thicker hair. Medium and coarse wavy hair can be frizzy so avoid texturising techniques that will enhance a fluffy appearance – such as razor cutting. Club cutting can help by keeping all hair lengths the same. Coarse wavy hair can be resistant to styling, so may benefit from being texturised or thinned out but avoid using a razor on the hair.
Curly hair Curly hair	Soft curly hair can have a combination of textures to consider. It may be frizzy in appearance and have lots of body. Tight curly hair can also have combined textures and will spring up after the hair has been cut when it is dried – particularly fine curly hair. When cutting curly hair consider the amount of tension you place on the hair during the cutting service, use a wide-toothed comb and use freehand cutting techniques.
Very curly hair 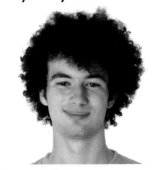 Very curly hair 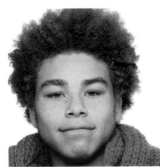 Wiry curly hair	Soft very curly hair is often fragile, so be careful if using razors or clippers. Comb the hair gently using a wide-toothed comb and use a conditioning spray to prevent client discomfort. If the client does not want to encourage the curls, then clipper cuts would be the most effective recommendation Wiry curly hair is also very fragile but can have less of a defined curly pattern. Avoid techniques that texturise the hair and use mostly club-cutting and freehand techniques. Take care with tools on the fragile hair.

Classification	How it can affect the service
Head and face shape 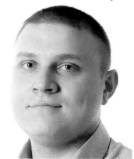 Round 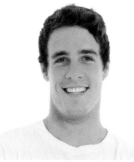 Oblong 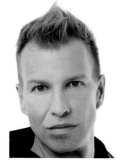 Square	The head and face shape can affect the choice of style. For round face shapes, avoid styles that add more roundness, such as too much width or height. For oblong face shapes, avoid height but add width if you can, and suggest a fringe to give the illusion of shortening a long face. The shorter the haircut, the more **prominent** the oblong shape will appear. **Prominent** Sticking out. For square face shapes, avoid square styles, such as 'flat tops', that will accentuate this feature. The head shape should be considered within the overall shape of the style. The ideal head shape is rounded from the crown to the **occipital bone** and then dips in slightly towards the nape. **Occipital bone** The bone between the crown and the nape area that normally sticks out a little bit. Some crowns are flatter than others and very short styles could make the back of the head look too flat. Others have very pronounced crown areas and need the cut to make the shape look flatter.
Prominent features 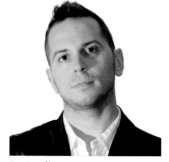 Protruding ears 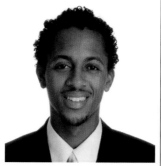 Prominent nose and high forehead	Facial features can affect the choice of style. For clients with **protruding** ears, you can suggest styles that cover the entire ear or are not cut too short around the ear. For strong nose features or jaw-lines, avoid centre partings that encourage the eye to follow down from the parting to the nose and chin. For high foreheads, suggest the haircut has a fringe or some hair styled forward over part of the forehead. **Protruding** Sticking out.
Neck shape 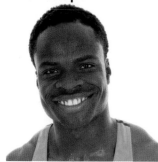 Thick neck	When considering the length of the haircut at the neck area, you should look at the shape of the neck. Thicker necks might suit a slightly longer cut.

Classification	How it can affect the service
Hairline 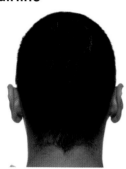	If the hair is being cut short at the nape area, you need to consider the natural hairline shape. Along with a nape whorl, you can have hairlines that grow in different directions each side, or grow into the middle from both sides. This might affect the length you want to cut to or the shape of the end result.
Facial hair 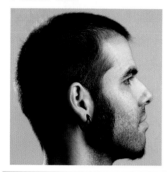	When you are cutting the hair, you will need to consider where the head hair stops and any facial hair starts. Some clients will choose their style to look like two separate features while others may want their head and facial hair to blend together.
Male pattern baldness 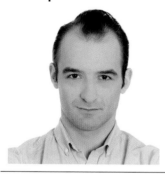	If your client wants to cover the hair-loss area, then suggest leaving the overall style slightly longer, particularly on the top. Some clients prefer to have the hair cut short around the thinning area, to make the rest of the hair look a little thicker.
Piercings 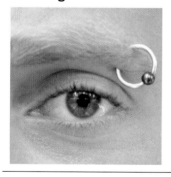	Check the skin, eyebrows and ears for piercings that could cause an injury if you accidentally caught them with the comb.

HANDY HINT

Male pattern baldness is known as the 'Hamilton pattern' due to the progressive patterns it follows that were identified by Dr J. B. Hamilton.

HANDY HINT

If during the consultation you identify an infectious condition, you must not continue with the service. Instead give your client some advice about how to deal with the problem or suggest he visits his GP. Try to keep these conversations discreet so the client is put at ease, and explain that you will welcome him back when the infectious condition has cleared. Remember that it is not your responsibility to diagnose a skin condition and there could be legal implications for the salon if you were to misdiagnose.

Classification	How it can affect the service
Adverse skin conditions 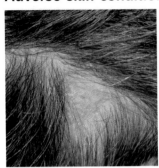	Some scalp disorders might require consideration in the style recommended, as your client might want them covered up. Always ask about scalp disorders during your consultation and check for infections and infestations which would prevent the service from being carried out. Refer to chapter CHB9 for more information.

Activity

Draw the different face shapes and add sketches of hairstyles that will enhance each facial shape. Or cut out images from magazines/research on the internet and create a stylebook for different face shapes.

HANDY HINT

Using barbering tools on hair that has product on it can blunt scissors and cause clipper blades to 'clog up' with hair and become ineffective at cutting the hair; they may snag hair and cause client discomfort.

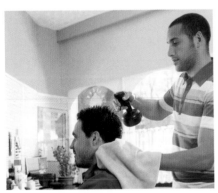

Wetting hair before cutting

HANDY HINT

When checking dry hair before the service, you are looking at a styled head of hair which might have products on it, or may have been styled to change the natural fall and make the hair feel thicker. Always recheck the hair type, natural movement and fall of the hair when it has been shampooed.

Activity

Look into a mirror and using a dry wipe pen, draw around your face shape. This will help you to understand face shapes. Ask a colleague to do the same and compare the shapes.

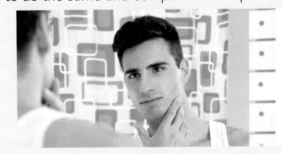

Tools, equipment and products

The tools and equipment you are likely to use during these services are:

- combs
- scissors and thinning scissors
- razors
- clippers
- clippers with grade attachments.

Prepare the client's hair before the service

You should always work on clean hair. If the service requires a dry hair cutting technique and the hair is oily or has products on it, then you'll need to shampoo it to cleanse and remove products and then dry the hair for the cut.

You'll need to consider whether you are going to use a wet or dry hair cutting technique before you start the service and prepare the hair accordingly.

Scissors

Scissors are held with your thumb and your ring finger – not your middle finger. Your little finger supports the scissors, often on the finger rest attached to the scissors; your first and middle fingers support the shanks. You move only your thumb when you cut the hair, as this gives you the greatest control when cutting.

Your scissors are likely to be the most expensive item in your tool collection. Dropping them with the blades open or pointing downwards can affect the position of the blades and be very costly. Care of scissors should include the following:

- use them only for their intended purpose – cutting hair
- do not carry them in the pockets of your clothes
- carry them in a safe manner and store them after use
- ensure they are fit for purpose
- use the correct type of scissors for specific styles
- clean and sterilise them after each client
- remove all hair cuttings and oil them regularly
- have them professionally sharpened when required.

For most basic cutting techniques, you will use scissors with an average blade length of 12.5–15cm (or 5–6in), depending on the size of your hands. However, barbers' scissors tend to be longer than those used by stylists. Choosing the right scissors for you to work with comfortably is important. As you become more experienced you are likely to want a selection of scissors for a variety of techniques, and you will probably buy more expensive scissors as your skill level increases.

Correct use of tools and equipment

When cutting men's hair, you can use scissors, clippers and/or razors, so it is important that you use them correctly, know how to clean and maintain them and store them safely.

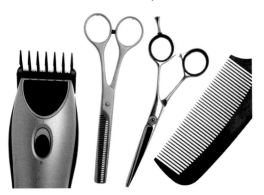

HANDY HINT

Refer back to chapter CH3 for more information on the types of scissors, clippers, trimmers and razors available.

HEALTH & SAFETY

Control your tools and use them safely to minimise damage to your client's hair and scalp to avoid accidents and maintain client comfort.

HANDY HINT

Scissors are available for left- and right-handed people. You must buy scissors to suit your cutting needs.

HANDY HINT

The thumb and finger holes in scissors vary in size; try them for size before buying and ensure they are comfortable but not so loose that you could lose control over the cut.

HANDY HINT

Shorter-length scissors are good for chipping into the hair; longer-length scissors are ideal for scissor-over-comb techniques and are used by many barbers.

WHY DON'T YOU...

Practise holding your scissors correctly, moving only your thumb. Rest the non-moving blade on your other hand.

HEALTH & SAFETY

Refer to the health and safety and salon policies chapter for more in-depth information on sterilising and disinfecting.

Tool	Correct use	Maintenance	Correct storage
Scissors (and thinning scissors) Thinning scissors	Always carry them with the blades closed. Do not drop them as you might damage the blades.	Clean the hairs from the blades with warm soapy water. Sterilise scissors in an autoclave, sanitise in a UV light cabinet or disinfect in a Barbicide solution. Oil the blades after cleaning and sterilising.	Keep them away from young children and store them in a barber's cutting pouch or scissor case.
Clippers Mains electricity clippers Rechargeable clippers	Keep the blades well oiled throughout use. Ensure the blades are properly aligned and adjust the blades to achieve the correct cutting length. Use on dry hair.	Remove the cut hairs from between the blades after every haircut (using a small clipper brush). Spray the blades with a chemical disinfectant and wipe the body of the clippers with chemical disinfectant wipes. Oil the blades after cleaning.	Unplug mains electricity clippers from the mains and look for any knots in the wires. Hang on a designated hook or place somewhere safe, where they cannot fall to the floor and get damaged. Place rechargeable clippers back on the battery charger base to ensure they are charged and ready for the next client.
Razors	Always hold the razor carefully to ensure that you and your client are not accidently cut with the razor blade. If you accidently drop the razor – let it go – do NOT try to catch it! Wear gloves when using a razor.	Remove the razor blade carefully and dispose of it in the sharps bin. Clean the body of the razor with warm soapy water and chemical disinfectant wipes.	Ideally, store your razors without the blade attached. Attach a new blade as you need it. Store the razor in a suitable scissor pouch/case.
Combs and attachments (grades)	Cutting combs are used to section the hair. Clipper grades are attached over the clipper blades and designed to create a variation of longer cutting lengths when clipper cutting.	Remove all loose hairs from the comb and grades, wash them in warm soapy water and sanitise them in the UV light cabinet.	Keep all grades together and store them according to your salon policy.

Techniques

During this part of the chapter we will look at the techniques used, such as:

- club cutting
- scissor over comb
- clipper over comb
- freehand
- thinning
- fading.

You will look at how to cut men's hair using these techniques, while following a guideline to achieve a range of different looks.

You will learn how to use these techniques to achieve uniform and square layers, graduated looks, flat tops, and how to fade into the neckline and how to cut the hair around the ear area.

Club cutting

Club cutting is also known as blunt cutting, and is the most popular cutting technique. It involves cutting the hair straight across, while holding the hair with tension between your fingers. This technique will reduce the length of the hair and layers but will retain the thickness of the hair. Club cutting can be carried out on wet and dry hair.

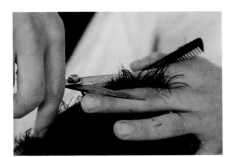

Holding the hair for club cutting

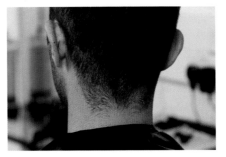

Check the neckline suits your client's requirements

HANDY HINT
Always follow your workplace, suppliers' and manufacturers' instructions to ensure the safe use of electrical equipment.

HANDY HINT
Clipper blades should be correctly aligned and checked before each service to ensure the blades are level and they cut evenly and without pulling on the hair.

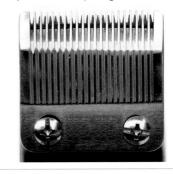

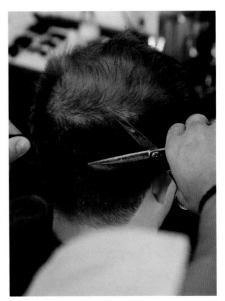

Scissor-over-comb technique

Scissor over comb

When you are using the scissor-over-comb technique, run the comb up the hair and use it to lift and support the hair to be cut. The hair is cut with the scissors over the comb. This technique gives a graduated effect to the cut and blends short hair into the neck. This technique is most effective on dry hair.

Using clippers

Clippers can be used with or without a clipper grade attached. If using clippers with a grade, you will need to decide the size of the

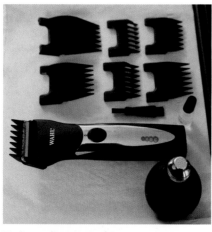

Various clipper grades

grade required and this will depend on your client's requirements. Clipper grades vary in size from grade 1 to grade 8, gradually getting about 3mm bigger (as a guide) with each grade:

■ grade 8 – 24mm (approximately 1 inch)

■ grade 6 – 18mm (approximately ¾ inch)

■ grade 4 – 12mm (approximately ½ inch)

■ grade 3 – 9mm

■ grade 2 – 6mm (approximately ¼ inch)

■ grade 1 – 3mm.

Activity

Using the measurements given in the list, work out the size of the following grades:

• grade 5
• grade 7.

HANDY HINT

Some clippers have a lever on the side that moves the teeth of the clippers wider and creates a half grade. If you used a grade 1 attachment and widened the teeth, you could create a 1.5 grade which will be about 4.5mm. If you used a grade 2 attachment and widened the teeth, you could create a 2.5 grade which will be about 7.5mm.

A common grade for the 'short back and sides' is a grade 2; grade 1 can be used for the back and sides but it is often used to blend a grade 2 down into the hairline, keeping the hairline very short and maximising how long the cut will last before it needs cutting again. Grades 3 and 4 can also be used around the back and sides of a cut, but are also used to blend in the grade 2 up into the occipital area of a scissor cut.

Grades 5 to 8 are mostly used on the top and crown areas for short, layered effects. Some men have a clipper cut all over the head and any grade can be used for this depending on the overall length required, or a variation of grades can be used so the hair gradually gets shorter towards the back and sides and hairline.

Activity

Using the measurements in the grade's list and in the Handy Hint, work out the size of the following grades:

• grade 4.5
• grade 6.5
• grade 8.5.

If using the clippers all over the head, start with the largest grade and blend down to the smallest grade. If you are using just one grade size all over the head, make sure the clippers are moved across the head in different directions – front to back, side to side, etc. This is because the hair will grow in many different directions and if you follow one direction only, the hair might be cut at varying lengths.

If you are using clippers with a grade at the back and sides and a scissor cut on the top and crown, you can start with the clipper grade cut first and then blend with your layer cut. It is very likely that you will need to use a clipper-over-comb or scissor-over-comb technique to fully blend these two techniques. Clippers are used on dry hair only.

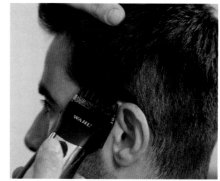

Clipper with a grade at side

Clipper over comb

Clipper over comb can be used to blend in scissor or clipper cuts. This technique helps to remove any bulk or definition lines from the varying clipper grades, or where the scissor cut meets a clipper cut. It is a popular technique used on dry hair to blend and fade into the hairline.

To use this technique, follow the comb with the clippers through the back and sides, angling the comb at +45° or –45° to create longer or shorter effects.

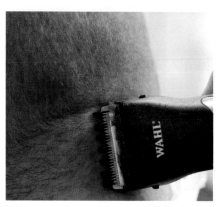

Clilipper with a grade at back

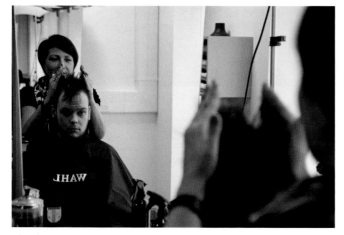

Checking the balance of the cut

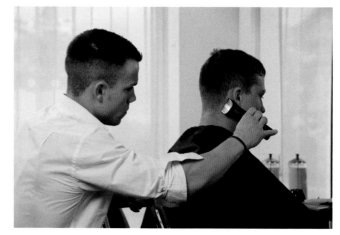

Shaping the neckline

Freehand technique

When using the freehand technique, you must not hold the hair with any tension but instead comb the hair into position and cut. This technique can be used when you do not need any tension, such as when cutting fringes, or allowing for the natural fall of the hair and cutting around the ears. Freehand cutting can be used on wet or dry hair but is particularly good on dry hair.

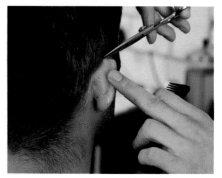

Using freehand for cutting around the ears

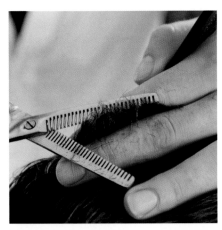

Thinning out the hair

Thinning the hair

You can use thinning scissors to remove unwanted bulk from the hair but maintain the length. When using thinning scissors, you must cut into the section of hair towards the mid-lengths and ends – avoiding the root area. Thinning out the root area can cause hair to stick up and show signs that it has been thinned out. Hair should be dry while this technique is carried out, otherwise you might remove too much 'bulk'.

Fading

Fading is used to blend short haircuts into the nape of the neck. If hair has been clipper cut or if scissor over comb has been used, blend the hair from the occipital bone down to blend in with the nape area and fade out to the hairline. This technique can enable the hairline shape to appear more natural-looking. Fading techniques are carried out on dry hair.

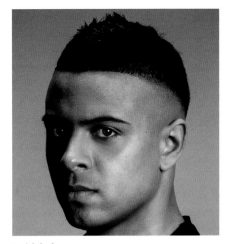

Bald fade

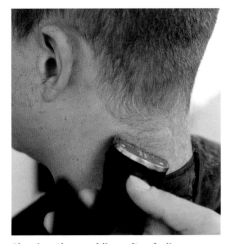

Shaping the neckline after fading

Activity

Practise these cutting techniques on a training head.

Guidelines

The guideline is the most important part of the haircut. If you are cutting the hair and you lose your guideline – STOP! The guideline determines the finished length of the cut and the overall shape and balance. Without a guideline you cannot work methodically through the haircut or maintain accuracy. Even the most experienced barbers will follow a guideline and use accurate sectioning.

Activity

Use a training head and practise establishing and following guidelines as described in chapter CH3.

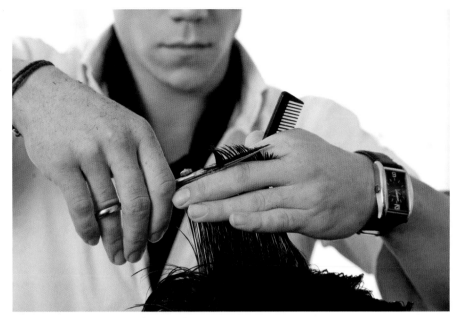

Internal guideline crown to back

Barber following the guideline when cutting

When you have cut your guideline, every section you cut afterwards will follow this guideline to the same length, so you must hold the hair at the same angle on both sides of the head. Always ensure that your cutting sections are clean and that you take manageably sized sections. Make sure you maintain your balance, otherwise the haircut might be uneven.

HANDY HINT

If you cannot see your guideline, stop cutting, go back a few sections and find it. Or you can section the hair the opposite way to work out where you have cut up to.

Angles

The cutting angles that the hair is held at will vary for every haircut and style.

WHY DON'T YOU...
Refer to chapter CH3 for more information on cutting angles.

Look	Cutting angle	Cutting angles and techniques
One length	The hair is pulled directly down at a 0° angle.	Club cutting Freehand
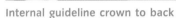		

Look	Cutting angle	Cutting angles and techniques
Uniform layers 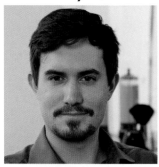	Use 0° for the baseline. For the layers the hair is pulled out at a 90° angle throughout the entire haircut. 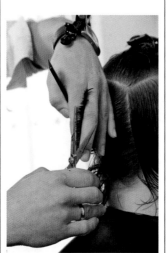	Club cutting Freehand 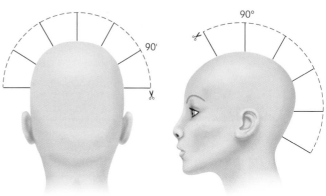
Graduation 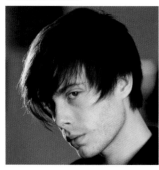	The inner layers of the hair lengths are longer than the outline shape and generally pulled out at 45°. 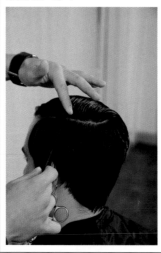	Club cutting Freehand Texturising Tapering Scissor over comb 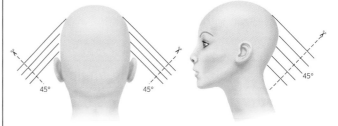

Look	Cutting angle	Cutting angles and techniques
Fringes 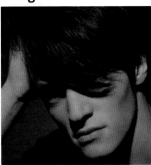 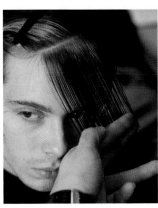	Often cut freehand to allow for the natural movement and fall of the hair growth patterns, but fringes can be cut under tension and pulled down to 0°.	Freehand Club cutting 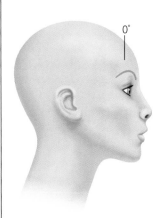

Activity

Research using style magazines or internet images of men's hairstyles and label the cutting angles used.

Activity

Practise sectioning and pulling the hair out at the angles described in the diagrams.

Cutting hair with tension

When you are cutting hair with tension, you must remember that wet hair stretches more than dry hair, so make sure that the end result is not shorter than you expected. You must always keep the same tension to ensure an even result. This includes keeping an even moisture balance during the cutting service, so that the hair is not of mixed porosity or elasticity. This could cause tangles, damage to the hair or uneven cutting results.

WHY DON'T YOU...
Refer to chapter CH3 for more information on cutting hair wet or dry.

Cutting hair wet or dry

Whether you cut the hair wet or dry will affect the technique you use and the end result. Hair should be checked while it is dry to identify the fall of the hair and rechecked after shampooing.

HANDY HINT

Keep hair damp when cutting to ensure the elasticity is even throughout.

HANDY HINT

Curly hair will spring up when dry – use less tension when cutting curly hair. This can be achieved by using the wider tooth end of your comb.

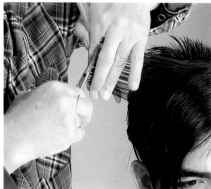
Wet cut

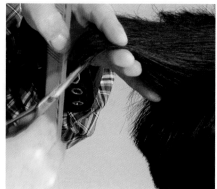
Dry cut

The importance of cross-checking the cut

It is important that your client's body position is balanced and upright throughout the haircut. If your client has his legs or ankles crossed, then the balance of the baseline cut could be uneven. Equally you must ensure that you have an even distribution of body weight.

Cross-checking the haircut during the service and at the end ensures an accurate finish. You can cross-check the haircut at any point during the service to check for balance and even cutting lengths. Using the mirror will help you to check for balance.

HANDY HINT

Cross-checking the cut ensures it is accurate, evenly balanced and has an even weight distribution throughout.

HANDY HINT

As hair only grows about 1.25cm (½ inch) each month, it is important that you do not cut the hair too short.

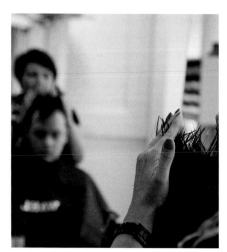
Cross-checking in the mirror

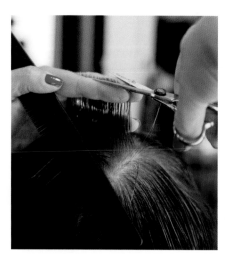
Cross-checking horizontally

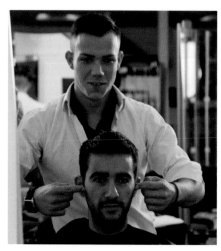
Cross-checking sideburns in the mirror

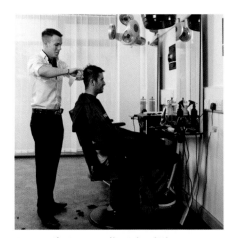

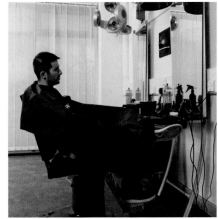

Ensure that your client is sitting straight

Poor sitting position could result in an uneven haircut

Using products

At the end of the cutting service, style the hair using styling products and add finishing products at the end. It is important to use products cost-effectively so that the salon does not waste money. Advise your client on how much to use, if he buys products from you to style his hair – you don't want him wasting his money either or using too much product and overloading the hair.

Providing advice and recommendations

It is essential that you provide suitable aftercare advice to your client on maintaining the look you have created. You should advise on products and how to use them, what equipment would best enable him to recreate the look, when to return for his next haircut, and even suggest colouring services that might enhance the style.

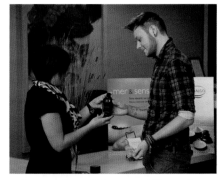

Ask your client if he would like to buy any products or equipment

Styling and finishing products to maintain the look

If your client has had a full cut-and-blow-dry service, you should have talked about the products that you used during the styling service and explained why and how you used them. If the service was a wet cut, discuss how your client should finish the look himself.

Advise your client on which styling and finishing products would enhance and support his finished look. Explain how particular styling products will aid the drying and styling process, help control the hair and provide longevity to the finished result. You should advise him on how much product to use and how to apply it. If the product could cause a build-up on the hair, advise him on how to remove the product effectively.

You could suggest the following products to help your client style his hair in between salon visits.

Product	Use
	Wax Use on dry hair to finish; adds pliable hold.
	Grooming cream Use on wet or dry hair; gives a firm hold with a matt finish.
	Clay Use on wet or dry hair to support the shape and offer a medium shine.
	Pomade Use on dry hair; this is a wax-free substance offering a flexible hold and creating a wet look.
	Fibre Use on dry hair for a firm hold that leaves hair pliable.
	Gel Use on wet or dry hair to create a textured 'gloss' look.

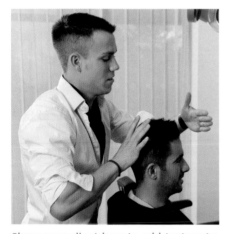

Show your client how to add texture to the style

Tools and equipment to maintain the look

Throughout the styling service you should advise your client on which tools to use at home to recreate his look, and during the blow-dry service demonstrate what you are doing and why. This gives your client a thorough understanding of what he will need to do when he is styling his hair at home. Talk to him about how to create body or movement if required, or how to prevent it. Remember to discuss the health and safety side of styling and the use of electrically heated styling equipment, such as straightening irons, and how this could cause damage to the hair.

Time intervals between services

You should advise your client on when to book his next cutting service. To help guide him, explain that it depends on how quickly his hair grows. You should suggest that he returns to the salon when the style grows out of shape and when he has trouble maintaining the style, as this might indicate it is ready for a cut.

Recommending further services

Having discussed the cutting service with your client, you may wish to recommend colouring services; this will enhance the image created. Adding colour and highlights to a haircut helps to add texture and definition to the shape. Without doubt, colour enhances and complements every style you create.

Provide cutting services using basic barbering techniques – review

Prepare for cutting services

To prepare for the cutting service:

- protect your client throughout the service – follow your salon requirements
- prepare your work area and tools in advance
- prepare the client's hair in readiness for the service
- make effective use of your time throughout.

Work safely and hygienically

Throughout the hair cutting service remember to:

- maintain your responsibilities for health and safety
- keep your work area clean and tidy
- keep your client free of hair cuttings
- sweep the floor during and after the service
- check the positioning of your client throughout
- maintain a good body posture
- remove loose hair cuttings from your client to maintain their comfort
- work to commercially viable times.

Consult with clients

Carry out a consultation, identifying the client's wishes and confirming the look required. At this stage you will be deciding on the tools you will need and the techniques you will be using to create the look required. Check the hair and skin for any factors that may affect the service and clarify whether the chosen look is achievable. Once you have agreed the service requirements, prepare the hair for the service.

Select products, tools and equipment

After consultation and preparation of your client's hair, complete the preparation of your work area and set up all the tools and equipment you will need for the service – make sure they are clean and sterile before use. If using clippers, oil the blades and check they are balanced.

Carry out cutting services

To carry out cutting services:

- consult with your client
- create and follow your guideline
- use cutting techiques to achieve the desired result
- adapt techniques depending on the factors identifed
- establish an accurate distribution of weight, balance and shape of the hair
- create your neckline shape
- remove any unwanted hair outside the desired outline shape
- balance and shape sideburns (if required)
- make final visual checks on the haircut and cross-check the result
- minimise risk of damage to tools and equipment.

You'll need to know your salon's commercially viable times to ensure you carry out the service within these time frames.

Step by steps

Activity

Practise the following looks below on a training head:

- uniform layered cut
- square layers
- graduation
- flat top

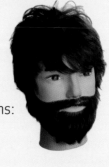

Remember to include the following in your designs:

- an around the ear outline
- cutting over the ear
- fading into the hairline

Creating a uniform layer look

When cutting the hair to create a uniform layer look, you will need to make a guideline section for the length of the hair and one for the internal layers of the hair. The hair is cut at 90° all over.

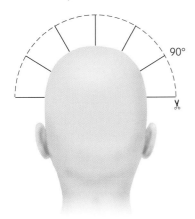

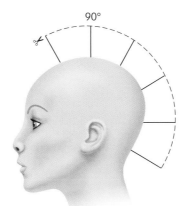

Uniform layer angles

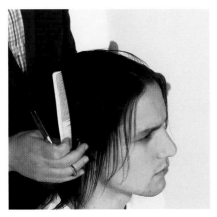

STEP 1 – Start with a vertical section on the top of the head from the front hairline to the crown.

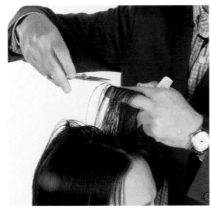

STEP 2 – Elevate the hair straight out from the head and cut a square line.

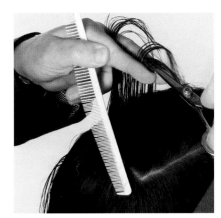

STEP 3 – Next, create a rectangular area in the top, using the initial section as a guide and work a horizontal section cutting a square line straight out from the head.

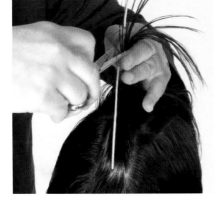

STEP 4 – Create a vertical section over the crown and, using the top section as a guide, elevate the hair straight up and cut a square line.

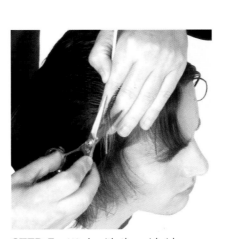

STEP 5 – Work with the mid-side areas following the round of the head.

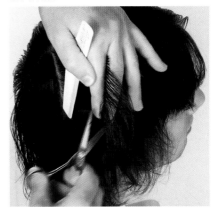

STEP 6 – Using the previous section as a guide and working with parallel sections, continue with this process to the round of the head at the back, ensuring a flat edge.

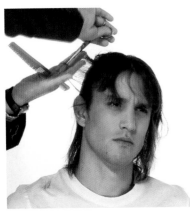

STEP 7 – Next, work on the internal layering of the perimeter using the existing internal shape as a guide.

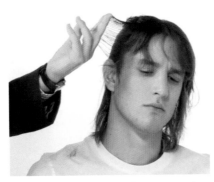

STEP 8 – Take a vertical section in the front hairline which incorporates the mid-section. Continue the existing line into the hairline.

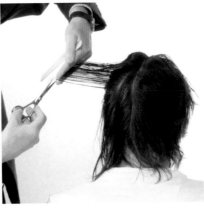

STEP 9 – Work the round of the head using over-direction to maintain the square shape.

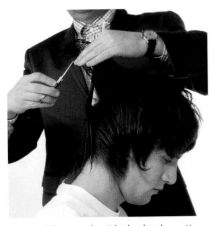

STEP 10 – Work with the back section hairline. Begin from an initial vertical section which incorporates the mid-section and continue with the existing line into the hairline using elevation to maintain the square line.

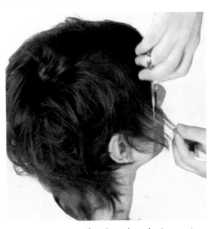

STEP 11 – Use freehand techniques to enhance the natural texture and movement of the hair.

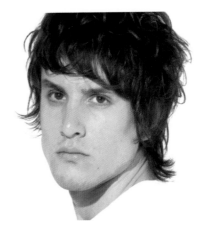

STEP 12 – The final look.

Activity

Create a mood board of varying uniform layer looks and write up how to achieve one of the images.

Creating a long square layer look

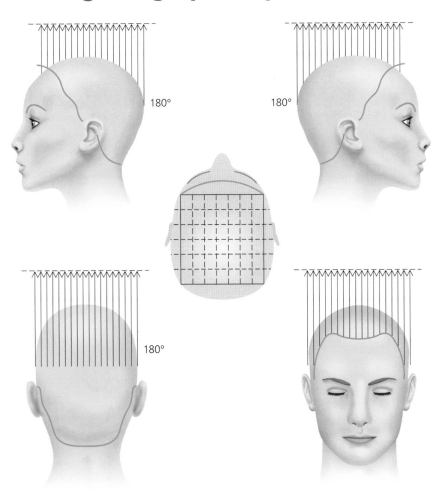

Square layer angles

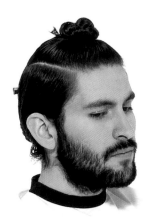

STEP 1 – Create a section in the top along the parietal ridge on both sides and then across the back where the head rounds to create an oblong. This sectioning will help define the back and sides from the corner of the round of the head.

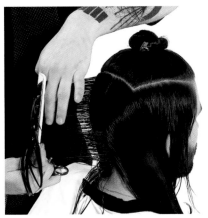

STEP 2 – Take a vertical section in the centre-back from crown to nape. Pull the hair to 90° to the head and cut a square line flat to the head and parallel to the section. Cut this guide in sections starting at the top with manageable finger-width panels. Ensure that your fingers are at the same angle all the way down, despite the head shape.

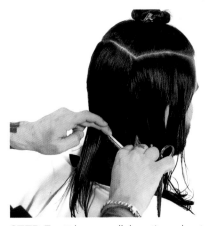

STEP 3 – Take a parallel section, elevate to 90° using the previous section as a guide and cut a square line with slight over-direction to the previous section. This will produce a square both vertically and horizontally. As each section is taken, ensure that the head is in the correct position for an accurate angle.

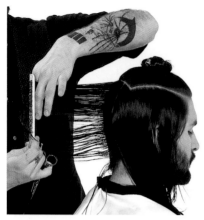

STEP 4 – Continue with parallel sections and the same process with slight over-direction to the previous section. Work to where the head rounds. Repeat the same process on the second side. Stand in the same position and use the same angles and body position for an accurate square shape.

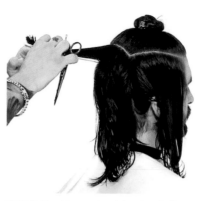

STEP 5 – Cross-check horizontally through both sides with the same elevation.

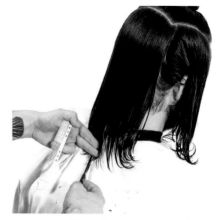

STEP 6 – Clean the perimeter outline with a pointing technique for a soft finish and to maintain maximum length.

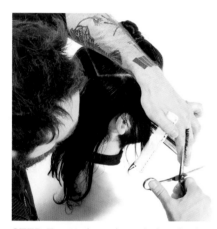

STEP 7 – Work on the right-hand side. Take a vertical section from the parietal ridge from the top of the ear, elevate the hair to 90° to the head and cut a square line.

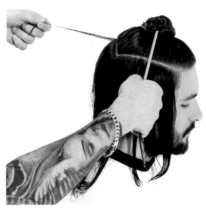

STEP 8 – Check that the lengths in the back and the side are the same.

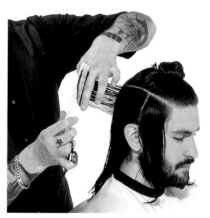

STEP 9 – Work with parallel sections towards the back with the same process and slight over-direction to the previous section to ensure a square internal side section. Work forwards with the same process from the top of the ear to the front hairline. Repeat the same process on the second side.

Activity

Create a mood board of varying square layer looks and write up how to achieve one of the images.

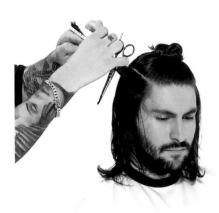

STEP 10 – Cross-check both sides horizontally.

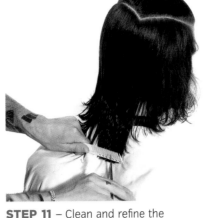

STEP 11 – Clean and refine the perimeter sides and connect to the back with a pointing technique.

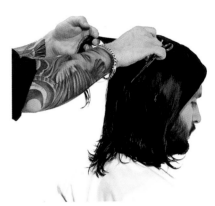

STEP 12 – Elevate a horizontal section of the crown to 45°. Over-direct to the existing square shape in the back and cut a square line. Continue with parallel sections all the way to the front hairline and cross-check.

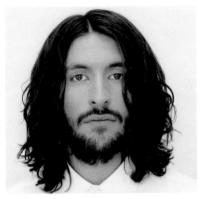

STEP 13 – The final look.

Creating a graduated layer look

When you create a short graduated haircut, the hair must gradually get shorter towards the nape and neck area. The top can be cut in a similar way to the uniform layers and held out at 90°, but the sides and back of this style must be cut at 45°.

Graduated look with clippering techniques

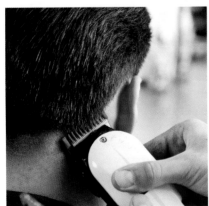

STEP 1 – Starting at the nape area using a clipper grade 1, pull away to create graduation from the nape.

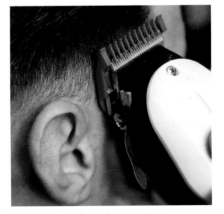

STEP 2 – Follow the previous technique around the sides, not going higher than the temples.

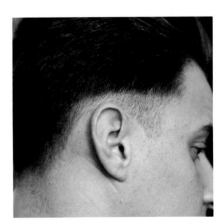

STEP 3 – This is the shape created.

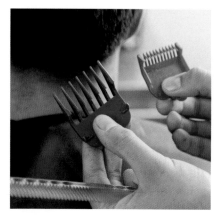

STEP 4 – Switch from a grade 1 to a grade 2.

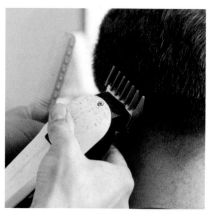

STEP 5 – Using the grade 2, remove the weight line around nape and temple area.

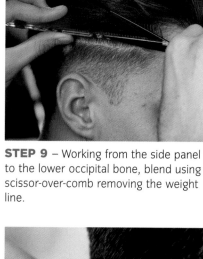

STEP 6 – Check the balance of the shape created in the mirror.

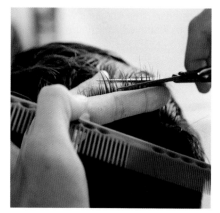

STEP 7 – Starting from the crown working forward, club cut through the top.

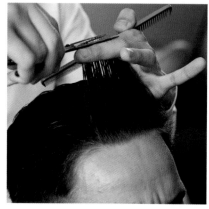

STEP 8 – When you get to the front, slightly angle towards the crown to create graduation and more length around the front.

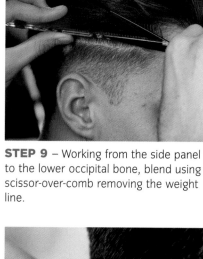

STEP 9 – Working from the side panel to the lower occipital bone, blend using scissor-over-comb removing the weight line.

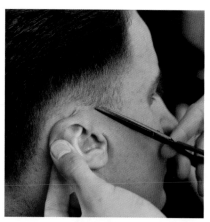

STEP 10 – Point cut to create shape around the ear.

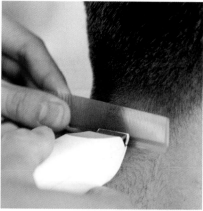

STEP 11 – Taper the neckline angling the comb to create graduation.

Activity

Create a mood board of varying graduated layer looks and write up how to achieve one of the images.

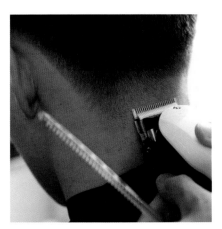

STEP 12 – Adjust the clipper level to grade 0 to create skin fade around the edges.

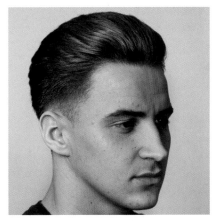

STEP 13 – The finished look.

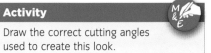

Activity

Draw the correct cutting angles used to create this look.

Creating a flat top look

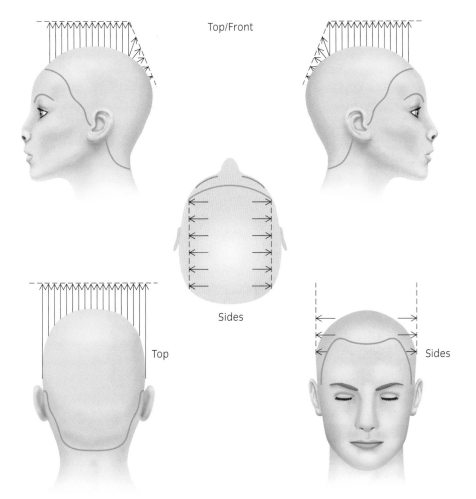

Flat top angles

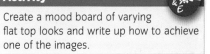

Activity

Create a mood board of varying flat top looks and write up how to achieve one of the images.

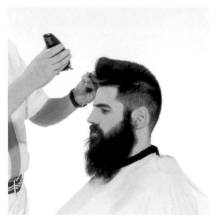

STEP 1 – Begin in the top front with medium clippers creating the guide for the shape. This is a visual and technical guide for the entire process.

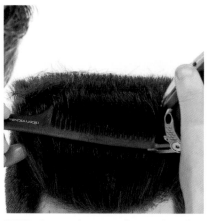

STEP 2 – Work across the comb with the clippers in the central panel first. The teeth of the comb run at 90° to the clippers in order to create a consistent, equal length.

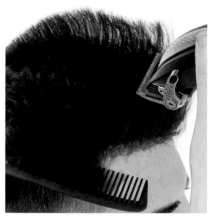

STEP 3 – Work with the same process back towards the crown using the previous section as a guide and include the temple areas.

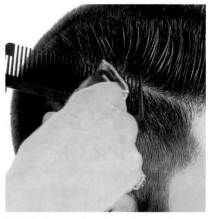

STEP 4 – Work in the sides on the parietal ridge, down the top and comb away the corners. Then create a guide just below the sectioned-away hair with clippers.

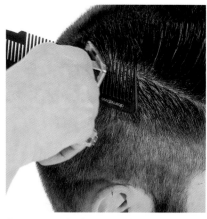

STEP 5 – The hair is pulled square to the side of the head at approximately 45°. Continue to create the guide to just past the round of the head.

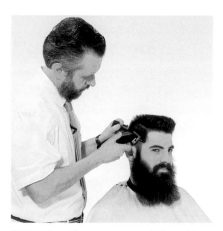

STEP 6 – Clipper-over-comb from the top down horizontally using the initial guide.

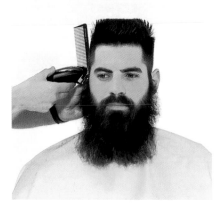

STEP 7 – Adjust the clipper blades to the longest setting without a guard. Work from the perimeter up, blending the sides to the initial guide and following the horizontal panels to the round of the head in the back.

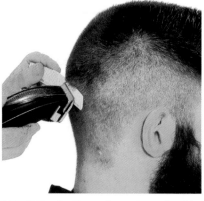

STEP 8 – Further refine using a flexible barbering comb to ensure good colourisation of fade. Refine the corner placement at the round of the head and the perimeter.

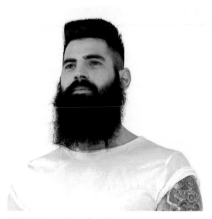

STEP 9 – The final look.

Cutting graduations

Activity

Research on the internet (or in style magazines) styles with fringes.

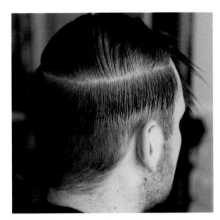

STEP 1 – Section the hair above the crown out of the way.

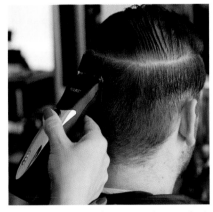

STEP 2 – Using clippers with a grade 2 attachment, clipper the back and sides.

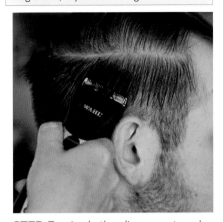

STEP 3 – Angle the clippers outwards to create graduation.

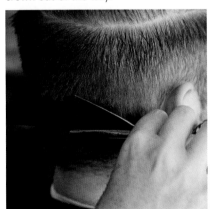

STEP 4 – Blend the back-clippered hair with scissor over comb.

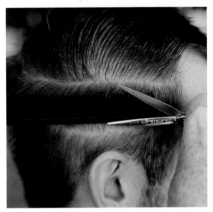

STEP 5 – Repeat with the side sections.

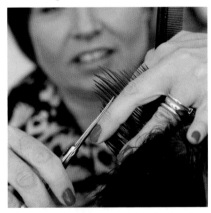

STEP 6 – Pull the layers out at 90° for the crown.

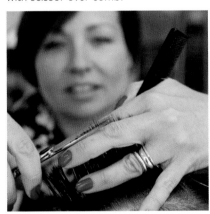

STEP 7 – Follow the 90° angle through the top and sides.

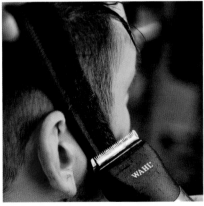

STEP 8 – Fade out the clipper cut into the sideburns/facial hair.

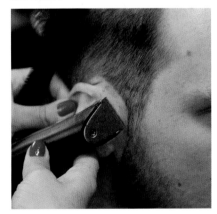

STEP 9 – Tidy the hairline around the ears and neckline.

Working around the ear outline

When you are cutting a style above the ear, you need to cut the hair cleanly around the ear area. If the hair is left too long around the ear, then it might appear as if it needs cutting again just a week or two later. To help achieve a clean cut around the ears, hold/gently fold your client's ear forward towards the face (or ask your client to hold their ear if you prefer). While the ear is held gently forward you can freehand cut around the shape of the ear. Sometimes clippers are used without a grade, to carefully follow the hairline around the ear area and create a neat finish.

Clippering around the ear

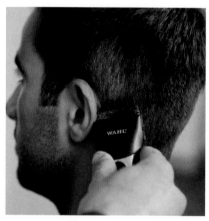

STEP 1 – Follow the hairline around the ears with the clippers.

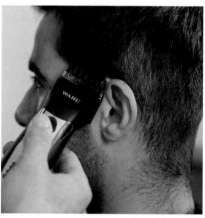

STEP 2 – In front of the ear, angle the clippers upwards but pull outwards to create graduation.

Cutting over the ear

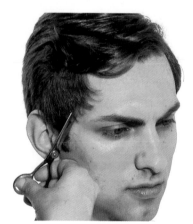

STEP 1 – In the front hairline, brush the hair forwards and cut in the comb to establish a natural-looking perimeter and avoid a hard line.

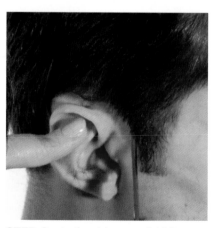

STEP 2 – In the side areas fold the ear and point a natural perimeter.

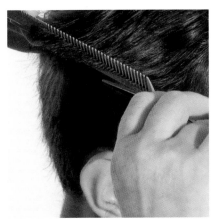

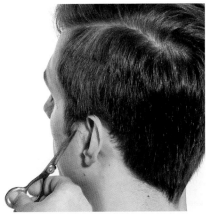

Activity

Practise cutting over the ear on a training head.

STEP 3 – Use the scissors-over-comb technique to blend the underneath with the mid-side areas and front.

STEP 4 – Refine the outline in the front and over the left ear with the same process as the right-hand side.

Graduation with clippering and fading techniques

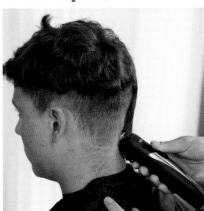

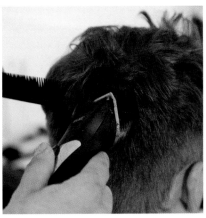

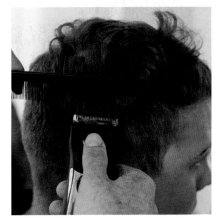

STEP 1 – Clipper the back and sides to just above the occipital bone.

STEP 2 – Use the clipper-over-comb technique to blend clippered hair.

STEP 3 – Continue this through the side into layers.

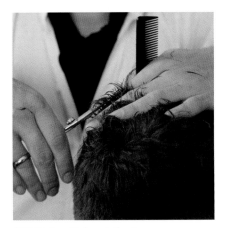

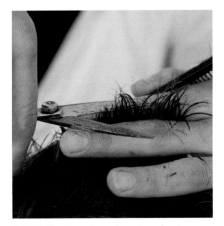

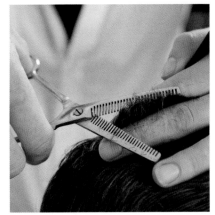

STEP 4 – Club cut the top.

STEP 5 – Continue layering the top section.

STEP 6 – Use thinning scissors to remove bulk.

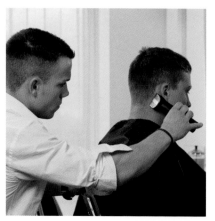

STEP 7 – Discuss the neckline shape with your client and shape it to suit your client's requirement.

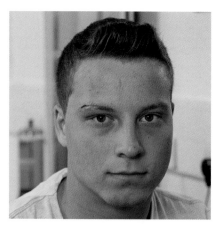

STEP 8 – Check that your client is happy with the end result.

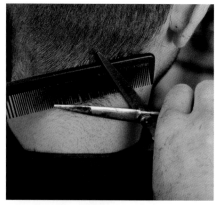

Tapering and blending into the natural hairline

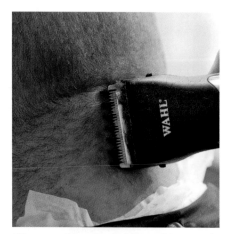

Clipper cutting the hairline with a grade 1 attachment

Cutting the neckline

When you have clipper cut or cut the hair into the neck with a scissor-over-comb technique, you will need to decide with your client how to fade into the neckline.

Tapered neckline

One of the more popular necklines is to blend the main haircut into the natural hairline. To create this effect, the hair is gradually cut shorter and blended into the natural shape of the hairline. You will need to consider the natural movement of the hairline, checking for any nape whorls or inward/outward nape growth patterns.

Faded neckline

To create this effect, the hair is clipper cut with a grade and gradually blended into a clipper cut without a grade, into the hairline.

Square neckline

To create a square neckline, the end result will be a blunt, clean finish. Use scissors or clippers to literally square off the edges of the hairline around the neck.

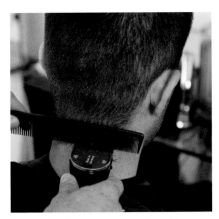

STEP 1 – Create a squared neckline with clippers.

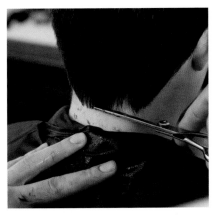

STEP 2 – Cut the baseline straight across with scissors.

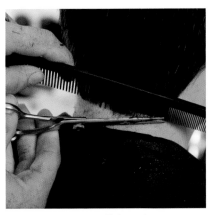

STEP 3 – Square off the edges.

Rounded neckline

To create a rounded neckline, use the scissors or clippers as for the square neckline but, rather than leaving square corners, round off the edges. Although this result is not as harsh as a square neckline, it is still a blunt finish to the cut.

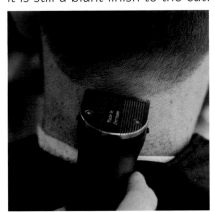

STEP 1 – Create the rounded shape at the back.

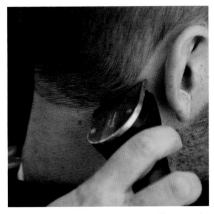

STEP 2 – Round the shape off towards the sides.

Eyebrow grooming

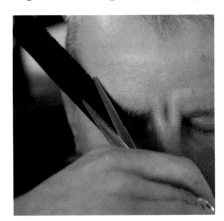

STEP 1 – Using either clipper- or scissor-over-comb techniques, remove excess length.

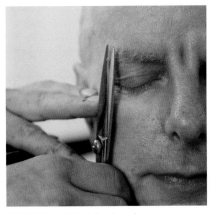

STEP 2 – Using freehand, remove any stray long eyebrows.

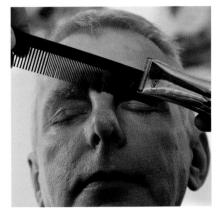

STEP 3 – Comb up and down the eyebrow to cut any stray long eyebrows.

Answers in the back of the book.

1 Which one of the following is the best way for a barber to avoid cross-infection?

  a Using clean towels and gowns

  b Wearing an apron whilst working

  c Cleaning surfaces before each client

  d Supplying wet wipes to clients

2 Which one of the following is the best way of consulting with clients?

  a Smiling and checking the progress of the cut in the mirror

  b Maintaining eye contact and asking questions throughout the service

  c Using open questions to obtain information and closed questions to confirm requirements

  d Using closed questions to obtain information and closed questions to confirm requirements

3 Which one of the following is the best way to position the client to achieve a balanced style during a haircut?

  a With the neck supported by a head rest

  b With the legs supported by a foot stool

  c With legs crossed and back firmly supported by the chair

  d With legs uncrossed and back firmly supported by the chair

4 Which one of the following factors can affect the length of the finished style when cutting wet hair?

  a Elasticity

  b Porosity

  c Density

  d Texture

5 Which one of the following should be avoided when a client has a widow's peak or a cowlick?

  a Short napes

  b Clipper cuts

  c Fringes

  d Razoring

6 Which one of the following is the best way to sterilise scissors?

  a UV cabinet

  b Autoclave

  c Barbicide

  d Chemical wipes

7 A common clipper grade used for short back and sides is number 2; which one of the following hair lengths is achieved by using a number 2?

  a 24mm

  b 18mm

  c 12mm

  d 6mm

8 Which one of the following techniques is best used when working with the natural fall of the hair?

  a Club cutting

  b Clipper over comb

  c Scissor over comb

  d Freehand

9 Which one of the following best describes the technique of fading?

  a Cutting outline shapes in the hairline

  b Blending short layers in the nape area

  c Blending long layers at the crown with short layers at the nape

  d Using freehand around the ears and around hair growth patterns

10 Which one of the following is the best product to use for creating a wet look, textured gloss?

  a Pomade

  b Fiber

  c Gel

  d Clay

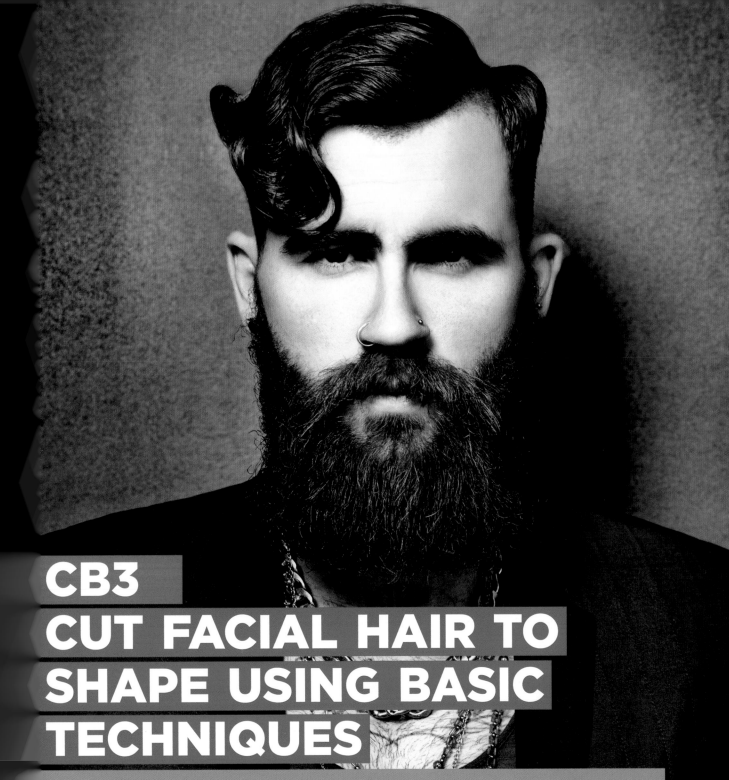

CB3
CUT FACIAL HAIR TO SHAPE USING BASIC TECHNIQUES

For years, beards and facial hair were considered signs of sandal-wearing hippies or men who were too lazy to groom themselves properly. However, more recently, facial hair and 'celebrity designer' beards have become increasingly popular; barbershops have noticed an increase in clients visiting the salon to have either facial hair trimmed and styled or to achieve that 'clean-shaven' look. Whatever your client's choice, facial hair grooming is now a very popular service at the barbers, and these are skills that you must master.

From this chapter you will:

■ know how health and safety affects facial hair cutting services

■ understand the factors that influence facial hair cutting services

■ know the tools, equipment, products and techniques used to cut facial hair shapes

■ be able to provide facial hair cutting services using basic techniques.

HEALTH & SAFETY

Refer to the health and safety and salon policies chapter for more information on the health and safety Acts you need to follow when cutting facial hair.

HEALTH & SAFETY

Refer to the health and safety and salon policies chapter for more information on environmental and sustainable working practices.

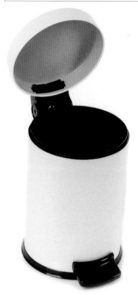

Waste bin with lid

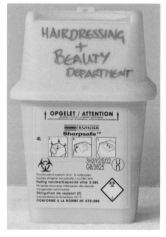

Sharps bin

HANDY HINT

As with all services, your personal hygiene, protection and presentation are important during facial hair cutting services.

Health and safety

Your responsibilities for health and safety

Your responsibilities for health and safety include:

- following your salon procedures and all of the health and safety Acts
- preparing a clean working environment
- maintaining your personal hygiene and presentation
- carrying out a consultation with your client
- gowning and protecting your client for the facial hair cutting service
- behaving in a suitable manner that does not cause risk of injury to you and those around you.

Environmental and sustainable practices and disposal

Always follow environmental and sustainable working practices when cutting facial hair.

Dispose of any soiled cotton wool (and plasters) in the designated salon waste bin with a lid to prevent any cross-contamination.

Hair clippings on the floor make for a slippery surface, so sweep the floor after every client and, if necessary, during the service.

Dispose of used razor blades in the sharps bin. Collection of these bins can be arranged by your local council and sometimes with your local pharmacy.

Activity

What would the risks and potential consequences be if a razor blade were disposed of in the salon waste bin?

Activity

Identify your salon requirements for protecting the client's eyes and clothes from hair clippings.

Personal presentation

You must always ensure that you are prepared for the working day ahead! Arrive at work clean and showered, wearing deodorant, with fresh breath, dressed in clean clothes and with your own hair and/or facial hair well groomed and well presented. You should avoid wearing any accessories that might get caught in your client's hair or put you at risk of contact dermatitis.

Hazards and risks

When you cut facial hair, you will be using sharp tools and cutting very close to, if not onto, your client's skin; you need to be aware that this increases the risks to you and your client. Wear gloves when using a razor. Care must be taken when using and transporting these tools to avoid the risk of injury. Sharps must be disposed of in a sharps bin.

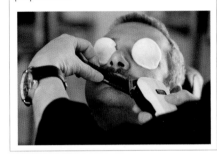

Hazard	Potential risk
Sharp objects Razors and scissors	Risk of injury to self and client
Infected clients Razor bumps	Cross-contamination
Electrical appliances – clippers Frayed wire	Risk of electric shock if faulty or used incorrectly
Spillages Water spillage	Risk of slipping over/injury
Hair on the floor – slippery surface Hair cuttings	Risk of slipping over/injury

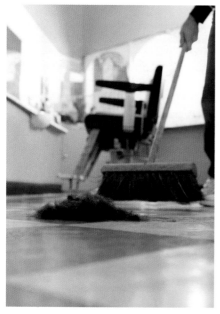

Keep your work area clean and tidy

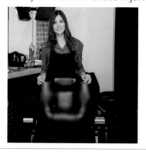

HANDY HINT

Barber's chairs are much heavier and more bulky than salon chairs. If you need to move them, do so carefully so that you do not hurt your back or cause injuries.

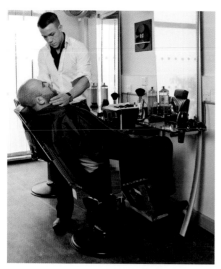

Ensure the client is comfortable

Safe working practices

The safety considerations that must be taken into account, are:

- keeping a clean and tidy work area
- using the right kind of barber's chair
- ensuring that you and your client are comfortably positioned, and that you use your tools safely
- protecting your client from hair clippings and dispose of clippings and waste safely.

Activity

In pairs or small groups, discuss the safety considerations for facial hair cutting services and why these are important.

Clean and tidy work area

Ensure that your work area is ready for your client's arrival. Workstations and barber's chairs must be hair-free, cleaned with warm soapy water, and wiped or sprayed with disinfectant. Your cutting tools must be sterilised before and after use; this is particularly important if you are using razor blades or cutting very close to the skin.

Barber's chair

It is important that you use the correct type of barber's chair when cutting facial hair, because you need access to the whole of the client's face and neckline, and you and your client need to be comfortable throughout the service.

Positioning

The comfort of you and your client is paramount during this service, as both of you need to stay still during the service. Any sudden movements could cause your client to get a cut from the scissors/razor.

Your body and tool position

You should always stand with your body weight evenly distributed; this will ensure that you are evenly balanced and that you are not putting undue stress on your back. You should place your work area and trolley to your preferred side of working and never over-stretch to reach for your tools.

Your client's positioning

When your client is seated comfortably in the barber's chair, you must check that his legs are not crossed and that both feet are either on the floor or supported by the footrest. You need to ensure that your client is positioned comfortably and, just as importantly, sitting squarely and not off balance. When your client's body position is suitable, recline the chair and adjust it to a suitable position/height for you to work. During the facial cutting, you will need to ask your client to move his head in various directions, so that you can cut around the neck area and follow the contours of the face and neck.

Protect client from hair clippings

Facial hair is often very coarse and can travel great distances in the air as it is being cut! You should ensure that your own clothes are protected and try to avoid the tiny hair cuttings entering your eyes.

Make sure that your client is well protected and that you remove loose hair clippings from him on a regular basis throughout the service. These can penetrate into the skin and cause infections, such as boils. Both you and your client are at risk of infection from loose hair clippings.

Preventing cross-infection and infestation

Although many of the tools that you will use will be similar to those used for cutting head hair, you are cutting very near to the skin and lip, so you need to take extra care.

Methods of cleaning, disinfecting and sterilising

You must clean and disinfect or sterilise your cutting tools after every service to maintain a good reputation, ensure a professional image and to prevent cross-infection and infestation. You must ensure that you protect yourself and your client from the risk of cross-contamination.

Make sure all your towels and gowns are contamination-free, and scissors and combs are sterile. To sterilise your tools effectively if you encounter any infections or infestations, you must boil wash all towels and gowns. Use heat, such as boiling water or an autoclave, for scissors and combs and remember that a UV light will only maintain sterilisation but is not an effective method of removing infectious germs or infestations from your tools.

If you are using razor blades, you must use a fresh blade for every client, unless of course the razor blades are not disposable. These types of razors must be sterilised in an autoclave, sanitised in a UV cabinet or disinfected with a chemical solution or wipe.

Before and after using electrical or rechargeable clippers, you must remove all the hair clippings from in between the blades, spray the blades with a clipper disinfectant solution and oil them before storing them away/using them again.

> **HANDY HINT**
> Protect clients from hair clippings to ensure that they are comfortable at all times and to prevent any stray hairs from entering the skin or eyes.

> **HANDY HINT**
> If you are cutting facial hair, tuck tissue or cotton wool in the top edge of the towel to prevent the coarse hair from falling down the client's clothes. Use cotton pads on his eyes to protect him from stray hair cuttings.

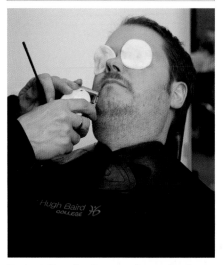

Protect the client's eyes from clippings

> **HANDY HINT**
> For a barber, poor posture can lead to fatigue and back injuries.

> **HEALTH & SAFETY**
> When using electrical appliances, you must follow the Electricity at Work Regulations and always be mindful of trailing wires, as these can cause trip hazards.

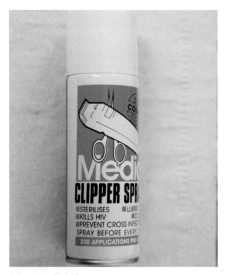

Clipper disinfectant

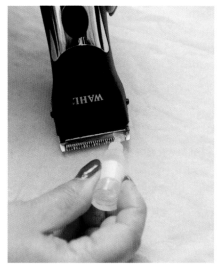

Clipper oil

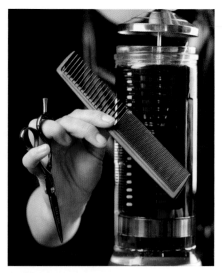

Barbicide

Working safely and hygienically

In order to work safely and hygienically, you need to do the following:

- follow health and safety Acts
- use protective materials and protect your eyes and those of your clients
- check tools prior to use and ensure they are clean and sterilised
- keep work area clean and tidy throughout the service
- position self and client correctly
- use tools with care
- remove hair cuttings throughout the service as well as at the end.

Before any facial hair cutting commences, you must check beneath the facial hair for open wounds or hidden cold sores that might not be visible due to hair growth and for signs of infection or infestation. Some clients might have facial hair to hide scar tissue, acne, facial moles or other potential skin disorders. These might pose a risk to you, or cause discomfort to your client if they are caught with a comb.

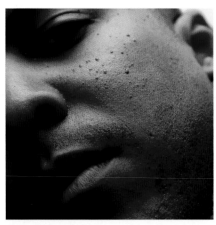

Check skin for scars, moles, acne or skin disorders

If you were to accidentally cut your client's skin or the lip, you should administer some minor first aid. First put on some gloves to prevent cross-contamination, stem the blood flow with clean, dry cotton wool, remove all loose clippings from the surrounding area and, if necessary, apply a suitable plaster, checking first that your client does not have an allergy to plasters. Remember to record the incident in the accident book.

Communicating well with clients

As we have mentioned in previous chapters, it is very important that you are polite to your clients and speak to them in a friendly manner. Engaging in neutral conversation about topics such as recent football results and which teams they support might help to relax your clients. You should be clearly spoken and show positive body language at all times. When speaking with clients or your colleagues, ensure you are respectful to them and respond to their needs.

You should use client-friendly terminology and speak in a reassuring and confident manner. Make sure you really listen to what your client is asking of you and respond by nodding and maintaining eye contact to prove you are listening. Before your client arrives, it is good practice to read your client's record card and during/after the visit record any changes or update it with today's service.

Consultation techniques and the importance of questioning

The consultation with your client for a facial haircut is no different to any other consultation; you still need to identify the service objectives. There are over 40 different styles of beards and moustaches; you will need to confirm which one of these your client desires and assess the potential of his hair to achieve the look required.

A series of open questions, starting with 'what', 'how', 'when' and 'why', will help you to obtain specific answers from your client about his requirements. Finish the conversation with closed questions to confirm both of your understandings.

To help your client choose a style for his facial hair, you can use magazines, mobile devices, or print off photos of celebrities with facial hair from the internet. Always listen carefully and hear what your client is asking you to achieve for him. Repeat any instructions back to clarify what has been agreed and discussed.

Activity

Use the internet to search for sites about beards and moustaches. How many websites on beards and facial hair can you find?

VALUES & BEHAVIOURS

Refer to the values and behaviours chapter for more information on client care and effective communication.

HANDY HINT

Revisit chapter CHB9 for more in-depth information on consulting with your client.

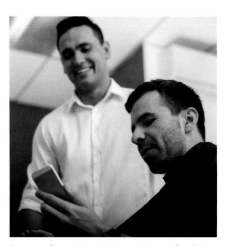

Smart phones are a great consultation tool

HANDY HINT

When speaking to your client and colleagues, you should demonstrate mutual respect. Speak to them confidently and politely, expressing yourself clearly and portraying positive body language.

WHY DON'T YOU...

Ask a colleague to pretend to be your client. Ask them to visualise a style and then ask the relevant questions to identify the image and look they require.

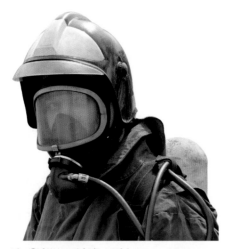

Jonny Depp and other celebrities have brought beards back into fashion

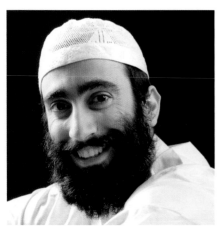

Firefighter with breathing apparatus

Some men maintain a beard for religious purposes

Factors that may influence services

Beards and facial hair have become an important fashion accessory for men, with more and more celebrities supporting these looks. R&B and hip hop music artists, movie stars, models and sportsmen have brought beards and designer stubble looks back into fashion and the media.

Although the factors that you need to consider for cutting facial hair are very similar to those for cutting head hair, there are some important differences. Facial hair is generally cut much shorter in length than head hair and therefore can grow out of style much more quickly. You will need to ensure that your client's requirements will suit his lifestyle, so that the shape and style of the beard or moustache will last and can be maintained, as and when required.

It is becoming increasingly acceptable to wear facial hair in the workplace and it does not look out of place with a suit, or with jeans and casual wear. The 'unshaven look', however, is not easy to achieve and requires a lot of care and attention. Some of the designer-stubble styles need maintaining every couple of days, and the initial days/weeks of growing facial hair might make your client look scruffy, so planning when to grow a beard also needs to be discussed. Before the chosen style is decided, check that your client has the time to maintain the desired look.

Some jobs can affect whether men can have beards. Firemen for example will need to ensure that any breathing apparatus fits snugly around their mouth and airways and a thick beard could prevent this. When consulting with your client about his facial hair requirements, you must discuss whether this might impact on his job and make judgements as to which style would be most suitable.

The following factors will need to be considered, as these can influence your client's decision on the chosen design and style:

- facial hair classification
- facial hair characteristics
- head and face shape, and facial features
- hair style and client's wishes
- adverse skin conditions
- facial piercings
- skin elasticity.

Facial hair classifications

Hair classification	Impact on service
Straight facial hair 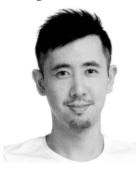	Fine/thin – may result in a patchy end result. Avoid very short beards. Full beards may take several visits to the barber for the desired result to be achievable. Medium – although straight, this type of hair can be easy to work with as it often has body and volume. Coarse – as this type of hair can be extremely straight you need to ensure you go over the facial hair in all directions to ensure the result is even throughout.
Wavy facial hair 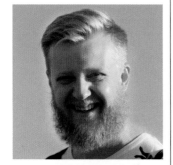	Fine/thin – due to the 'S' pattern in this type of hair, ensure you go over the facial hair in all directions. Medium – can be a little frizzy. The hair may need to be conditioned prior to the service commencing. Coarse – very frizzy and is likely to need to be conditioned prior to the service. This type of hair may also be abundant and you will need to go over the facial hair cut in all directions to ensure an even finish.
Curly facial hair 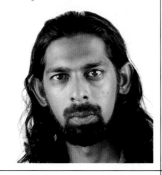	Loose curls – this type of facial hair may be of combination texture and therefore difficult to ensure an even finish. It may be thick and full, so full beards are achievable – but ensure you have cross-checked the end result fully. Tight curls – as for loose curls.
Very curly facial hair 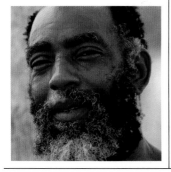	Soft – this type of hair is very fragile, so take care with your tools. The hair is often tightly coiled, so again cross-check thoroughly. Wiry – as for soft very curly hair but this type of hair has more of a 'Z' pattern shape and the curls may be less defined.

Facial hair characteristics

Hair characteristics include the following:

- density
- texture
- elasticity
- porosity
- condition
- growth patterns.

Texture and density

Clients who request a full beard but have sparse or no hair around the mouth should be advised to have a disconnected beard and moustache, so that the look balances.

It might not be possible to achieve a thin or fine moustache if the facial hair growth is naturally very dense or abundant. You might need to cut the facial hair with clippers, as cutting dense hair could take too long using a scissor-over-comb technique.

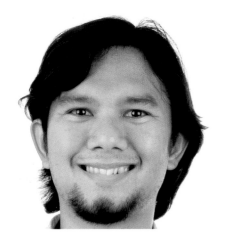
Fine facial hair

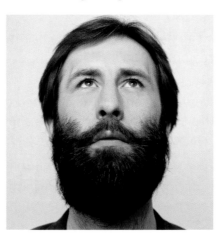
Medium facial hair

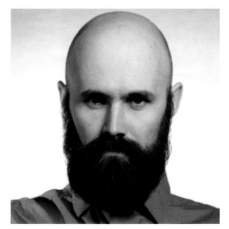
Coarse facial hair

Elasticity, porosity and condition

If facial hair is of poor elasticity or porous then extra care will need to be taken with your tools as the hair is more fragile. Be careful not to snag the facial hair and cause any discomfort for your client.

Hair growth patterns, distribution and quality

As with hair on the head, facial hair can have varied growth directions and this can cause the results to affect the finished shape, look uneven or grow out unevenly and untidily. A whorl growth direction needs to be cut or clippered in several directions, to ensure all the hairs are cut to the same length. You will need to consider the distribution of hair, as one side of the face might have more hair than the other. Also the quality of the facial hair might not suit certain styles, so check both sides of the face when you are consulting and discussing the style requirements.

Head and face shapes

It is important that the facial hair/beard complements the current hair style. A 'bald' head and a big beard could look out of place, so always ensure the two are balanced.

If your client has a round face, suggest a squarer cut and finish for the beard or moustache. For square faces and jaw-lines suggest a rounded beard or curved moustache.

Facial features

Cutting the facial hair of clients with dimples can sometimes cause you difficulties in achieving a balanced result. To ensure the end result is even, ask your client to poke their tongue in the dimple area to push the cheek area outwards when you cut/clipper the hair.

Clients with heavy-set chins generally prefer a fuller beard and moustache to balance the chin feature.

Clients with small mouths tend to suit smaller/thinner moustaches, and those with large noses suit a thick or wider moustache which will minimise the look of the larger feature.

If your client has any facial scarring, this can be disguised more easily with a beard or moustache.

Hair style and client's wishes

Most clients choose facial hairstyles to complement their haircut. Always look at their current hairstyle and offer advice on facial hairstyles that will blend or match. Always consult with your client to identify their wishes and to ascertain whether their desired result is achievable.

Adverse skin disorders

Some adverse skin disorders or contra-indications could affect the service. If the skin condition is infectious or contagious you must not proceed with the service.

You will need to be mindful of the adverse skin and scalp conditions mentioned in CHB9 when cutting facial hair. Always check in the beard growth for any signs of infection.

Facial piercings

Always check the face and eyebrow area for any piercings; you must be extremely careful not to catch these with the comb or your cutting tools.

HANDY HINT

When discussing the facial hair design, you should always consider your client's age and the suitability of the chosen style.

HANDY HINT

Facial hair grows at the same rate as head hair – about 12.5mm/1.25cm or roughly ½ inch a month. Advising your client when to rebook for their next facial hair cut will depend on the length of the facial hair style.

HANDY HINT

The effects of continual close cutting to the skin can result in barber's itch and the risk of developing ingrowing hairs. You should advise your client on aftercare to prevent or remedy these ailments. Regular exfoliation of the skin can often help.

HANDY HINT

For more detail on hair characteristics and adverse skin disorders, see chapter CHB9.

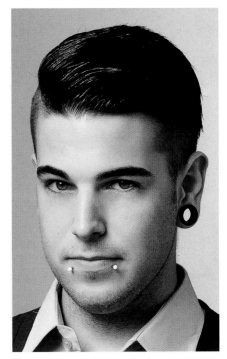

Piercings can catch on tools

HANDY HINT

Always carry your scissors in a pouch or case and **palm** them when not in use.

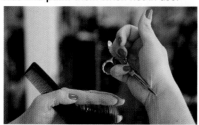

Palm

Holding your scissors with the blades closed in the palm of your hand.

Tools, equipment and products

The tools and equipment you are likely to use during these services are:

- combs
- scissors
- clippers
- clippers with grade attachments
- trimmers and T-liners.

Safe use and maintenance of cutting tools

Tools and equipment	How to use safely	Maintenance
Combs	Before service – use the comb to untangle the beard and moustache before cutting. During service – used with scissor- or clipper-over-comb techniques to guide the hair when cutting to the correct hair length – either end of the comb can be used, depending on the hair length required.	Before and after every service – clean with hot soapy water and remove all hair clippings, then disinfect in a chemical Barbicide solution or sanitise in a UV light cabinet.
Scissors	During the service, use scissor-over-comb techniques to achieve the desired lengths and trim the hair to shape.	Before and after every service – clean with hot soapy water and remove all hair clippings, then disinfect in a chemical Barbicide solution, sterilise in an autoclave or sanitise in a UV light cabinet. Oil blades after sterilising.
Clippers	During the service, use clipper-over-comb techniques to achieve the desired lengths. Clippers can also be used pointing the blades directly onto the skin to achieve a shaved line and to remove hair back to the skin.	Before and after every service, remove the hairs from the blades, spray with a disinfectant and oil the blades.

Tools and equipment	How to use safely	Maintenance
Clipper grade attachments 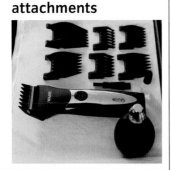	During the service, use clippers with various grades attached to achieve different lengths.	Before and after every service – clean grade attachments with hot soapy water and remove all hair clippings, then disinfect in a chemical Barbicide solution or sanitise in a UV light cabinet.
Trimmers and T-liners 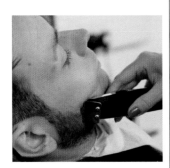	During the service trimmers and T-liners are used to create small precise lines in the beard line or moustache.	Before and after every service – remove the hairs from the blades, spray with a disinfectant and oil the blades.

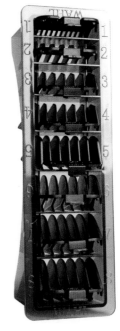

Activity

What action would you take if you dropped the electrical clippers and the blades were now making a terrible noise when switched on?

HANDY HINT

Clipper blades should be correctly aligned and checked before each service to ensure the blades are level and they cut evenly without pulling on the hair.

Clipper blade attachments

Clippers can be used with or without a clipper grade attached. If using clippers with a grade, you will need to decide the size of the grade required and this will depend on your client's requirements. Clipper grades vary in size from grade 1 (3mm) to grade 8, gradually getting about 3mm bigger with each grade (as a guide).

Activity

If grade 1 = 3mm and each grade increases by 3mm, what is the size of the following grades?

- grade 2
- grade 4

- grade 5
- grade 8.

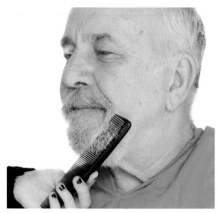

Assess the facial hair before cutting

Preparing facial hair for shaping services

When your client arrives, you should protect him with a clean cutting gown and towels placed at the front and back of the shoulders. If you are cutting the head hair and facial hair, then you should shampoo the hair prior to the service. If you are carrying out a beard and moustache cut, then the face should be washed with a facial soap and water. If the facial hair is a full beard, you could apply a conditioner to the hair to soften it slightly. However, due to the coarseness of the hair, the conditioner will not work as well as it does on head hair. If you are trimming a moustache only, then a facial wipe would suffice to cleanse the facial hair. Comb all beards and moustaches through with a wide-tooth comb to untangle the hair and to allow all of the hair to be cut.

Techniques

In this part of the chapter we will look at the techniques used, such as:

- scissor over comb
- clipper over comb
- clippering with grade attachments
- freehand.

Scissor over comb

Scissor over comb is a popular technique that is used for beard and moustache-trimming and shaping. It allows for graduation in the shape but you will need to be very accurate with your cutting.

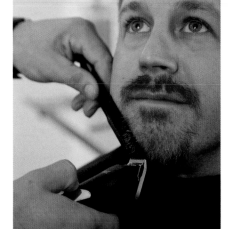

Scissor over comb

When you are using scissor-over-comb techniques, ensure that the beard has been washed and towel-dried thoroughly, place your comb on the skin and work upwards from the neck area towards the lower lip. You can use either side of your comb, or angle the comb at 45° to achieve shorter or longer lengths, depending on your client's requirements.

Some barbers prefer to use this technique to demonstrate their skills and personalise the look, but this is not always possible on thick or dense hair, so clipper-over-comb techniques might be used instead.

Clipper over comb

Clipper over comb is used in a similar way to scissor over comb, but produces quicker results. Using the clipper-over-comb technique still requires accuracy with your hand and comb balance, otherwise the result will be uneven.

Clipper over comb

Clippering with grade attachments

In the same way that you might clipper the back and sides of a haircut with clipper grades attached to clippers, you can do so for beard-trimming. When the desired length has been agreed, attach the appropriate clipper grades and work through the facial hair from the neck upwards. When you have cut the beard or moustache to length, remove any unwanted hair outside the outline of the shape by removing the clipper grades and cutting the hair against the skin.

Clipper grades range from grade 1 – the shortest – up to grade 8 – the largest. Each grade leaves the hair longer by about 3mm, starting from 3mm up to 24–25mm – refer to Chapter CB2 for more information.

Freehand

Use freehand to finalise the detail of the shape; to create a blunt line above the lip, shape and blend into the sideburn area or enhance the outline shape of the beard or moustache. Take extra care when you are cutting near the ears and especially around the lip area, as the skin might not be as easy to see through the hair growth and you might cut your client.

Providing advice and recommendations

As with every service that you provide, you must offer aftercare advice to your client. This should include which products to use at home (including products for exfoliation), recommendations for any equipment for home maintenance, how to maintain the current look, which additional services are available for your client and when he should return for his next appointment.

Products

You should recommend to your client that he regularly exfoliates the skin outside the facial hair shape to prevent any ingrowing hairs or the increased risk of 'barber's itch'. Show your client how to carry out this exfoliating treatment, suggesting how often and demonstrating the products that are available for him to purchase and use at home in between salon visits.

If your client suffers with dry skin and very coarse beard hair, you can recommend shampoos and conditioners to be used on the beard; this will work for full beards only. Equally, for clients with less facial hair or those that close shave more regularly, you can suggest a gent's skincare range to help moisturise the face.

Equipment and maintenance

If the style requires minimal trimming on a regular basis, it is likely that your client will want to maintain this himself in between visits.

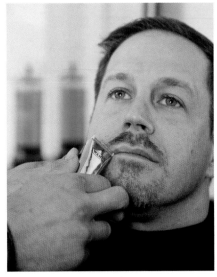

Freehand using mini-clippers

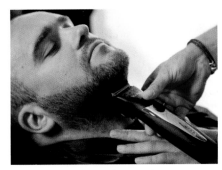

Clippering with grade attachments

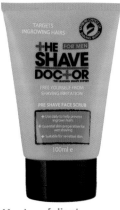

Men's exfoliant

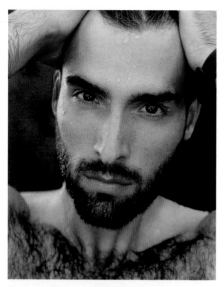

A clean-shaven neckline

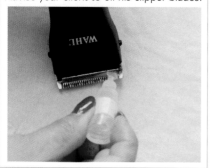

Suggest which clippers or razors he should use if he is removing most of his facial hair. Demonstrate the areas of the cheek or neck that he should clipper cut, explaining how to do it and advise how often he should do it.

The hairiness of men varies from person to person. Men with very hairy chests might need guidance on where to stop shaving the neck hair before it becomes removal of chest hair. A clean-shaven neckline can help to lessen the overall look of a hairy chest.

Additional services

Shaving styles for men are very individual and personal; some clients like to personalise their beards. This might be in the form of colouring or bleaching their facial hair. If your salon offers this service, discuss with your client any ideas you have for making his beard individual to him.

Recommending when to re-book

The recommendations you make will very much depend on the style you have created. Maintaining a more rugged look requires more regular upkeep, otherwise the rugged look quickly becomes a scruffy look. These styles might need grooming every three days or so. A full-beard style might last from three to five weeks depending on the length of the beard and the rate of hair growth; you will need to personalise this part of the service to suit every individual look and every individual client. As with head hair, facial hair growth is about 1.25cm per month.

Provide facial hair cutting services

In this part of the chapter you will look at how to provide the facial cutting services and how to cut facial hair to create many different looks.

Prepare for cutting services

As your client arrives you must follow your salon requirements for gowning and protecting your client to ensure their clothing, skin and eyes are protected from hair cuttings. You will also need to prepare the facial hair for the service.

Work safely and hygienically

Throughout the facial hair cutting service remember to:

■ maintain responsibilities for health and safety

■ use your time effectively and work to commercially viable times

- prepare your tools in advance of the service and keep your work area clean and tidy
- take care with your cutting tools and follow MFIs, supplier and workplace instructions
- prevent cross-contamination by working safely and hygienically
- sweep the floor during and after the service
- dispose of waste in an environmentally friendly manner
- check the positioning of your client throughout
- maintain a good body posture
- remove loose hair cuttings from your client to maintain their comfort.

Consult with clients

Always carry out an in-depth consultation with your client to ascertain what the client would like. Establish any factors that may affect the service – checking the hair classifications, hair characteristics, the head and face shape, the client's wishes and their style requirements. Ensure you check for any ingrowing hairs, adverse skin conditions and facial piercings, and check the client's skin elasticity.

Before you commence the cut confirm with your client, in client-friendly language, the look you have both agreed.

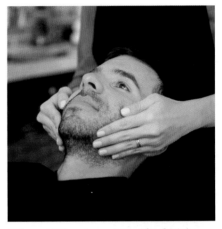

Offer additional services, like facial massage

Select products, tools and equipment

From the outcome of the consultation select the appropriate products, tools and equipment you will need for the service and complete the preparation of your work area.

Carry out cutting services

Remove excess bulk

When you are cutting a full beard, it is advisable to remove all excess bulk from the beard first, so that you can see the natural hairline of the facial hair. When this is done, you can cut in your outline shape, with either clippers or mini-clippers.

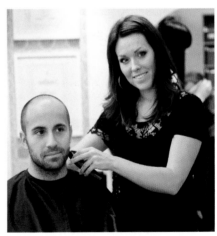

Work in a methodical manner

Establish and follow guidelines

When cutting the beard or moustache, you must work in a methodical manner – establish a cutting guideline and ensure you follow it throughout. It is important to always use your mirrors to make sure the cut is even and balanced, and regularly cross-check your cut.

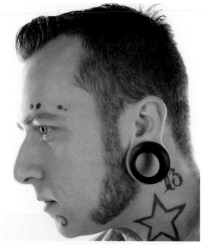

Sideburns

Outline shapes

With so many beard and moustache designs and styles to choose from, make sure you do not forget to discuss with your client the finer details, such as the hairline and outline finish.

Beards generally mean chin and cheek hair. Therefore the hair on the neck is often cut back to the skin or much shorter than the beard length itself. You will need to check the following with your client: does he want a full beard? Where does he want the cheek and the neck hair to stop and be blended out to? If he has sideburns, does he want them blended into the beard or left longer?

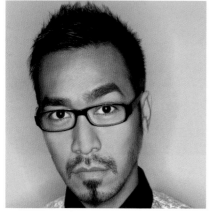

Partial beard

Does he want a partial beard – facial hair that is neither a full beard nor a moustache?

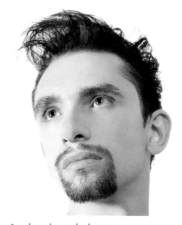

Anchor beard shape

Would he like an anchor beard shape – a beard shaped like an anchor from the centre of the bottom lip and around and up the chin?

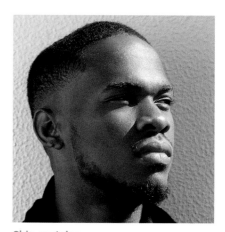

Chin curtains

Does he want a chin curtain – beard hair that travels from ear to ear along the chin but does not meet up with the lower lip or have an accompanying moustache?

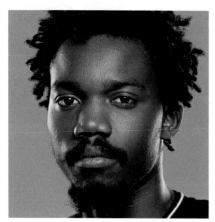

Goatee

Does he want a goatee – a narrow beard which sits under the mouth and around the chin and is not attached to a moustache?

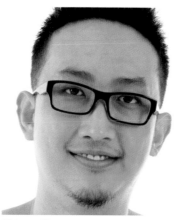

Chin puff

Would he prefer a chin puff – a narrower version of the goatee?

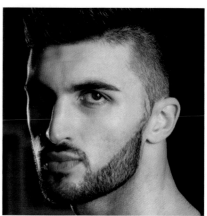

Stubble

Does he want stubble – a neatened, several-day full-beard growth?

With so many beard and moustache options to choose from, ensure you discuss with your client the cheek hair, neck hairline, sideburns and moustache shapes and hairlines. When you have agreed where you are cutting to along the natural hairline, make sure you remove all the hair outside of this outline shape.

Activity

Research the following facial hair shapes and create a facial hair style book.

- Pharaoh – a beard starting from the base of the chin, it can be any length.
- Curtain rail – a narrow beard following the **mandible**.
- Lipline moustache – a horizontal moustache about the width of a pencil.
- Mexican moustache – a moustache following the natural line of the upper lip and extending down towards the chin.
- Pencil moustache – a narrow moustache following the natural line of the upper lip.
- Rooftop moustache – a moustache that extends from under the nose to form a straight '**chevron**' shape.

Mandible

Jawbone.

Chevron

V-shaped stripe.

Step by steps

HANDY HINT

Remember that the angles in which the cutting tools and the head are positioned will affect weight distribution, balance and degree of graduation of the facial hair.

Goatee-tapered beardline using scissor-over-comb

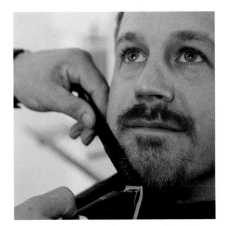

STEP 1 – Remove the excess length with the clipper-over-comb technique.

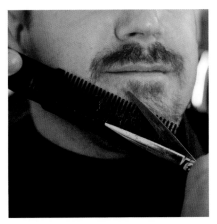

STEP 2 – Shape the goatee beard and cut to the desired length with the scissor-over-comb technique.

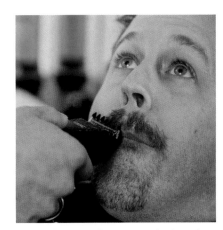

STEP 3 – Trim the moustache length with clippers and grades.

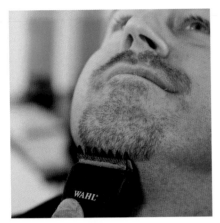

STEP 4 – Trim the goatee using clippers and grades.

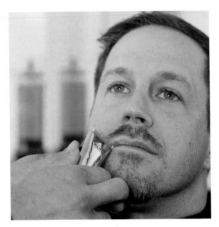

STEP 5 – Use mini-clippers to create the lipline shape.

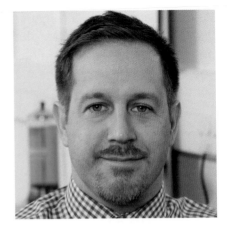

STEP 6 – Check your client is happy with the finished result.

HANDY HINT

Cross-check the cut to ensure the finished look is symmetrical and even in shape and density. Check the weight distribution, and balance.

HANDY HINT

Ask your client to move their head for you so you can follow all the contours of the neck and face shapes and remove any unwanted hair outside the desired outline shape.

Activity

Practise cutting a goatee beard on a practice head block.

Full beard using clippers with grades using clipper-over-comb

You can cut full beards by using uniform layers on longer beards, or scissor- or clipper-over-comb techniques on shorter, full beards as shown below.

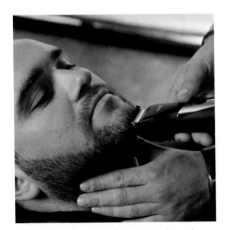

STEP 1 – Remove the excess length from the beard.

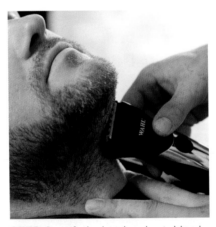

STEP 2 – Lift the head and cut, blend or remove the length under the chin.

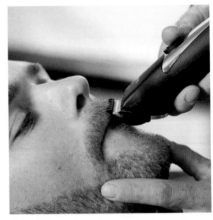

STEP 3 – Trim the moustache to the agreed length.

HANDY HINT

Make final visual checks to ensure the finished cut is accurate.

HANDY HINT

Work with the natural growth patterns of facial hair and consider the weight distribution within the facial haircut.

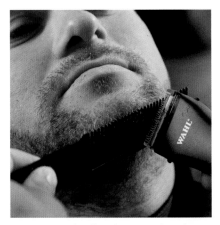

STEP 4 – Blend and personalise the facial hair with clipper-over-comb techniques.

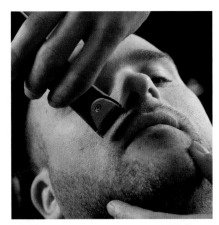

STEP 5 – Personalise the moustache outline.

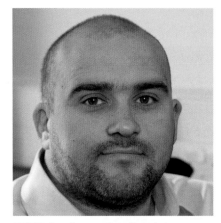

STEP 6 – Ensure the client is happy with the finished look.

Freehand traditional moustache

HANDY HINT

At the end of every facial haircut, ask your client if he would like his eyebrows trimmed! Some clients are surprised by this question, but reassure them that eyebrows are also facial hair, and trimming them enhances the whole image of the beard and moustache.

Activity

Practise cutting a full beard on a training head block.

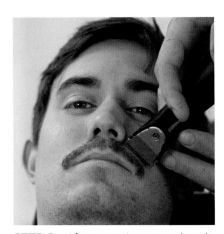

STEP 1 – After removing excess length with scissor-over-comb techniques, create the top lipline shape with mini-clippers.

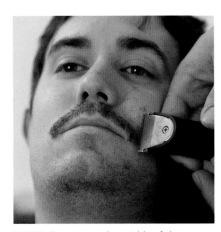

STEP 2 – Agree the width of the moustache and use clippers, blade down onto the face.

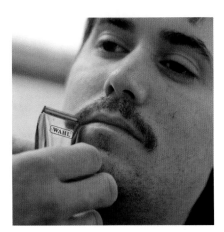

STEP 3 – Check the balance on both sides.

STEP 4 – Create the bottom lipline and shape to personalise the moustache.

Current fashion moustache and beard

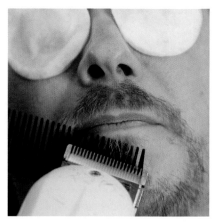

STEP 1 – Before commencing, lift the chin upwards for ease of working.

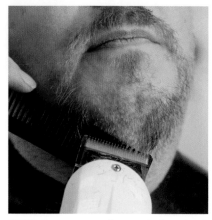

STEP 2 – Remove the excess length of the beard with the clipper-over-comb technique.

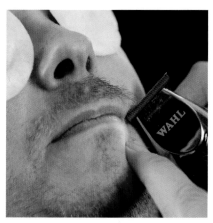

STEP 3 – Remove the beard length under the lipline using the clipper-over-comb technique.

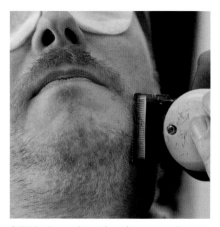

STEP 4 – Adjust the clipper grade length and remove the unwanted facial hair.

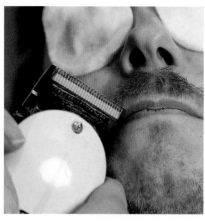

STEP 5 – Tilt the clippers to the side and create the lipline moustache length required.

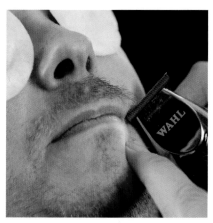

STEP 6 – Using the mini-clippers, define the lipline shape.

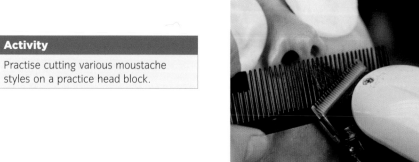

STEP 7 – Using the clipper-over-comb technique, remove the moustache length.

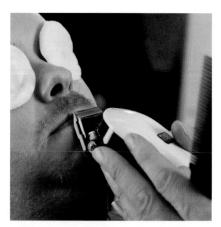

STEP 8 – Check the moustache length is defined before you show the client the end result.

Straight line top-lip moustache using clippers

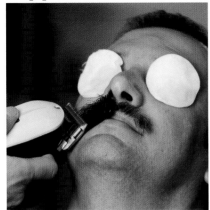

STEP 1 – Cut the length of the moustache with the clipper-over-comb technique.

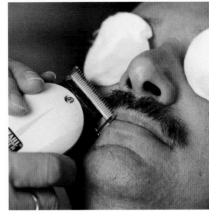

STEP 2 – Remove the outline length from the bottom of the lipline using a freehand technique with clippers.

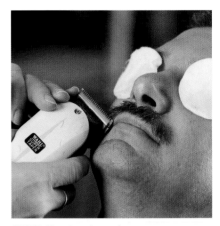

STEP 3 – Continue the process.

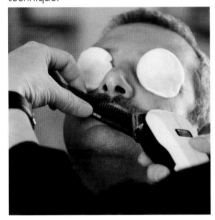

STEP 4 – With the new shape in place check the internal lengths are cut to the agreed length using clipper-over-comb techniques.

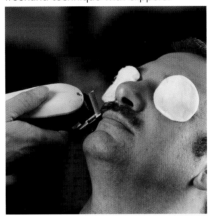

STEP 5 – Agree the width of the moustache and cut using a freehand technique with clippers.

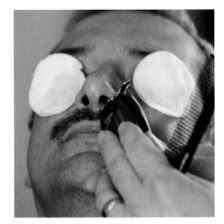

STEP 6 – Check the moustache for balance on both sides, tidy up any loose hairs and show the finished result to your client.

Eyebrow grooming

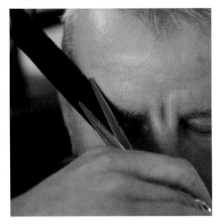

STEP 1 – Using either clipper- or scissor-over-comb techniques, remove excess length.

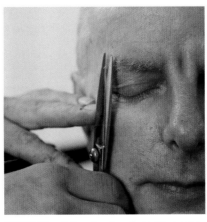

STEP 2 – Using freehand, remove any stray long eyebrows.

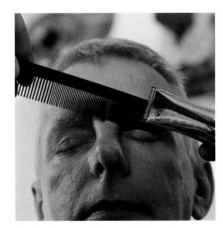

STEP 3 – Comb up and down the eyebrow to cut any stray long eyebrows.

Answers in the back of the book.

1 What is the most likely consequences of disposing of a used razor blade in the salon bin?

a Staff could suffer cuts and infections

b Staff could be at risk of losing their job

c The contents of the bin might spill

d The contents of the bin might infect others

2 Why should a barber's chair be used when cutting facial hair?

a To minimise the risk of cross-contamination of tools

b To ensure that the service can be carried out hygienically

c To keep the client comfortable and expose the whole face and neck

d To make sure the client is happy with the service and will pay the agreed price

3 What is the most likely result of failing to remove hair clippings from the face during the service?

a Infestations

b Allergies

c Infections

d Dermatitis

4 What are the limitations of using a UV light to sterilise tools?

a It does not remove infectious germs

b It does not disinfect

c It only lasts for twenty minutes

d It takes too long to clean

5 Why is it important to check underneath facial hair before starting the service?

a To give advice on skin care

b To check for skin disorders

c To minimise the risk of sensitivity

d To minimise the risk of cross-infection

6 How can very coarse, tightly curled facial hair impact the cutting service?

a It will always need razoring

b It always will need thinning

c It may need more careful cross-checking

d It may need more treatments to avoid patchiness

7 Which one of the following facial hair styles would best suit a client with a heavy-set chin?

a A full beard

b A thin moustache

c Chin curtains

d Short stubble

8 Which two of the following skin disorders are contagious?

1 Cold sores

2 Cysts

3 Skin tags

4 Impetigo

a 1 and 2

b 2 and 3

c 3 and 4

d 4 and 1

9 What is the best advice to give a client whose moles have increased in size?

a Refer to a pharmacist

b Refer to a trichologist

c Refer to the manager

d Refer to a GP

10 What is the cause of the common facial cyst?

a Fungus

b Bacteria

c Infected follicles

d Blocked sebaceous glands

CH4 COLOUR AND LIGHTEN HAIR

Colouring is one of the most exciting, creative, profitable and challenging services in hairdressing. It is also one of the most popular services offered in salons. Colouring the hair adds texture, style and creativity to individualise a look. The service you offer and the skills you develop in colouring will be among the most important you learn. The theory you learn in colouring will be useful throughout your hairdressing career, so maximise your potential by mastering these colouring skills.

After reading this chapter you will:

- know how health and safety affects colouring and lightening services
- understand the factors that influence hair colouring and lightening services
- understand the products and techniques used in colouring and lightening services
- understand the science of colouring and lightening services
- be able to colour and lighten hair.

Health and safety

You've already looked at your professional and salon/stylist image in the health and safety and salon policies chapter, but let's revisit these areas specifically for the colouring service.

Your responsibilities for health and safety

When colouring or lightening hair you may be using permanent colours, lighteners and **hydrogen peroxide** in various strengths, so health and safety is very important. Always carry out thorough consultations with your clients, checking the hair and scalp condition and carrying out all relevant tests. You must follow the manufacturers' instructions and protect both your client and yourself.

You must always adhere to all the health and safety Acts; but during a colour service you must pay particular attention to the Control of Substances Hazardous to Health Regulations (COSHH).

When mixing, using and applying colours, ensuring you follow:

- the manufacturers' instructions (MFIs)
- local by-laws
- your salon's policies and procedures.

This includes wearing personal protective equipment (PPE) and:

- **S**toring chemicals and substances correctly
- **H**andling chemicals and substances correctly
- **U**sing chemicals and substances correctly
- **D**isposing of chemicals and substances correctly.

SHUD derives from the rules of COSHH.

PPE and protective products

Always wear your personal protective equipment (PPE). It is important to protect your hands from contact dermatitis and to protect your clothes from damage when colouring. Remember to clean off any products from your skin immediately, dry your hands and apply a moisturiser or barrier cream to them for extra protection against dermatitis.

Hydrogen peroxide

The solution that activates the colouring product to allow the colouring process to take place.

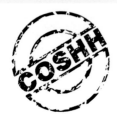

HANDY HINT

SHUD – what you **SHOULD** do when using chemicals.

HEALTH & SAFETY

Refer to the health and safety and salon policies chapter for a recap on the health and safety Acts you must follow when colouring and lightening hair.

HANDY HINT

Remember - PPE is your personal protective equipment, not your client's!

PPE for the stylist and the assistant

This includes:

- gloves to protect your hands from chemicals and staining
- aprons to protect your clothes from chemical damage.

If you suffer with asthma or allergies, you should:

- wear a particle mask when mixing or using colours and lightening powders to prevent inhaling substances
- wear eye protection when mixing colours and lightening powders to prevent chemicals from entering the eyes.

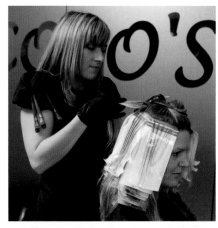

Gloves and apron on!

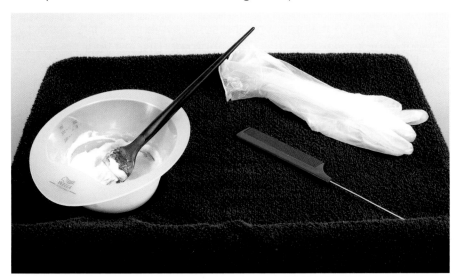

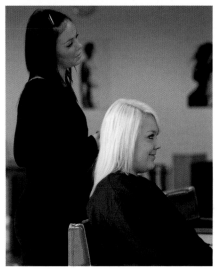

Gowned client

Protection for your client

Protective clothing is used to protect your client's clothing and to protect your clothes and hands.

Protect your client suitably for the service required.

Always use:

- a fresh clean towel
- a fresh clean gown
- a plastic/disposable cape or another fresh clean towel (this may vary depending on your salon requirements).

A client must wear a gown during a chemical service to protect their clothes; and to prevent skin staining, some salons apply barrier cream around the client's hairline and ears when applying dark shades of colour directly onto the scalp.

HANDY HINT

When you are ready to start the colour service, always check that your client is balanced and comfortable. Ensure your client's feet can either reach the floor or a footrest and that their back is supported against the back of the chair.

HANDY HINT

Bad news always travels more quickly than good news! Look after your clients when colouring their hair and respect their belongings.

Personal hygiene and presentation

Make sure all areas are hygienic and ready for the client. Poor standards of health and hygiene can offend your clients, spread germs and cause cross-contamination. Always seek guidance from your manager before going to work if you have a potentially infectious condition.

Always make sure you are well presented. Your own hairstyle and colour should be an advertisement and selling point for the salon. You should always have clean styled hair and represent your salon's image.

> **Activity**
>
> List four ways to maintain your personal hygiene. List five things about your appearance that are important. Discuss your answers with your supervisor or tutor.

Legal requirements regarding age restrictions

In November 2012 a new European Union (EU) directive came into force prohibiting certain colours and chemicals being used on any person under the age of 16.

The two restricted chemicals used in hair colours are:

- HC Orange No 2
- 2-hydroxyethylamino-5-nitroanisole.

Manufacturers using products containing these chemicals are required to ensure their labelling includes the phrase, 'This product is not intended for use on persons under the age of 16'.

Colours that are mixed with hydrogen peroxide are also not permitted for use for clients under the age of 16.

> **Activity**
>
> Research your salon's product range to identify which products state, 'This product is not intended for use on persons under the age of 16' in the manufacturers' instructions.

HANDY HINT

When mixing chemicals and products, always wear your PPE and mix in a well-ventilated area. Remember to follow COSHH and SHUD, and safely measure your peroxide and other liquids at eye level to ensure accurate measurements.

Hazards and risks

Almost anything can be a hazard in the salon and it is your responsibility, along with your employer, to prevent these hazards becoming risks to the safety of yourself and others. Maintaining a clean and tidy salon helps to reduce hazards.

A hazard is something with the potential to cause harm. A risk is the likelihood of the hazard's potential being realised. Chemicals are a hazard! If chemicals are not stored, handled and used correctly then they pose a risk to you and those around you.

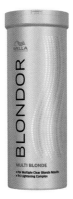

Powdered lightener

Activity

Observe a colour service and list all the potential hazards as you see them.

Dangers associated with powder lighteners

Inhaling the fine powders from lightening products can cause **respiratory problems**, particularly if you suffer from asthma or other lung-related health issues. To prevent any health issues, you should wear a particle mask and always mix the product in a well-ventilated area.

Inhaling

Breathing in.

Respiratory problems

Breathing problems.

Safe use of electrical equipment

Before using electrical items, ensure you check them visually for any cracks in the main body or plug. Check that the wires are tangle-free and not frayed. If you identify any problems or faults with electrical equipment, remove it from the salon, label it as faulty and report it to a senior member of staff.

HANDY HINT

Take care with powder lighteners – inhaling substances can cause respiratory problems.

Client preparation and safety considerations

When your client arrives, sit them comfortably at your workstation and carry out a thorough consultation.

During the consultation you need to identify:

- the age of the client (if you are not sure whether they are over 16)
- the client requirements
- their previous hair history
- any barriers to the service
- their hair and scalp condition
- whether the result will be achievable
- the best product, service and technique to use.

Safety procedures include:

- gowning and protecting your client and wear your PPE
- checking the hair and scalp for any factors that may affect the service
- preparing the hair for the service

- protecting the client's skin – using barrier cream where appropriate
- applying products cleanly to avoid spreading to client's skin, clothes and surrounding areas
- taking precautions to avoid inhalation of powder lighteners.

Dermatitis

When using colouring and lightening chemicals you are at more risk of developing dermatitis. Always protect your skin and wear gloves when:

- mixing chemicals
- rinsing tint bowls and brushes
- using colouring products
- removing colouring products from your client's hair
- mopping up spillages.

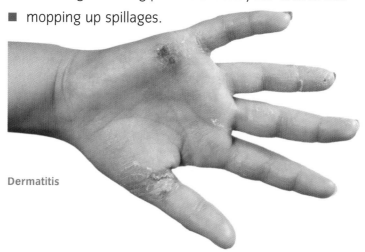

Dermatitis

Safe working practices

Safe working practices include:

- following all safety considerations
- positioning client and stylist correctly
- preventing any cross-contamination
- maintaining a hygienic, clean and tidy work area
- promoting environmental and sustainable working practices whilst working.

Positioning of client and stylist

You could be standing for long periods of time when colouring hair, so to ensure that you are comfortable throughout you must stand correctly. Your client may be sitting in one position for a couple of hours, so always check that they are comfortable too.

Keep an even balance through your body and avoid favouring one leg when you stand for long periods of time. Ensure your trolley is prepared in advance of the service and if right-handed, position your trolley to your right-hand side and vice versa if you are left-handed.

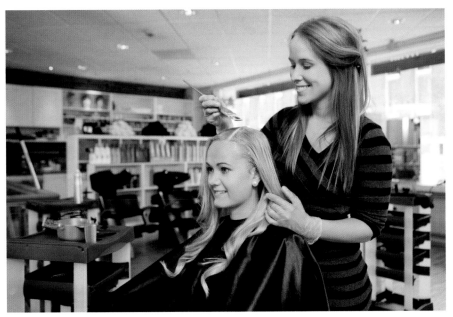

Trolley on right-hand side, stylist and client positioned appropriately

Sustainable working practices

When using chemical products we must consider the effects they have on the environment. Make sure you dispose of your colouring waste in an environmentally friendly manner.

Using products cost-effectively and minimising waste

Wasting products costs your salon money and in the long run this may cost you money too! The more money the salon makes, the bigger likelihood of a pay rise for you. Waste products also affect the environment.

Always mix your colours and lightening products following the instructions and consider the service you are carrying out, and the density and length of the client's hair.

At the end of the service, immediately remove waste products and dispose of them in the dedicated salon waste bin. Rinse any unused chemicals down the sink with plenty of water, following local by-laws and MFIs.

Activity

Using your maths skills, mix the correct amount of product to suit the length and density of the client's hair.

HEALTH & SAFETY

Refer to the section in the health and safety chapter about environmental and sustainable working practices for more information.

Activity

List three reasons why it is important to use products economically.

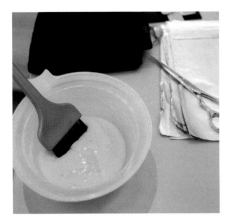

Mix the correct amount of product to suit the length and density of the client's hair

Preventing cross-infection and infestation

To prevent cross-infection and infestation you should maintain a clean and tidy work area, work safely and hygienically and clean, disinfect and sterilise your tools, equipment and work area after every client.

Clean and tidy working areas

A clean, well-prepared workstation will help you to sustain a hazard-free area and prevent cross-contamination. Work efficiently and maintain a professional image. Report any problems with tools and equipment to a senior member of staff, and inform the relevant person of any products that need re-ordering.

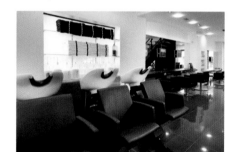

Clean and tidy salon

Always ensure your workstation and shampoo areas are clean and tidy. Wipe clean work surfaces and the basins, and then sterilise them with an anti-bacterial spray. At the end of the colour service, make sure any waste materials are disposed of in a lidded bin, tint bowls are cleaned and put away and all stains are removed from the basin, so the area is ready for the next client.

Working safely and hygienically

When colouring hair and using chemicals such as lightening products and hydrogen peroxide it is essential that you work safely. Spilling products on your skin can cause allergic reactions or burns, and incorrect storage such as leaving lids of bottles can put others at risk. Always mix colours in a ventilated area, follow the MFIs, wear your PPE and protect your client.

HEALTH & SAFETY

Always cover and protect any cuts or open wounds to prevent cross-contamination and further harm.

HEALTH & SAFETY

Refer to the health and safety chapter for more in-depth information on working safely and hygienically.

VALUES & BEHAVIOURS

Refer to the values and behaviours chapter for more in-depth information on sterilising and disinfecting.

HANDY HINT

Clean equipment with detergent and water, sterilise in an autoclave or an ultraviolet light and disinfect with chemical liquids such as a Barbicide solution.

Activity

Working in small groups or pairs, list all the safe and hygienic practices you can think of. Consider the safety of the salon, your client, yourself and others.

Methods of cleaning, disinfecting and sterilising

When mixing colours it is really important that your tint bowls and brushes are clean. If they are stained with previous colours, it may affect the resulting colour of your client's hair.

Tint bowls and brushes should be washed in warm soapy water and rinsed until the water runs clear. Test that the bristles of the tint brush are clean by wiping them on disposable paper towels, and checking that colour is not present – particularly near to the base of the bristles. Towels and gowns should be washed after every service.

Disinfect or sterilise bowls, brushes, work surfaces, combs, clips, re-usable colour-meches (if used) and all tools and equipment used in readiness for the next client.

Importance of questioning clients

The consultation process is a very important part of the service. Ask plenty of open questions to identify the client's requirements: what they are hoping for and their vision of the end result.

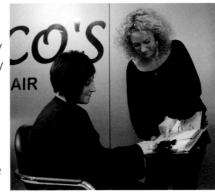
Consultation is very important

You should use visual aids, such as colour charts or magazines, to clarify that you both have the same vision. This will enable you to choose the most suitable products, techniques, tools and equipment to achieve their desired result.

Confirm desired result

Ensure that you use positive body language together with open and closed questions to identify your client's needs. When giving your client effective aftercare advice, maintain eye contact and speak politely and clearly.

Colouring services are one of the most popular services in the salon – clients colour their hair for many reasons and you'll need to identify which colouring service best meets the needs of your client.

Why do clients colour their hair?

- to cover white hair
- to darken
- to lighten
- to change the tonal colour
- to add texture and enhance the style
- to change their look.

Confirming the likely costs, duration and expected outcomes of the service

At the end of the consultation you and your client should be confident that the desired result is achievable. Before making a start, ensure that your client has been informed of the likely cost and duration of the service. This should include the development time and confirmation of the expected result.

Commercially viable service times for colouring

You need to complete your assessments and services within commercially viable times. This is important to enable you to work effectively in the salon once you are qualified. Your salon would have calculated the cost for each service, including material and labour costs; all services must be completed within an allocated time frame.

WHY DON'T YOU...
Compare these colouring service times to your salon requirements and note any variation.

Guide times for typical colouring services

Colouring service	Guide to service time
Temporary	This type of colour service is included in the hairdressing service time, as temporary colour is applied as normal mousses, setting lotions or water-based colour rinses
Semi-permanent/ quasi-permanent	Application time around 15–30 minutes including consultation, shampooing and product application Additional development time around 20 minutes (see MFIs) Total service time 35–50 minutes
Regrowth permanent	Application time around 30–40 minutes including consultation, product preparation and application Additional development time around 30–50 minutes (see MFIs) Total service time 60–90 minutes
Full-head permanent colour	Application time around 50–60 minutes including consultation, product preparation and application Additional development time around 30–50 minutes (see MFIs) Total service time 80–110 minutes
Pulled-through highlights	Application time around 30–40 minutes including consultation, technique application, product preparation and application Additional development time around 30–50 minutes (see MFIs) Total service time 60–90 minutes
Full-head highlights	Application time around 90 minutes including consultation, product preparation and application Additional development time around 30–50 minutes (see MFIs) Total service time 120–140 minutes
Partial head highlights	Application time around 60 minutes including consultation, product preparation and application Additional development time around 30–50 minutes (see MFIs) Total service time 90–110 minutes

Activity

Using your salon price list, work out the cost and duration of Wendy and Nicky's services.

You can work individually, in pairs or small groups.

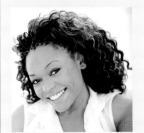

Wendy

Wendy wants a half head of woven highlights, with a cut and blow dry.

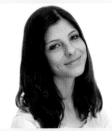

Nikki

Nikki wants a full-head quasi-permanent colour and a finger dry.

HANDY HINT

Allocating time frames to each service means that the charge to the client covers all relevant costs, enabling the salon to reach profitability and be commercially viable.

Factors that may influence services

You need to look at the following factors during your consultation. Many factors affect natural and artificial hair colour, causing damage or the colours and tones to fade from the hair. Make sure you consider these factors when you add colour, as they determine the types of product, service and technique you may use.

These factors include the:

- hair classifications – straight, wavy, curly or very curly hair
- hair characteristics – condition, porosity, elasticity, density and texture
- length of hair
- temperature
- existing hair colour
- percentage of white hair
- test results
- strength of hydrogen peroxide
- skin tone
- time interval from last perm or relaxer
- recent removal of hair extensions.

HANDY HINT

You will be using your maths skills when you:
- estimate the length of hair
- estimate the percentage of white hair
- work out the strength of hydrogen peroxide required.

HANDY HINT

For more information on hair characteristics and classification, see chapter CHB9.

HANDY HINT

You will be using your maths skills when you:

- estimate the length of hair
- estimate the percentage of white hair
- work out the strength of hydrogen peroxide required.

Pre-soften

A technique where 6% liquid peroxide is applied to the hair before the tint application to open the cuticle. For more information on pre-softening hair, see 'Covering white hair' (later in this chapter).

Hair classifications

Hair classifications refer to how straight, wavy, curly or very curly your client's hair is.

Straight hair

Fine or thin straight hair tends to be very soft, shiny and sometimes oily. Oily hair will need to be pre-shampooed prior to the colour application to ensure there are no barriers to the colour.

When colouring hair that is coarse and straight, highlighting and lowlighting techniques can help to add texture to a hairstyle, so recommending this technique may benefit the client depending on the hairstyle worn.

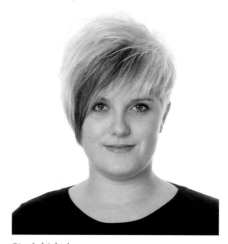

Straight hair

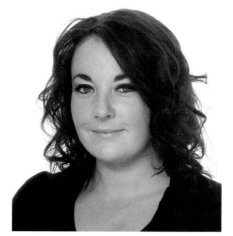

Wavy hair

Wavy hair

Wavy hair can sometimes be frizzy too; you'll need to consider this, especially if you are contemplating using a lightening product on the hair. Coarse wavy hair can be resistant. If white hair is present too, you may need to **pre-soften** the hair to ensure coverage of the white hair.

Curly hair

Loose and tight curls tend to have a combination texture. This may affect the condition of the hair, so consider what products would ideally suit the hair's condition and texture. This type of hair can often be thick and abundant, so more product may be required. If you are carrying out woven highlights, it can be more difficult to secure the colour meches or foils near the root, so you may wish to straighten the hair before you start the service. Some curls can also be frizzy, so you may recommend avoiding lightening products where possible.

Curly hair

Very curly hair

Hair that is very curly, whether soft or wiry, tends to be very fragile and is likely to tangle easily. Curly hair and very curly hair are more susceptible to cuticle damage because of their shape. The curly pattern causes bends in the hair and this in turn raises the cuticles. Curly hair can be highly porous, as the natural hair oils (sebum) cannot travel the length of the hair shaft as easily as they can on straight hair. It is very important to use pH-balancing products on curly hair to help keep the cuticle closed and maintain a pH of 4.5 to 5.5.

If you are weaving the hair or carrying out pulled-through highlights you may need to shampoo and dry the hair into a smoother style, otherwise these techniques may cause your client discomfort. Always consider which products will best suit the fragile hair.

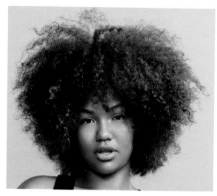

Very curly hair

Hair characteristics

Hair characteristics refer to the hair's condition, porosity, elasticity, density, texture and growth patterns.

Hair characteristic	Influence on service
Condition	The hair's condition may be very strong and resistant, so, for example, pre-softening may be required if covering white hair or a stronger developer if using a quasi-permanent colour. If the hair's condition is poor and weak, non-chemical colours should be used and recommended.
Porosity	Porous hair will restrict your choice of products, as lightening products may cause damage. Resistant, non-porous hair may require longer development times for permanent hair colouring products. Uneven porosity may result in an uneven colour, so you need to consider what products and services will be suitable.
Elasticity	If the hair is weak in elasticity then you will need to avoid using chemicals on the hair. Semi-permanent products will add shine to the hair. Conditioning treatments prior to the service will help prepare the hair for future services.
Density	The density of your client's hair will determine which techniques you use, how much product is required and how long the service may take to complete. You may need to adapt the size of your sections or weaves. Fine weaves in abundant hair result in a subtle colour and thick weaves on finer hair could create a heavily highlighted effect, which may not suit the client's requirements.
Texture	Texture is the fineness or thickness of each hair. A client may have fine hair but a lot of it, or coarse, thick hair that is sparse. The texture of the hair may affect the amount of product required, the time the service takes to complete and the size of your sections when colouring the hair.

Hair characteristic	Influence on service
Growth pattern	Not many hair growth patterns affect the colouring and lightening services but it is advisable to work with any strong hair movement – rather than try to fight it.
	Identifying the growth patterns will help you work with natural partings in the hair and identify how the client wears their hair.
	Trying to hold a foil in place during woven highlights on a cowlick or going against a widow's peak can cause the stylist problems. Adapt your sectioning patterns to work with any hair growth patterns or strong movement in the hair.

Length of hair

The length of your client's hair will determine which techniques you use, how much product is required and how long the service may take to complete.

Temperature

Warmer or cooler temperatures can have an effect on colouring development times. Warmth speeds up development times and lightening products develop more quickly under heat. Cooler temperatures, on the other hand, increase development time.

Accelerators generate heat, adding to the heat naturally arising from the head. If you are completing a full-head colouring service, you may need to start your application at the mid-lengths and ends of the hair because these are furthest away from the source of heat (ie the head). After allowing the mid-lengths and ends to develop for 20 minutes, start the root application, so that the whole head colour develops evenly.

Accelerator

An electrical appliance used to provide heat, accelerating or speeding up development.

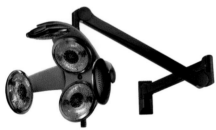

Accelerators reduce development time by about 50%.

HANDY HINT

- Cool temperatures increase colour development time.
- Warm temperatures reduce colour development time.

Activity

Using your salon brand of colouring and lightening products, identify how using heat/accelerators affects the development time and note your answers. Using your maths skills, identify how much time could be saved each day by using heat, if a stylist carried out an average of three colours per day.

Existing hair colour

You must consider the existing hair colour to identify the following:

- Is the colour of the hair natural or artificial?
- How many shades of lift are required to achieve the target shade?
- Can you use tint to achieve the required lift or do you need to use a lightening product?
- What is the tone of the hair?
- Is the target shade lighter, darker or the same depth as the existing shade?
- Has the previous colour faded?

Percentage of white hair

This is important because the percentage of white hair can affect the products used and services available to the client. When colouring white hair, you must consider the following:

- Is there white hair? Is it strong and resistant? Do you need to pre-soften the hair?
- Does your client want a semi-permanent colour? Will it blend enough white hair?
- Does your client want a quasi-colour? Will it cover enough white hair?
- Does your client want a permanent colour to cover 100% white hair?

Test results

You must consider the results of all hair and skin tests carried out to ensure the client will not suffer an allergic reaction and that the hair is suitable for the service.

HANDY HINT

For more details and information on the necessary tests, see chapter CHB9.

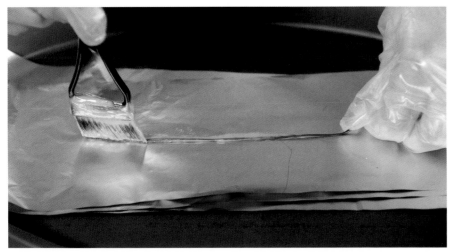

Colour test on a strand of hair

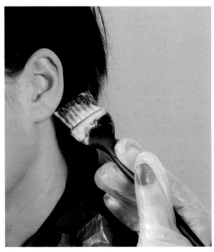

Skin test

Strength of hydrogen peroxide

Hydrogen peroxide and developers can be used to lighten or darken the hair depending on the strength used. (Refer to the table 'Strengths of peroxide and their uses' later in the chapter.)

Skin tone

You need to check that the client's chosen hair colour will complement their skin tone. To help identify whether a client's skin tone is warm or cool, you should look for some tell-tale signs.

In general, natural redheads, reddish golden browns, deep browns and golden blonde hair colours have warmer complexions. Their skin may be paler with pink, peach, copper or gold undertones. People from Latin America, Africa or Europe with freckled complexions generally have warm tones. Depending on the hair's depth, colours such as caramel, copper and yellow-gold suit warm skin tones.

For cooler skin tones – skin that is pale to medium with little colour in the cheeks – look for hair colours that are naturally bluish-black, dark brown or medium ash blonde. Cool red colours, such as burgundy, suit true olive skin, such as some Asian and Mediterranean skin, as the hair is naturally dark. Naturally lighter hair would require lighter cool ash shades.

Time interval from last perm or relaxer

Previous services can affect the condition and the result of your colouring service. If your client has recently had a perm or relaxing service you should not use colouring chemicals on the hair for a couple of weeks, longer if the condition does not allow. However, a semi-permanent colour may be applied directly after a perm or relaxer service and could replace any tone that has been lost due to the chemicals in the perm or relaxer.

Recent removal of hair extensions

Clip-in hair extensions rarely cause any damage to the hair, so colouring services are not affected.

If your client has recently had woven or bonded extensions removed, the hair and scalp may be too delicate for a colouring service. Extensions can damage the hair if the client does not follow the correct aftercare advice or if they are left in too long.

For bonded hair extensions a releaser solution or **acetone** is applied to the resin bond to dissolve it and release the extension from the hair. Some manufacturers allow colouring products to be applied immediately after the removal of hair extensions, as long as the hair

HANDY HINT

Red or flushed complexions will look redder if you colour the hair with red or warm tones. Pale complexions will look even paler if you colour the hair with darker tones.

HANDY HINT

Always check the manufacturers' instructions for guidance on when you can colour or lighten the hair after a perm or relaxer service.

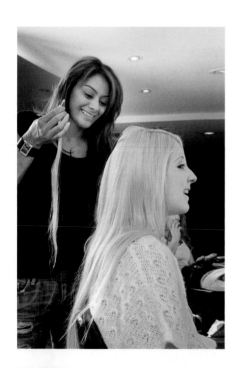

Acetone

A chemical solvent.

is cleansed with a detoxing shampoo (to remove the acetone from the hair) prior to the colour application.

Ideally, after the removal of hair extensions, additional chemical services should be avoided for a week or two if possible, even longer if the hair is damaged or the scalp is sensitive. Always check with your supplier and manufacturers' instructions before applying a colour service.

You must consider all of these factors to ensure that the colour suits the client and doesn't affect the hair by damaging the cuticle and the inner cortex. The cuticle must be smooth and in good condition to be able to sustain further chemical treatments. The cuticle is opened during chemical services to allow the colour to penetrate into the cortex. If the cuticle is rough and raised, the hair is porous, which could affect the colouring result or cause further damage to the hair.

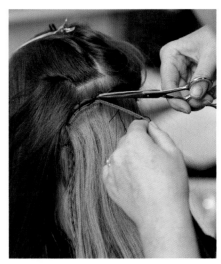

Removal of sewn-in extensions

Products, tools and equipment

Colouring and lightening products

When colouring and lightening hair there is a vast range of products to choose from:

- temporary colours
- semi-permanent colours
- quasi-permanent colours
- permanent colours
- lightening products.

Choosing suitable colouring products

You must choose the most suitable products for your client's requirements, and the products you choose to colour your client's hair will depend on the reason they are having their hair coloured. The table that follows shows which products are most suitable for your client's requirements.

WHY DON'T YOU...
Carry out a survey on ten clients to identify their reasons for colouring their hair. Compare their answers to the examples listed in the tables that follow.

Colouring product	Lasting effects	Coverage of white hair	Levels of lift achievable	Hydrogen peroxide strengths (developers)
Temporary colour	1 shampoo	Blend only	None – add tone only.	Not applicable
Semi-permanent colour	6–8 shampoos	Blend only	None – darken or add tone only.	Not applicable

Colouring product	Lasting effects	Coverage of white hair	Levels of lift achievable	Hydrogen peroxide strengths (developers)
Quasi-permanent colour	12–24 shampoos	50% as a guide	None – darken or add tone only.	The developer used in quasi-permanent colours is actually a weak peroxide – as a guide 3% or 10 volume
Permanent colour	Permanent	Up to 100%	Depending on the natural depth of hair and peroxide strength, lifts up to three shades. Also darkens and deposits tone.	3% or 10 volume 6% or 20 volume 9% or 30 volume 12% or 40 volume
High-lift tint	Permanent	Blend only	Depending on the natural depth of hair and peroxide strength, lifts up to four to five shades. Also deposits tone.	9% or 30 volume 12% or 40 volume
Lightening products (bleach)	Permanent	Blend only	Depending on the depth of hair and peroxide strength, lifts up to six shades. Also removes tone.	For on-scalp techniques, 6% only and for off-scalp techniques: 6% or 20 volume 9% or 30 volume 12% or 40 volume
Toners	Semi-permanent	Blend only	None – they are used to remove unwanted tone only.	Varied options – you can use 6% or 20 volume but generally 3% or 10 volume developer is used, or a true semi can be used.

HANDY HINT

For more information on peroxide strengths and calculations, for example '10 volume' or percentages, see 'Strengths of peroxide' under 'Products, tools and equipment' later in the chapter.

Non-commitment colouring services

Temporary and semi-permanent colours are referred to as non-commitment colours. They are pH 4.5–5.5, so their acidity is the same as that of the hair and skin and therefore do not affect the cuticle or the cortex.

Temporary colouring products

You apply these products directly to the hair before or after styling. They're available as mousses, lotions, gels, sprays, rinses, creams and even hair mascaras. They stain the hair and are used in the same way as styling products. Mousses, gels, lotions, rinses and creams are usually applied to wet hair, and sprays and hair mascaras to dry hair. Temporary colours are removed from the hair with the next shampoo.

The following table shows why your clients may or may not choose a temporary colour service.

Reasons to have temporary colour	Reasons not to have temporary colour
No commitment	Only lasts one shampoo
Lasts only one shampoo	No lift possible
Adds shine	Colour may be uneven or last longer in porous hair
Adds tone	
Neutralises unwanted tone	
No harsh chemicals	
Enhances current look	
Introduction to colour	
Quick fashion effect	
No development time	

Always follow the MFIs when using colouring products and wear PPE to prevent staining the skin and damaging your clothes.

> **HANDY HINT**
>
> Hair mascaras are used to paint colour onto the hair, to add texture and create a highlighted effect.

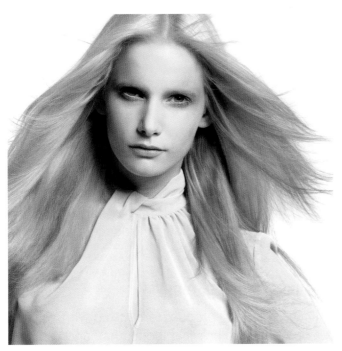

Temporary colour 'painted in' to hair

Semi-permanent colouring products

These conditioning colours generally come in liquid or cream form and can be applied directly to pre-shampooed hair. Apply them either from the bottle or by measuring the product into a bowl and applying with a sponge or brush. Semi-permanent products are rinsed from the hair after the development time. Following the manufacturers' instructions, apply a conditioner if required.

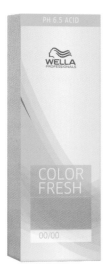

Semi-permanent colour

The following table shows why your clients may or may not choose a semi-permanent colour service.

Reasons to have semi-permanent colour	Reasons not to have semi-permanent colour
No commitment	Lasts only six to eight shampoos
Introduction to colour	Vibrancy of colour gradually fades with each shampoo
Full-head coverage	No lift possible
No regrowth	Colour can only blend white hair
Lasts only six to eight shampoos	Colour may be uneven or 'grab' in porous hair which means the colour molecules will attach to the cuticles and last longer than they are intended to
Adds shine, tone and depth	
Neutralises unwanted tone	
Can be used for colour correction services	
No harsh chemicals	
Skin test is not always required (but always check MFIs)	
Mostly hypoallergenic	
Enhances current look and refreshes existing colour	
Quick service and fashion effect	
Blends up to 20% of white hair	

Commitment colouring services

Quasi, permanent and lightening products are alkaline; therefore they lift the cuticle during development and affect the cortex. As these colours have a long-lasting effect on the hair, they demand a commitment to colour. These colours introduce a developing agent or peroxide to the colour.

Quasi-permanent colouring products

Quasi-permanent colouring products are mixed with a developer (mild or weak peroxide) to pre-shampooed hair and can be applied either straight from an applicator bottle or using a bowl and brush/sponge.

The following table shows why your clients may or may not choose a quasi-permanent colour service.

Reasons to have quasi-permanent colour	Reasons not to have quasi-permanent colour
Adds depth and tone	No lift possible
Covers up to 50% white hair	Overuse can lead to a regrowth area
Lasts 12–24 shampoos	Skin test is required
Introduction to permanent colour	Contains chemicals
Weaker chemicals used	Colours gradually fade
Used for colour correction	
Fashion colours	
Refreshes faded colours	

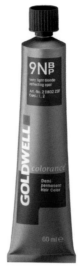

Quasi-permanent colour

Permanent and high-lift tints

Permanent and high-lift tints are generally supplied in 60ml tubes and are always mixed with peroxide. You apply them to clean, dry hair using a bowl and brush.

The following table shows why your clients may or may not choose a permanent or high-lift colour service.

Reasons to have permanent/high-lift colours	Reasons not to have permanent/high-lift colours
Adds depth and tone	The result is permanent
Lightens by up to three shades for permanent colours	Skin test is required
Lightens by up to four or five shades for high-lift colours	Contains chemicals
Permanent colours can cover up to 100% white hair	Vibrant tones gradually fade
Used for fashion effects (foils)	Committed to colour
Permanent result	Regrowth occurs every four to six weeks
Used for colour correction	
Fashion/vibrant colours	
Change of image	
Adds texture	
Covers regrowth	

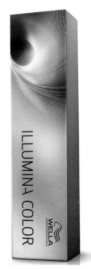

Permanent colour

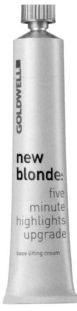

High-lift tint

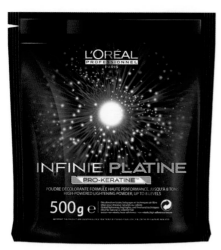

Lightener powder

Consistency

Density or thickness.

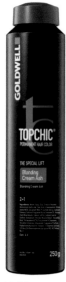

Lightener cream

Choosing lighteners and toners

Although normal tints and high-lift tints lighten the hair, they're not 'lightening products'. When referring to lightening products, we are referring to bleach products. These products come in many varieties.

Lighteners can be a bleach powder, cream or a gel, and they're always mixed with peroxide. You apply them to clean, dry hair using a bowl and brush.

Bleach powder

Bleach powder can be a blue or white powder and is most commonly used for highlighting methods and off-scalp techniques. However, some lightening powders can be used on the scalp but always read the manufacturers' instructions to be sure.

Lightening powders are normally mixed to a preferred **consistency** rather than measured. Add lightening powder to a bowl and mix with the peroxide to make a paste but always check the manufacturers' instructions to ascertain whether there is a mixing ratio.

Lighteners are available with neutralising tone – this means you can remove golden and warm tones from the hair whilst lifting with a lightener.

Bleach gel

Gel bleaches are normally used for scalp applications. This thicker type of lightener contains a booster or activator which is pre-mixed with the gel and the peroxide to obtain maximum lift while limiting the harm to the hair's condition. There are many varieties available, so you must refer to the MFIs for methods of mixing and applying the products.

The following table shows why your clients may or may not choose a lightening colour service.

Reasons to use a lightener	Reasons not to use a lightener
Lightens by up to six shades	The result is permanent
Removes depth	Contains strong chemicals
Removes tone	Committed to colour
Removes tint from the hair	Regrowth occurs every four to six weeks
Fashion effects (foils)	
Permanent result	
Change of image	
Adds texture	
Covers regrowth	

Toners

Toners are generally used to remove unwanted tone after a colour service. For example, if the end result of a colour is too yellow then a violet toner can be applied. Toners can be in the form of liquid temporary colours, a true semi-permanent colour, a quasi-permanent colour and sometimes even a permanent colour with a low-level hydrogen peroxide or developer.

Activity

Using your salon brand of products, identify all the products and colours that could be used to neutralise and tone hair.

Monitoring development

As most lightening products do not have a fixed development time, it is imperative that you visually check the result at regular intervals, and carry out a strand test to check if the colour result has been achieved.

Hydrogen peroxide

Ammonia is a key ingredient in quasi-permanent and permanent hair colours. At room temperature ammonia is colourless with a pungent smell. It can be highly irritating to the skin and respiratory system.

Ammonia
An alkaline gas.

Ammonia, which is mixed with the tint, activates the **oxidation** process. Ammonia swells the cuticle of the hair, allowing penetration of the hair colour into the cortex.

Oxidation
A chemical process that combines a substance with oxygen.

Hydrogen peroxide is often written as H_2O_2. It is a colourless liquid which is unstable and readily breaks down into water and oxygen. Hydrogen peroxide is an acid, about pH 3–4. It is the most common chemical used in hairdressing to provide oxygen. Its purpose is to lighten the natural and artificial colour pigments, and to develop the colour of oxidation tints.

When peroxide is mixed with the ammonia in the tint, the oxidation process begins to work. The ammonia swells the cuticle and the peroxide provides the oxygen to oxidise the hair's colour pigment inside the cortex.

Strengths of peroxide

Peroxide comes in varying strengths; some weaker strengths are referred to as developers. Peroxide strengths are expressed as volumes or percentages.

Volume strengths of peroxide describe the parts of free oxygen that may be given off during development. For example, '20 volume'

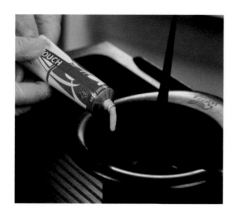

gives off 20 parts of free oxygen. When expressed as a percentage, it describes the percentage of pure peroxide. For example, in 6% peroxide, 100 grams of solution would be made up of 6 grams of pure peroxide, and 94 grams of water. So:

- 10 volume strength is equal to 3% solution
- 20 volume strength is equal to 6% solution
- 30 volume strength is equal to 9% solution
- 40 volume strength is equal to 12% solution.

Strengths of peroxide and their uses

Percentage of peroxide	Volume of peroxide	Uses
1.5% 3% 4%	As a guide, we refer to these weak solutions as '10 volume' and 'developers'	To darken, to add tone and quasi-permanent colours
6%	20 volume	One shade of lift, to darken, to add tone, to cover up to 100% white hair
9%	30 volume	Two shades of lift with a normal tint, or three shades of lift with a high-lift tint
12%	40 volume	Three shades of lift with a normal tint, or four to five shades of lift with a high-lift tint

Developer strength for quasi-permanent colours

To decide on the developer strength, consider the vibrancy of the depth and tone, and how long the colour will last. As a guide, 3% (10 volume) is used by most manufacturers. However, some also offer 1.5% or 4% strengths. The benefit of 1.5% developers is that the colour is more subtle and will not last as long, giving the client freedom to change their colour more often. Using 4% developer will give a longer-lasting effect and red/violet tones will be more vibrant.

Mixing ratios

Tubes of colour and tint generally come in 60ml tubes and a minimum quantity of a ¼ tube (15ml) is often used. To help you mix accurately, these ¼ tube (15ml) measures are marked on the side of the tube.

Quasi-permanent colours are mixed at a 1:2 ratio of colour to developer. Therefore, 15ml (¼ tube) of tint would be mixed with 30ml of developer.

Normal tints are mixed at a 1:1 ratio of tint to peroxide. Therefore, 15ml (¼ tube) of tint would be mixed with 15ml of peroxide.

High-lift tints (those that give maximum lift for blonde colour results) are generally mixed at a 1:2 ratio of tint to peroxide. Therefore, 15ml (¼ tube) of tint would be mixed with 30ml of peroxide.

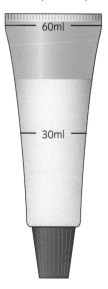

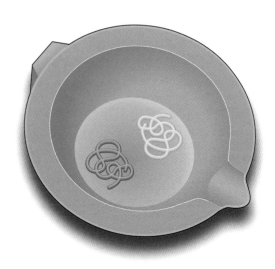

Activity

Using your salon's range of colouring products, identify how many millilitres of tint and peroxide (or developer) you would need for the following:

- ¾ of a tube of quasi-permanent colour
- a full tube of high-lift tint
- 1½ tubes of normal permanent colour.

Activity

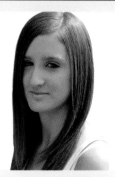

Jo

Jo would like a depth 9 and is currently a natural depth of 7. How many shades of lift are required? What strength peroxide would you use?

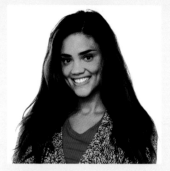

Samira

Samira would like a depth 7 with red tones and is currently a natural depth 4. What colour would you suggest? What strength peroxide would you use? Describe the colour in client-friendly words.

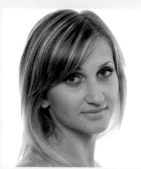

Anne

Anne would like a depth 6 and is currently a natural depth 8 with some highlights. What strength peroxide would you use?

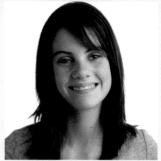

Donna

Donna would like a very light blonde and is currently a natural depth 5. What colour are you aiming for? Would you use a permanent, high-lift or bleach colour? What strength peroxide would you use? Would you suggest a full-head colour or a highlight technique?

Importance of following MFIs

Manufacturers provide you with instructions to ensure that you produce the best possible result for your client. They are also provided to ensure that you work safely and don't put yourself or others at risk. Always follow your MFIs when working with colouring and lightening products.

It is imperative that you follow your specific manufacturer's instructions relating to skin tests to ensure your clients are not at risk of an allergic reaction and to prevent any legal consequences.

Always mix your colours and follow the mixing ratios according to your manufacturers' instructions, as these will vary between manufacturers.

Make sure that you monitor and develop lightening products properly, if there is not a fixed time for development; check the process visually on a regular basis to ensure the end result is not overprocessed.

Follow the MFIs for the development of colours and time them correctly using a timer. This will ensure the correct development time, it allows the colour product to lift and deposit the tone, and enables you to achieve the best results for your client.

Tools, equipment and materials

The tools and equipment you'll need will vary depending on the colouring service chosen.

For regrowth and full-head applications you'll need:

- a brush – to brush through the client's hair and remove tangles
- a wide-toothed comb – to section the hair during the application
- section clips – to section the hair and to secure the towel around the client
- a tint bowl and brush – for the application of products
- weighing scales – if you weigh tint and peroxide in your salon
- a measuring jug – to measure the peroxide solution
- a timer – to time the development process accurately
- an accelerator – to reduce development time.

For highlighting applications you'll need all of the above and:

- a pintail comb – to weave the hair if you're completing woven highlights
- either foils, meches, wraps or clingfilm for woven highlights, or a cap or spatula for pulled-through highlights.

HANDY HINT

When reading, interpreting and following the instructions of the manufacturer you are using your English skills.

HANDY HINT

Use all products cost-effectively and economically to ensure you do not waste the salon's money or harm the environment with unnecessary wastage.

HANDY HINT

Prepare your materials in advance (for example, pre-cutting foils).

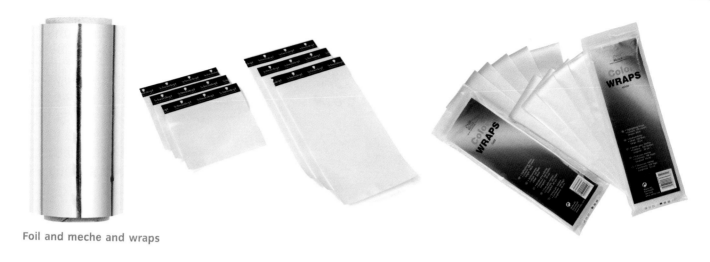

Foil and meche and wraps

Science of colouring and lightening services

Testing the hair – contra-indications

Questioning your client

Sometimes a service cannot be carried out because of contra-indications. You must ask your client whether they have had any adverse reactions to medication, products or services in the past. You must clearly write any answers to these questions on the client's record card in case of any future legal action that might take place. During the consultation check the condition and appearance of the hair and scalp to allow you to assess the options available.

> **HANDY HINT**
>
> You should draw on the knowledge you gained in CHB9, 'Advise and consult with clients'.

> **Activity**
>
> In pairs or small groups list the types of question you could ask the client to identify contra-indications and discuss how you would record them.

> **HANDY HINT**
>
> Always note previous treatments, known allergies, skin disorders, medical instructions or advice and **evident** hair damage on the client's record card.
>
> **Evident**
>
> Easily seen.

Recognising any contra-indications

Use the table below to identify how to find out about clients' contra-indications.

Contra-indication	How you can find out	What else you could do	How and why contra-indications affect the service
History of previous allergic reaction to colouring products	Ask your client if they have ever had an allergic reaction to colour before including home colours and professional products.	Carry out a skin test following the MFIs.	A client with a history of previous allergic reactions to colour is more at risk of future allergic reactions. You may need to offer an alternative colour service or advise that colours services are not carried out.

Contra-indication	How you can find out	What else you could do	How and why contra-indications affect the service
Other known allergy	Ask your client if they have any allergies, such as a nut allergy. Some products contain almond oils, so you wouldn't be able to use these on a client who is allergic to nuts.	Carry out a skin test following the MFIs.	A client with a history of other allergic reactions is more at risk of allergic reactions to colour. They may also be sensitive to some of the ingredients. You may need to offer an alternative colour service, or advise that colour services are not carried out.
Skin disorders	Ask your client if they suffer from any skin problems such as eczema or psoriasis.	Visually check the scalp, looking for skin disorders, infections, infestations and any cuts or abrasions.	Some skin disorders will prevent colour services from being carried out. Infections or infestations – no colour service to be carried out. Open cuts or wounds – no colour service to be carried out. Psoriasis or eczema may not affect the service unless the areas are open or sensitive for the client.
Incompatible products	Ask your client about their previous hair services and treatments, in and out of the salon, as they may react with professional products.	Visually check the hair for any signs of hair discolouration, and if in doubt, carry out an **incompatibility** test. **Incompatibility** Unsuitablity.	If your client has any product or service that is not compatible with the chosen service, then you cannot proceed with the colour. Alternative options may be available.
Medical advice or instructions	Ask your client if they're taking any medication or have been given medical advice that may affect the service result or the condition of the hair.	Visually check the hair to see if it appears healthy. Is there any new hair growth or damage?	If a doctor has advised against colour services, then always follow their advice and do not put your client at risk of injury or reaction, or risk the salon being sued.
Evident hair damage	Ask your client what they do to their hair on a daily basis, eg using straightening irons or curling tongs.	Visually check the hair for damage. Carry out porosity and elasticity tests.	If your client's hair is damaged, then do not use additional chemicals on the hair. Consider alternative milder colour options or alternative services while you treat the hair's condition.
Age restrictions	Ask your client their age to ensure they are at least 16 years old.	Ask to see photo ID if you are unsure of your client's age.	If your client is under 16 years of age and the MFIs state the colour is not intended for use on persons under the age of 16, do not carry out the service – offer alternative services.

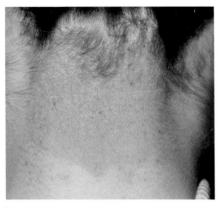

Eczema

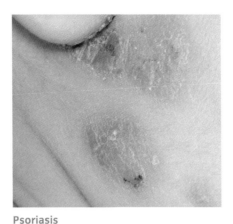

Psoriasis

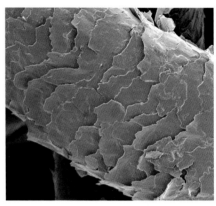

Microscope view: damaged cuticle

Hair and skin tests

During the consultation and the service itself you'll need to conduct some hair tests to confirm that the client's hair is suitable for the service required. You must follow the MFIs to ensure you adhere to health and safety procedures. The results of these tests must be recorded on the client record card and if any adverse reactions occur you must seek guidance from the relevant person. Remember to work within the limits of your authority and report all adverse reactions.

Record cards must be completed for the following reasons:

■ to record the service carried out

■ for future reference

■ to provide evidence in case of any future legal action

■ to maintain the professional image of the salon.

Types and purposes of hair tests and their expected results

The following table shows the hair tests to be carried out before and/ or during the service. It states:

■ when to carry out the hair or skin tests

■ how to carry out the hair or skin tests

■ why you should carry out the hair or skin tests

■ the expected result of the hair or skin tests

■ action to take if the results are adverse.

Test	When to carry out the test	How to carry out the test	Purpose	Action
Skin sensitivity test	24–48 hours before a colour service	Always follow MFIs as these may vary. As a guide, clean an area in the inner elbow or behind the ear. Then apply the client's chosen colour (possibly mixed with peroxide depending on MFIs) to the area and leave it exposed to dry. Or you can issue your client with a skin test patch and advise your client on the MFIs for home use. Check that your insurance company allows this method of skin testing.	To test for an allergic reaction or sensitivity to the product. A positive reaction is red skin and/or sore areas that may weep and itch. A negative reaction is no change to the skin area.	If no reaction occurs, proceed with the service. If a positive reaction, do not apply colour to the scalp as the client may suffer with a severe reaction such as anaphylactic shock. Retest with an alternative product in 24–48 hours' time.
Incompatibility test	Before the colouring or lightening service, if you suspect metallic salts are present in the hair	Take a small cutting of the client's hair and place it in a solution of 20:1 liquid peroxide and ammonium hydroxide (perm lotion). Leave for up to 30 minutes. If metallic salts are present the hair may change colour and the solution may bubble, fizz and/or give off heat.	To identify if any metallic salts are present, which would react with professional colouring products	Do not apply chemical products to your client's hair as they may experience scalp burns and/or damage to or disintegration of their hair. Offer an alternative service that is chemical-free and retest in two to three weeks' time.
Porosity test	Before any service on dry hair	Take a few hairs and slide your fingers along the hair shaft in the direction of point to root. Hair cuticle should feel smooth if the hair is non-porous and feel rough or raised if the hair is porous.	To identify whether the cuticles are smooth or rough	If the hair is very porous, do not use chemicals as this could cause damage to client's hair or the desired outcome may not be achieved. If porous on mid-lengths and ends only, consider a porosity leveller and/or treatment, and cut the hair prior to the service.

HANDY HINT

Not carrying out the tests could result not only in client dissatisfaction but also in significant harm and legal action.

HANDY HINT

Results from the hair tests could prevent colouring services from being carried out or affect your choice of products.

Test	When to carry out the test	How to carry out the test	Purpose	Action
Elasticity test	Before any service on wet hair	Take one or two hairs and mist them lightly with water, then stretch the hair a couple of times between your finger and thumb. Wet hair should stretch about 30% more than its original length and return when released.	To test the strength of the cortex	If the hair is weak and lacks elasticity, do not use chemicals as they will cause damage to the client's hair or the desired outcome may not be achieved. Offer treatments and conditioning colours, such as semi-permanent colours.
Colour test	Before a colour or lightening service	Apply the chosen colour to a section of the hair (either a test cutting or on the head). The desired result should be achieved, or further development may be required.	To see whether the desired result is achievable	If the desired result is not achieved with the colour test, identify why and try an alternative product, retesting before applying the colour.
Strand test	During the colouring or lightening service	Wipe off the colour or lightener from a few strands of hair. If permanent colour is developed, then the desired result should be achieved. If the bleach is regularly checked, the level of lift should be achieved without damage to the hair. Further development may be required if the colour result has not been achieved.	To see whether the colour result has been achieved, or whether the lightener development is sufficient	If the colour is not achieved, leave the hair to develop for longer (if condition allows). If the colour is too light, remove the lightener immediately, apply a conditioning treatment and then tone with a semi-permanent toner (do not use chemicals).

Activity

List three tests carried out before a chemical service, and state their purposes.

List one test carried out during a chemical service, and state its purpose. Discuss your answers with your supervisor.

HANDY HINT

If the test results show any signs of damage or breakage to the hair, do not proceed with the service. Report this to a senior member of staff and advise your client to have penetrating conditioning treatments. Retest the hair a few weeks later.

Activity

Explain the services or options you would offer your client if:

- they suffered an allergic reaction to permanent tint
- they had porous hair
- they had weak elasticity
- the results of an incompatibility test produced heat and bubbling
- the colour test did not lift sufficiently to meet with the client requirements.

Activity

In small groups, discuss the information that should be detailed on a client record card after a colouring service. Compare your answers.

Skin sensitivity test instructions

MFIs for skin sensitivity tests can vary between manufacturers, so always read their instructions and follow them to the letter. Remember to ask for ID from your client if you are unsure whether they are under 16.

Completing client record cards

During and after the service, ensure the client details are correct, easy to read and up to date on the record card. Make sure you enter all of the service details, including client answers to any questions about their hair, and whether they're happy with the service outcome. Always keep client information confidential and follow the Data Protection Act.

HANDY HINT

You are using your English writing skills when completing record cards correctly.

How colour affects hair

What to consider when colouring hair:

- the principles of colour selection and the ICC (International Colour Chart)
- the natural hair pigment
- the effects of colour and lightening products on the hair's structure
- porosity and its effects on colour choice.

The principles of colour theory

Primary colours

The colour star is made up of the three primary colours: red, yellow and blue.

Primary colours cannot be made by mixing other colours together. However, by mixing the primary colours together, we can make

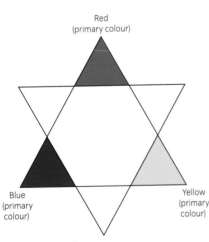

Red
(primary colour)

Blue
(primary colour)

Yellow
(primary colour)

Primary colours

secondary colours. All other colours are made by mixing primary and/or secondary colours together.

Secondary colours

Primary colours are mixed together to form the three secondary colours: orange (created by mixing red and yellow), green (created by mixing yellow and blue) and violet (created by mixing blue and red).

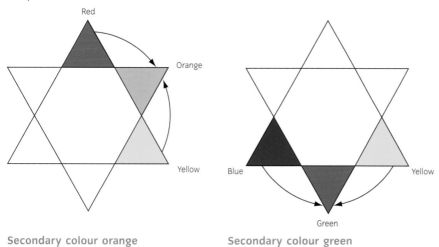

Secondary colour orange

Secondary colour green

Secondary colour violet

When you mix all the primary colours together you create a neutral brown colour.

To help you remember the order of the colour star, try to memorise 'Richard Of York Gave Battle In Vain'.

Richard	Red
Of	Orange
York	Yellow
Gave	Green
Battle	Blue
In **V**ain	Indigo/Violet

The colour star is used by artists and anyone else who mixes or uses colour. The principles of colour are the same for painting a picture as for colouring the hair. Our hair is made up of natural pigments, containing primary and secondary colours. When you add artificial colour to the hair, you rely on your understanding of the colour star.

The International Colour Chart

The International Colour Chart (ICC) is the numbering system that all manufacturers follow. Everyone uses the same numbers to describe a colour's depth.

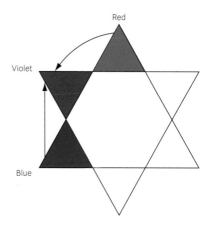

Neutral brown created by mixing all primary colours

WHY DON'T YOU...
Paint your own colour star and compare your secondary colours with your colleagues'.

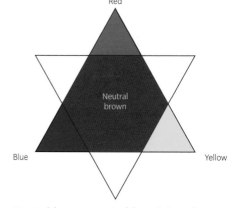

HANDY HINT
In hairdressing we refer to yellow as *gold*, orange as *copper* and indigo as *violet*.

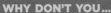

WHY DON'T YOU...
Mix the three primary colours together. Did you get a neutral brown? Compare the results with your colleagues'.

When you refer to your client's hair colour, you look at the depth and the tone of the hair. The depth is how light or dark the hair is, and the tone is the colour you see. If you describe someone as a redhead, you're describing their tone. If you describe someone as bleached blonde, you're referring to the depth of the hair.

Depths of hair

The natural depths of hair range from 1 (black) to 10 (lightest blonde).

The range of depths, from lightest to darkest, is as follows:

10	lightest blonde
9	very light blonde
8	light blonde
7	medium blonde
6	dark blonde
5	light brown
4	medium brown
3	dark brown
2	darkest brown
1	black

WHY DON'T YOU...
Work with a colleague to try to identify each other's natural hair depth.

Tones in the hair

Sadly, manufacturers don't follow the same numbering system when describing tones. They all use a number system which you'll need to learn. Once you have mastered the ICC, it'll be easier to learn the tonal colours that your salon uses. You'll need this understanding throughout your hairdressing career, but you can always refer to the colour chart.

The tone numbering system describes the colour you see. All manufacturers use a similar description of the tone, but the numbering system will vary. Depths and tones are usually written in numbers for the stylist's use and given descriptive names for the client's benefit. For example, the description for depth 8 (light blonde) may be written as 8/0, 8–0, 8.0 or 8N depending on the manufacturer. The 0 refers to the tone.

Examples of primary tones

Description of tone	Wella	L'Oréal	Goldwell
Natural	/0	/0	N – natural
Ash	/1 or /9	/1	A – ash
Blue ash	/8	/1	BV – blue violet
Green ash	/2	N/A	NA – green
Gold	/3	/3	G – gold
Red	/4	/6	R – red
Mahogany	/6	/5	RB – red brown
Brunette/mocha	/7	/8	B – brown

> **WHY DON'T YOU...**
> Work with a colleague to try to identify each other's tones. Is the colour warm or cool?

In the colour chart, the first digit after the depth is the primary or stronger tonal colour. For example 8/3 is depth 8 (light blonde) with a primary tone of 3 (gold): this could be described as a light golden blonde. Primary tones are often mixed together to create secondary tones: these are indicated by the second digit.

Examples of secondary tones

Description of tone	Wella	L'Oréal (as a guide)
Natural ash	/01	/01
Natural gold	/03	/03
Copper (red and gold)	/43	/4 or /46 or /44 or /64
Copper (gold and red)	/34	/4 or /43 or /34
Violet red	/46	/56
Mahogany red	/56	/26 or /45
Golden brown	/73	/35 or /53

For example, 6/43 is depth 6 (dark blonde) with a tone of /43 (red and gold). This colour could be called dark red gold blonde or dark copper blonde.

If the mixed tone were more gold than red, it would be shown as 6/34. This would still be a dark copper blonde, but the copper tone created would not be as vibrant as 6/43.

Colour tones

In hair, red, gold and copper colours are known as warm tones; blue, green and violet are known as cool tones.

By mixing more or less of each primary colour we create different shades. For example, if you mix red with yellow, you make orange

> **WHY DON'T YOU...**
> See how many shades of orange you can make.

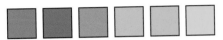

Variations of copper/orange colours

Neutralise

To make neutral or balance out.

(copper). If you add more red than yellow, the resulting tone would be a brighter copper than if you mixed more yellow than red. The various possible shades of copper can be seen on any colour chart.

Neutralising unwanted tones in the hair

The principles of the colour star not only work to create colours and various shades, but also to neutralise any unwanted tone in the hair. Colours opposite each other on the colour star will **neutralise** each other.

For example:

- red neutralises green
- green neutralises red
- yellow neutralises violet
- violet neutralises yellow
- orange neutralises blue
- blue neutralises orange.

If a colour result has a green tone, you'd need to add a red toner to neutralise it. If highlight results are a little too gold (yellow), you would neutralise the tone with a violet toner. When highlighting naturally copper- (orange-) toned hair, you should use a high-lift tint with a blue tone.

Neutralising tones work by mixing all three primary colours. When neutralising unwanted golden tones, use a violet toner because yellow is a primary colour and when you add violet (which is made with red and blue primary colours) all three primary colours have been mixed together, creating a neutral tone.

Unwanted green tones are neutralised in the same way. Green is a secondary colour made up of yellow and blue primary colours – when neutralised with red, all three primary colours have been mixed together to create a neutral tone.

This same principle works for neutralising orange tones. Orange (red and yellow) mixed with blue creates a neutral tone.

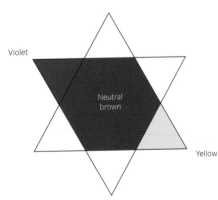

Violet / Neutral brown / Yellow

Neutralising golden tones

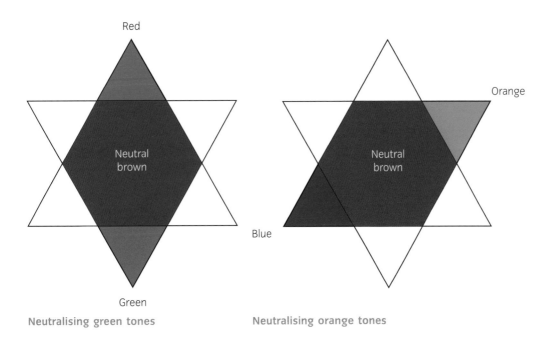

Neutralising green tones

Neutralising orange tones

Removing depths and tones

When you lighten hair you lose **pigments** in a certain order: red, orange and then yellow. Red tones are larger molecules and therefore can be removed from the hair more quickly. Yellow tones are tiny molecules and it can take much longer to remove these. The yellow pigments from depths 8, 9 and 10 are the hardest to remove. If you remove too many yellow pigments, you risk breaking and damaging the hair.

Pigment

The substance that colours our tissue (hair and skin).

Tones		Depths	
Very pale yellow		10	Lightest blonde
Pale yellow		9	Very light blonde
Yellow		8	Light blonde
Yellow/orange		7	Blonde
Orange		6	Dark blonde
Orange/red		5	Light brown
Red		4	Brown
Red		3	Dark brown
Red/blue		2	Darkest brown
Blue red		1	Black

Tones in the depths of hair

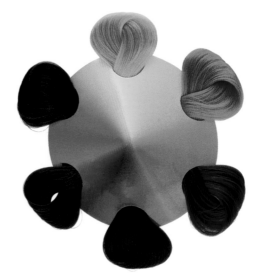

HANDY HINT

Recall the structure of the hair, and look at the pictures of colour molecules in the cortex under the microscope in chapter CHB9.

Activity

If you lighten the hair colour from depth 5 to depth 8, what colour pigments (tones) will you remove? What tones will your client be left with?

If you lighten the hair from depth 7 to depth 9, what colour pigments (tones) will you remove? What tones will your client be left with?

If you darken the hair from depth 5 to depth 3, what colour pigments (tones) will you have added?

Natural and artificial hair colour

The cortex contains all the natural and artificial colour pigments of the hair. It is the layer of the hair where all chemical action takes place. You can see the hair's colour through the transparent cuticle.

Natural hair colour varies from person to person, depending on the colour pigments. The pigments are called **melanin** and consist of two types:

Melanin

Pigments that give colour to the hair and skin.

- Eumelanin is made up of black to light brown colour pigments. These are large colour molecules with varying amounts of all three primary colours but predominately contain blue and red pigments.
- Pheomelanin is made up of blonde colour pigments. These are tiny molecules of colour spread throughout the cortex with varying amounts of red, yellow and orange colour molecules but predominately contain yellow pigments.

If you looked at two heads of hair, one dark brown and one light brown, both would have the same amount of colour pigment, but the amounts of blue, red and yellow melanin would vary. These different combinations give us depths and tones.

Effects of artificial and natural light on the hair

The salon's lighting system is very important to enable the client to see their colour result accurately, effectively and in the best possible light.

Natural daylight is the ideal way to show the hair's true colour. Natural light is referred to as white light, but it is made up of all the colours of the spectrum – red, orange, yellow, green, blue, indigo and violet. If you see white, that is because all seven colours are being reflected to your eyes from the object you are looking at. If you see one colour, such as red, the other six colours are being absorbed. If you see black, then no colour is being reflected into your eyes and all are being absorbed.

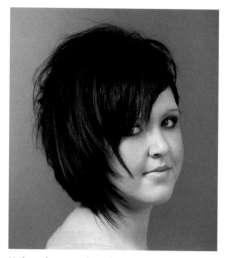

Hair colour under electric bulbs

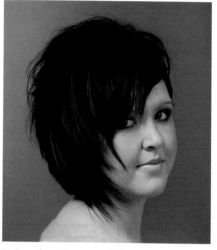

Hair colour in natural daylight

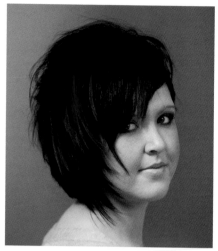

Hair colour under fluorescent tubes

Electric bulbs can make the hair look warmer in appearance and neutralise blue or ash tones because of the yellow tinge given off by the bulb. Fluorescent tubes can make the hair appear more ash in tone as they give off a bluish tinge and remove the warmth from the hair.

Effects of colouring and lightening on the hair

Clients may choose partial-head or full-head colour, or a highlighted effect. Whether you're colouring the hair with a temporary colour, a permanent colour or using lightening products, it is essential that you understand their effects on the hair's structure.

Effects of temporary colour

Temporary hair colours are not such a popular service as permanent colours, but they can be quickly applied for a short-term look.

Temporary colours contain large colour molecules which coat the outside of the cuticle and stain the hair shaft. If the hair is porous and the cuticle is raised, the colour might grab and coat the cortex, which can cause the colour to last longer and/or give an uneven colour result.

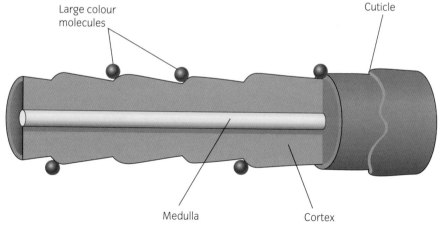

Effects of temporary colour molecules on the hair

Effects of semi-permanent colour

Semi-permanent colours are a great way to introduce colouring services to your clients. They're quick and easy to apply and develop, and the client is not committed to the colour.

Semi-permanent colours contain large and small colour molecules. The larger colour molecules coat and stain the outside of the cuticle, whereas the smaller molecules coat the inside of the cuticle and the outer layer of the cortex.

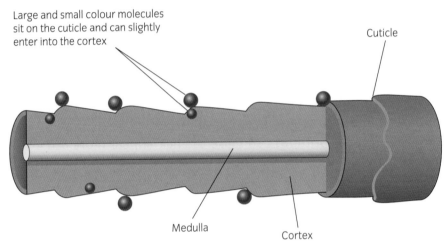

Large and small colour molecules sit on the cuticle and can slightly enter into the cortex

Cuticle

Medulla

Cortex

Effects of semi-permanent colour molecules on the hair

Effects of quasi-permanent colour

Quasi-permanent colours are popular services in salons. When used effectively the colour is not permanent so there is a minimal commitment.

Quasi-permanent colours contain small and medium-sized colour molecules. The small molecules coat the cuticle and lie in the cortex, whereas the medium-sized colour molecules penetrate into the cortex. The weak developer when mixed with the quasi-permanent colour oxidises and swells the cuticle slightly, allowing the deposit of depth and tone into the cortex.

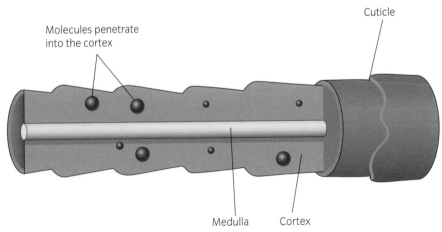

Molecules penetrate into the cortex

Cuticle

Medulla

Cortex

Effects of quasi-permanent colour molecules on the hair

Effects of permanent and high-lift colour

Permanent and high-lift hair colours are the most popular colour treatments in salons. They can be used to create many effects and variations, such as regrowth and full-head colour services, and highlighting and lowlighting effects. Combinations of these services can be used. For example, you can combine a half head of woven highlights with a full head of colour in between the packets.

These products can be used to lighten or darken the hair, depending on the strength of peroxide used. The stronger the peroxide used, the higher the lift, and the greater the effect on the cortex of the hair.

They contain small colour molecules that expand and join together during the development process. The peroxide, when mixed with the ammonia from the tint, swells the cuticle and allows the small molecules to enter into the cortex. This allows the tint to deposit the required depth and tone.

The products must be fully developed, to allow the colour to reach its desired depth, deposit the tonal colours and neutralise – colour molecules need time to swell and join in the cortex to become permanent.

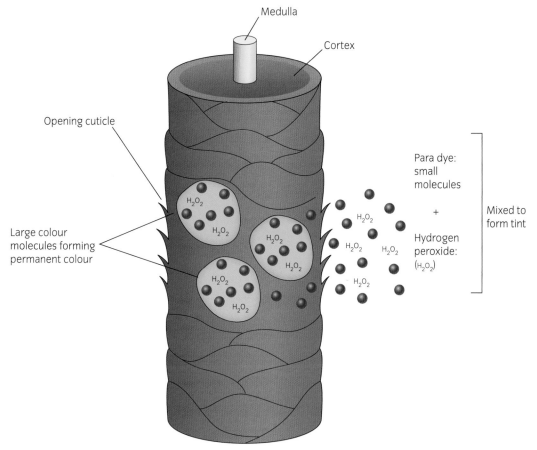

Effects of permanent/high-lift colour molecules on the hair

Effects of lightening products

Lightening products enable clients to achieve the lightest blondes and lighten artificial colour in the hair. They can be used to create varying effects, including regrowth, partial and full-head colour services, and highlights.

Hydrogen peroxide gives off oxygen: O_2

Melanin (the natural pigment of the hair) is oxidised by the hydrogen peroxide to form colourless oxy-melanin

Effects of lightening products on the hair

These products can be used with any strength peroxide for off-scalp techniques, such as highlights. Peroxide with a strength of 6% must be used for on-scalp techniques, such as regrowths. Lightening products can achieve up to five or six shades of lift.

The lift achievable and development time greatly vary depending on the peroxide strength and the depth of your client's hair in relation to your target shade. Lightening products affect the hair by oxidising the natural and artificial colour pigments in the cortex. These products are alkaline and contain ammonia. Ammonia, when mixed with peroxide, releases oxygen; the oxidisation process causes the melanin to become **oxy-melanin**.

Oxy-melanin

A colourless molecule.

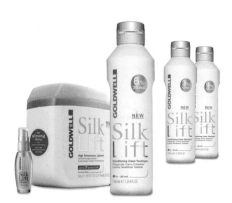

Pre-lightening products

Pre-lightening hair

Depending on the client requirements, a permanent tint may not produce the levels of lift required. Always remember that you cannot apply a permanent tint to lift permanent tint already on the hair – tint does not lift tint.

If there is permanent colour already on your client's hair and the desired colour choice is lighter then you will need to pre-lighten the hair with a lightening product first. Equally if the level of lift required by the client is not achievable using a permanent colour with 12% hydrogen peroxide, then you need to pre-lighten the hair with a lightening product first.

Porosity and its effects on colour choice and techniques

Due to the effects each colour product has, you must consider the condition and porosity of your client's hair before deciding on the colour choice and the techniques to be used. Porous hair will not withstand further harsh chemical treatments, and colouring or lightening products must not be overlapped.

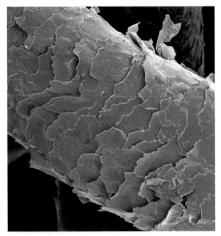

Microscope view: damaged cuticle layer

Activity

In pairs or small groups, discuss what colour services and products would be available to clients with porous hair. Explain why some products or services could not be offered.

Temperature

The temperature of the salon will affect your colour and lightening development times, as well as the outcome. Some manufacturers' instructions also state whether you should apply colours to the roots first or start with the mid-lengths and ends – this is because of the heat given off from the head area at the roots of the hair.

Restore the hair's pH

After all chemical services an **anti-oxidant** conditioner should be used to stop the oxidation process. This closes the cuticle and returns the hair to its natural state of pH 4.5–5.5. It prevents colours from fading, the hair from becoming dry/brittle and causing damage to the cuticle or cortex.

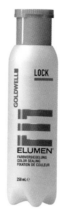

Post-colour care

Anti-oxidant

A substance that stops the oxidation process.

Techniques

Colour, lowlighting and highlighting techniques

After a thorough consultation and armed with all the product knowledge, you're now able to carry out the most suitable colouring service to meet your client's requirements. The colour and lightening techniques you will carry out are:

- full-head application of quasi-permanent
- regrowth application of permanent colour
- full-head application of permanent colour
- woven highlights and/or lowlights
- pulled-through highlights and/or lowlights.

Full-head application of quasi-permanent

Quasi-permanent colours are normally applied on pre-shampooed hair. As the product is more fluid than permanent colour and it's applied to wet hair, larger sections can be taken. The service is normally carried out either at the workstation or the shampoo area, and the colour applied from roots to tips and gently massaged through.

Once developed, the quasi-permanent colour must be rinsed off the hair, followed by a shampoo. An anti-oxidant conditioner should then be used to return the hair to pH 4.5–5.5.

Regrowth application of permanent colour

Regrowth applications are applied to clean dry hair and generally using the 'hot-cross bun' sectioning pattern. The colouring product is

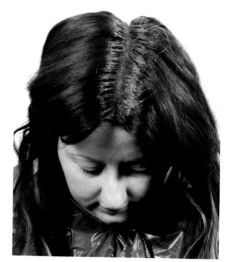

Applying a quasi-permanent colour at the shampoo area

Regrowth application of permanent colour

applied to the roots only and left to develop. Colour refreshing techniques may also be used to brighten up faded ends.

Full-head application of permanent colour

For a full-head application, the same hot-cross bun sectioning pattern is used. Depending on the colour choice and lift required the colour is either applied:

■ at the roots, mid-lengths and ends at the same time and then left to develop evenly, or;

■ to the mid-lengths and ends first, left to develop for about 20 minutes and then the colour is applied to the root area. Applying colour at the mid-lengths and ends first gives the colour a chance to develop before being applied to the warm root area which will develop more quickly – this technique is required for most high-lift colours and vibrant tones to ensure an even coverage.

Emulsifying

Colouring products must be thoroughly removed from the hair at the end of the development time using the following method:

1 Apply a small of amount of water to the hair.

2 Emulsify the product into the moistened hair using a rotary massage technique.

3 Rinse the emulsified product until the water runs clear.

4 Shampoo the hair using a shampoo for coloured hair.

5 Condition the hair using an anti-oxidant conditioner.

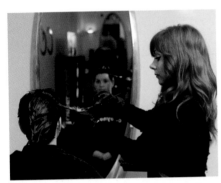
Full-head application, permanent colour

> **HANDY HINT**
>
> Tint removes tint. If you encounter any staining of colour around the hairline and ears, you can apply some tint from the bowl and massage gently into these areas (emulsify) prior to the colour removal process.

> **HANDY HINT**
>
> Colouring products must be thoroughly removed from the hair to prevent further development or damage to the hair and scalp. Emulsifying will enable the colour to be loosened from the hair and prevent staining to the skin and scalp.

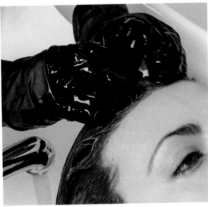
Massaging to emulsify the colouring product

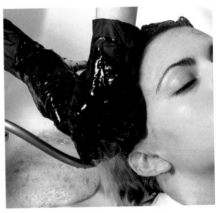
Rinsing until the water runs clear

Highlighting techniques

Permanent, high-lift and lightening products can be used for creating highlighting and lowlighting effects. These techniques are useful when clients want to see a proportion of their natural hair colour, or an additional colour, alongside a lighter highlight. The techniques available are pulled-through or woven highlights. Always consider the hair's length, density and texture before you make your choice.

Woven highlighting techniques

Woven highlights are produced using foils, meches or wraps. They're suitable for any hair length. It is very important to consider the client's requirements and expected results, and the density and texture of the hair when deciding on the quantity of hair to be woven.

The woven technique is very flexible as you can use various colours and products alongside partial or whole-head colouring techniques.

T-bar and half-head sectioning patterns are commonly used in salons for quick, cost-effective highlighting.

Woven highlights

Careful removal of developed meches

If you're using lighteners, some meches may need to be removed while others are still developing. To do this, secure the meches that are still developing and ensure that they do not move and cause seepage. Apply water over the meche's seals, or unfold the foils to loosen them. Remove the meches or foils carefully from the hair and thoroughly rinse the area.

At the end of the service, carefully remove all remaining meches or foils from the client's hair without causing discomfort. Once the materials are removed from the hair, remove the product in the usual manner.

Pulled-through highlighting techniques

Pulled-through techniques are becoming as popular as woven techniques and can be used to achieve quick effective methods of highlighting. There are several methods that you can use.

Balayage/dip-dye ombre

The hair is sectioned into the hot-cross bun sectioning pattern. Then, starting at the back, take a 1cm (½ in) wide section and backcomb the hair up towards the roots. Place the non-backcombed hair (mid-lengths and ends) onto a spatula, apply the chosen colour to the mid-lengths and ends, and pull the spatula through the hair.

> **HANDY HINT**
>
> For a non-pulled-through effect, this technique can be used. The non-backcombed hair is placed onto the foil, colour applied to the mid-lengths and ends and then left to develop.

> **Balayage / dip-dye ombre**
>
> 'Bayalage' means 'sweeping' in French. Techniques where colour is hand swept or painted onto the hair.

> **Activity**
>
> Using the internet, research the history of **balayage** and **ombre**.

Pulled-through meches

Another method of pulled-through highlights is to use clear meches that are held against the roots of the hair and the stylist makes holes in with a hook. The hair is pulled through the holes and then stuck to the adhesive.

Cap highlights

Cap highlights can be used if only one additional colour is required, and the hair is short. Always remember to add talcum powder to the inside of a cap before you pull it onto the head, otherwise it can cause discomfort for your client.

You should pull the hair through the holes to achieve the desired thickness of highlights.

At the end of the service rinse the product from the cap, apply conditioner to the hair to gently ease the cap from the head, shampoo the colour from the hair, and apply an anti-oxidant conditioner.

Spatula highlights

Spatula highlights can be a quicker way of creating a woven highlighted look. These are more suitable for one-colour highlighting on longer hair. Only permanent and high-lift tints can be used with this method, as bleach swells and would create an uneven, patchy result.

At the end of the service, rinse the product from the hair until the water runs clear, wash with shampoo and then use an anti-oxidant conditioner.

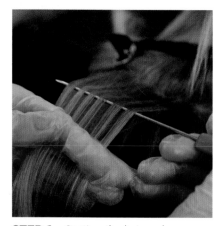

STEP 1 – Section the hair and weave a small section.

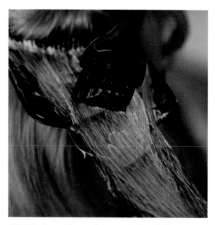

STEP 2 – Place the spatula at the root area and apply the product onto the spatula.

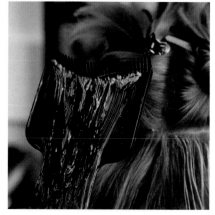

STEP 3 – Slowly pull the spatula away from the root area.

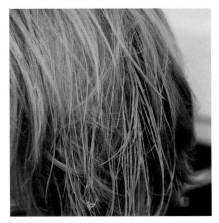

STEP 4 – Gently lay the coloured hair onto the non-coloured hair.

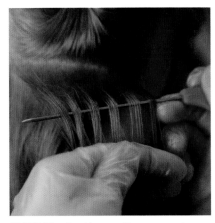

STEP 5 – Continue with your next weave.

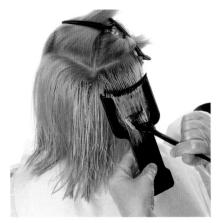

STEP 6 – Apply the colour carefully.

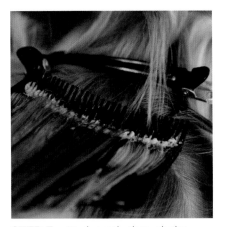

STEP 7 – Work neatly through the sections to the top of the head.

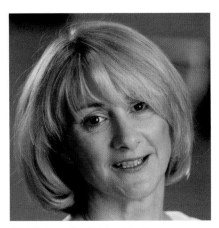

STEP 8 – The finished look.

Colour gun

A colour gun can give a highlighted effect on medium to long hair. You can combine several colours, ranging from fine to thick highlighting effects. Colour is applied directly from the gun onto the hair by placing the gun at the root area and moving it along each section of hair from root to point, squeezing the trigger to release the colour. Remove the product from the hair as you would for spatula highlights.

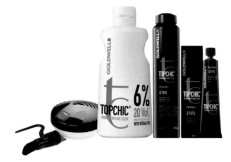

Goldwell P-CAT (Professional Colour Application Tool)

Activity

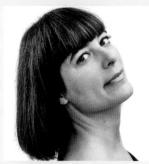

Katie

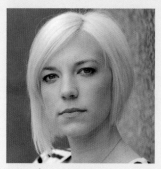

Hannah

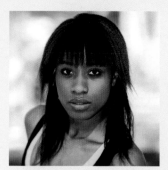

Maleah

Katie would like light blonde highlights but your test results show metallic salts are present in the hair. What action should you take? Would you proceed with the service? What further services would you recommend for Katie?

Hannah has heavily bleached hair, and the porosity and elasticity tests show the cuticle is rough and the cortex is weak. She would like to return to a medium brown colour. Which service would you recommend for Hannah?

Maleah has African type hair and would like a whole-head colour. This is her first colouring service. Her hair is in good condition but she has psoriasis and very sensitive skin. What tests would you carry out and, depending on the results, which services would you recommend for Maleah?

Choose one of the client case studies and prepare a trolley with the tools and equipment you would need to carry out the appropriate service.

Problems and their causes

You may encounter some problems when colouring the hair. The table below shows the causes and remedies to common problems.

Colouring problem	Cause of problem	Resolving the problem
Hair is too yellow	Underdeveloped Peroxide strength was not strong enough Wrong colour/product choice Did not consider tones present in the hair	Use a violet toner. Rebleach if hair condition allows.
Uneven colour result	Poor mixing of product Uneven application Porous hair prior to application Incorrect selection of colour for white hair Underdeveloped	Apply a quasi-permanent colour if suitable. Spot tint/bleach uneven areas.

Colouring problem	Cause of problem	Resolving the problem
Poor coverage on white hair	Resistant hair Did not pre-soften Incorrect choice of colour Incorrect strength of peroxide used	Pre-soften hair in future. Reapply product if hair condition allows.
Skin staining	Poor application Dry skin/hairline Did not use barrier cream	Use a stain remover. If not too late, emulsify colour at the basin.
Scalp irritation	Product too strong Allergy to product Possible cuts or abrasions	Remove product immediately. Rinse with cool water. Refer to GP if required.
Over processed result, or deterioration of hair condition	Overdeveloped Peroxide too strong Too much heat used Overlapped previous colour	Remove product immediately. Apply conditioning treatment to the hair.
Product seepage	Poor application Incorrect mixing of product Incorrect use of foils or meche	Spot tint to cover seepage of product.

Activity

Find out from your salon manager what the limits of your authority would be if you had to solve the colouring problems listed in the table above.

Covering white hair

Clients with high percentages of white hair tend to find that colour coverage can be less effective – white hair is often resistant to the colour because of the tightly compacted cuticle. To overcome this you may need to pre-soften the hair.

The technique involves applying neat (undiluted) 6% liquid peroxide to the hair, prior to the colouring service. It can be used prior to a full-head or regrowth application.

- Apply the liquid peroxide to clean dry hair using a bowl and brush.

- Using either a handheld hairdryer or by placing your client under a hood dryer, dry the solution into the hair.

- Do not rinse out the solution and, once dry, continue with the application process as normal.

- Record the process on the client's record card.

HANDY HINT

Take extra care when using lightening products on previously chemically treated hair. Ensure your application is not overlapped, as this will cause greater porosity, damage to the hair's condition, and potentially uneven colour results.

HANDY HINT

You may need the record card if the client is unhappy with the service or wants to take legal action. The record card provides evidence to support any defence and shows that professional standards were met.

This technique uses added heat from the hairdryer to open the cuticle, allowing the peroxide to enter the cortex, ready for the colouring process.

Carry out refreshing techniques

Hair depth can naturally lighten with sunlight, humidity and wind because hair is exposed to oxygen in the air. Hair tones can also be lost in sunlight or UV light, particularly red and violet tones, as their larger colour pigments sit nearer the surface of the hair.

As permanent colours can often fade between salon visits, clients may be advised to have their mid-lengths and ends refreshed along with a regrowth touch-up. Depending on the amount of depth and tone lost, the techniques and services you suggest will vary.

Methods to refresh colour loss

If your client has minimal loss of depth and tone, you should:

1 Complete the regrowth colour application.
2 Develop for the full development time.
3 Add 10–15ml of water to the hair and emulsify the product through the mid-lengths and ends.
4 Leave for 3–5 minutes.
5 Remove the colour in the usual way.
6 Record the process on the client's record card.

If your client has significant loss of depth and tone, you should:

1 Complete the regrowth colour application.
2 Develop for 10–15 minutes.
3 Mist the mid-lengths and ends with water.
4 Apply a quasi-permanent colour to the mid-lengths and ends.
5 Develop for a further 20 minutes.
6 Remove the colour in the usual way.
7 Record the process on the client's record card.

If your client has loss of tone only (for example, faded red tones), you should:

1 Complete the regrowth colour application.
2 Develop for 20 minutes.
3 Add 10–15ml of water to the hair, and emulsify the product through the mid-lengths and ends.
4 Develop for a further 10–15 minutes.
5 Remove the colour in the usual way.
6 Record the process on the client's record card.

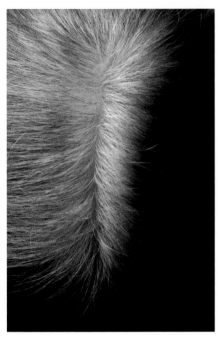

Refresh for colour loss required

If your client is changing the tonal colours of their hair, but maintaining the depth, complete the application as follows:

1 Complete the regrowth colour application.
2 Add 10–15ml of water to the hair and emulsify the product through the mid-lengths and ends.
3 Develop for the full development time.
4 Remove the colour in the usual way.
5 Record the process on the client's record card.

Lightening products used for regrowth and full-head services must be thoroughly removed from the hair at the end of the development time using the following method:

1 Apply a small of amount of water over the hair.
2 Gently emulsify the water into the lightening product, using a gentle rotary massage technique – be gentle with the hair because it will be in a delicate state, and the scalp may be tender.
3 Rinse the emulsified hair until the water runs clear.
4 Gently shampoo the hair, using a shampoo for coloured hair.
5 Condition the hair using an anti-oxidant conditioner.

> **HANDY HINT**
>
> Lowlights are colour effects darker than the client's natural depth colour; highlights are colour effects lighter than the natural depth colour.

Providing advice and recommendations

After every colouring service you should provide your client with effective aftercare advice. Your advice should include:

- how to maintain their hair colour
- time intervals between services
- present and future products and services.

How to maintain their hair colour

You may need to recommend lifestyle alterations to your client, to ensure both the colour and condition of the hair are preserved. This may include advising wearing a hat on sunny or windy days, or warning about the effects of chlorine on hair colour. Chlorine can cause hair to dry out and become brittle, the colour to fade and even a colour reaction. You might recommend shampoos that remove chlorine from the hair, and additional shampoo and conditioning products that will enhance the colour and improve durability.

Excessive use of electrical heat appliances will also cause the colour to fade and the hair to lose condition. You should advise your client appropriately and suggest regular conditioning treatments.

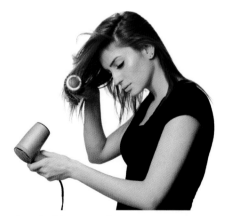

Electrical heat appliances can cause colour loss

WHY DON'T YOU...

Ask your salon manager or other stylist how long they would suggest a client waits before having the following services after a colouring service:

• hair extensions
• a **permanent blow-dry**
• a permanent wave.

Permanent blow dry

A semi-permanent blow-dry service designed to straighten the hair for up to three months.

WHY DON'T YOU...

Identify the products available in your salon that you could recommend to clients after a colouring service.

Time interval between services

Depending on the service carried out, you may need to advise your client on time intervals between other services or future colouring services.

Present and future products and services

Finally, you should advise your client when to return to the salon for additional services, or for their next colouring service. Explain how long they should expect the current service to last, and advise them on what to look for as a guide for when they should return. This may include white hair becoming noticeable around the hairline, a visible regrowth or colour fade. Make suitable suggestions for additional services such as their next haircut or treatments you have recommended. Suggest that your client books their next appointment while they're still in the salon. This helps the salon to maintain regular trade and revenue, and also allows your client to look forward to their next appointment.

Activity

If a client wanted to rebook for their next colour service, when would you suggest they rebook? How many weeks for:

• a regrowth tint?
• a full head of woven highlights?
• T-bar section of woven highlights?
• pulled-through capped highlights?
• balayage or dip dye?

How many times a year would your client visit for the above services? Use your salon price list to work out how much money the salon will generate from these clients and their services each year.

Colour and lighten hair

Prepare to colour and/or lighten the hair

Once you have decided on the product and service required, you need to prepare the client for the service. Make sure you have gowned and protected your client effectively.

Many colouring services are carried out on dry hair. If this is the case, check that the hair is clean enough and there isn't an overload of hairdressing products on the hair which may cause a barrier to the service. Always check the MFIs and, if applying a colour on pre-shampooed hair, then prepare the client for a shampoo first.

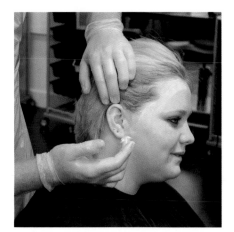

Barrier cream being applied to the client's hairline

Remember – surface conditioner is not normally applied before a colour because it closes the cuticles and causes a barrier to the service.

Work safely and hygienically

When carrying out the colour service, ensure that you maintain health and safety throughout by always keeping your work area clean and tidy, wearing your PPE, monitoring your own posture and the client's positioning and ensuring that they are gowned properly at all times.

Use working methods that:

- minimise waste and dispose of it correctly
- make effective use of your time
- minimise cross-infection
- ensure you use clean resources
- minimise the risk of harm and injury to yourself and others
- promote environmental and sustainable practices.

HANDY HINT

If you're completing a full-head colour/ lightening service and it is your salon policy to use barrier cream, ensure that the hairline is completely covered. Make sure that you have not coated the hair itself, as this would prevent the colour from taking.

HANDY HINT

Maintain your personal hygiene throughout the service and wear gloves to protect your skin when applying colours, checking the development and removing colour products from the hair.

HANDY HINT

Follow the instructions of your manufacturer, suppliers and salon.

Consult with clients on services and test results

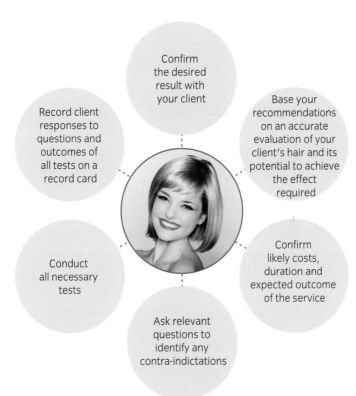

Confirm the desired result with your client

Base your recommendations on an accurate evaluation of your client's hair and its potential to achieve the effect required

Record client responses to questions and outcomes of all tests on a record card

Confirm likely costs, duration and expected outcome of the service

Conduct all necessary tests

Ask relevant questions to identify any contra-indictations

Select products, tools and equipment

Choose your products, tools and equipment based on the results of necessary tests, the consultation with your clients and any relevant factors that may influence the service. Seek assistance from the relevant person when contra-indications and or reactions to tests cause doubt over the suitability of the service.

Prepare and mix all products following MFIs and complete any final preparations to the client's hair, protecting their skin (where necessary), prior to the service.

Carry out the colouring and/or lightening service

1   Use colour and lightening techniques suitable for achieving the desired look while following MFIs.
2   Section hair cleanly and evenly to assist accurate application of products.
3   Apply products taking into account relevant factors influencing the service.
4   Apply products in a way that minimises the risk of the product being spread to your client's skin, clothes and surrounding areas.
5   Time the development of products following MFIs.
6   Confirm the required result has been achieved by taking strand tests at suitable times throughout the process.
7   Massage the hair and scalp to emulsify the colour, as necessary, prior to removal, following MFIs.
8   Remove colour and lightening materials from the hair with minimum discomfort to your client.
9   Leave the hair free of products after the desired effect is achieved.
10 Identify any problems during the service and resolve them within the limits of your own authority.
11 Refer problems that you cannot resolve to the relevant person.
12 Achieve the desired effect to the satisfaction of your client.
13 Complete the service within a commercially viable time.

Throughout the service and also at the end, provide your client with relevant advice on how to maintain their hair colour and the time interval between services. Make recommendations on present and future products and services that will benefit the client and enhance their hairstyle and/or condition.

Client satisfaction

At the end of every colour and before the client pays for the service you must check that they are happy with the service. Write the client response on the record card. Therefore, if the client is happy with the colour, you can repeat the service again next time.

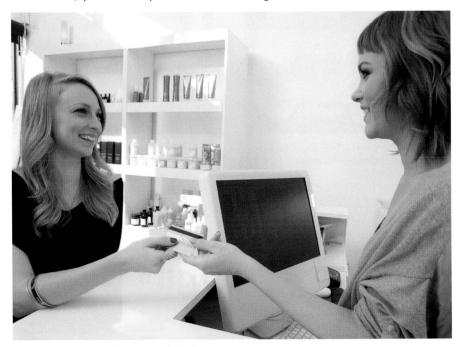

Ensure that every client is satisfied

Step by steps

How to carry out a temporary colouring service

Gown and protect your client for the service, and wear PPE to apply the colour to pre-shampooed/conditioned hair. Comb the product through to ensure an even application.

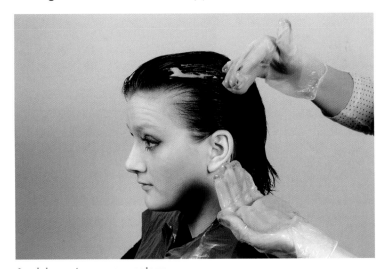
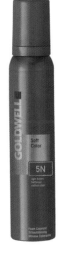

Applying a temporary colour

Semi-permanent colouring service

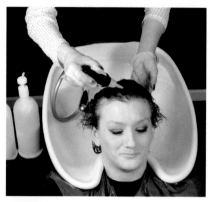

STEP 1 – Gown and protect your client and shampoo their hair.

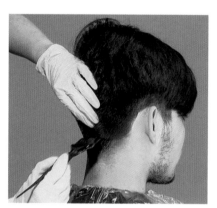

STEP 2 – Apply the semi-permanent colour evenly directly from the applicator bottle.

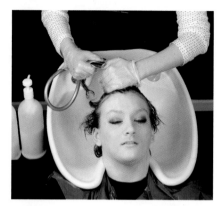

STEP 3 – Sit the client comfortably for the development time, add water to emulsify, then rinse thoroughly and condition the hair.

Quasi-permanent colouring service

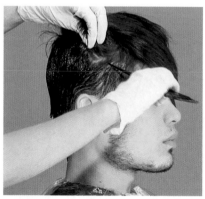

STEP 1 – After applying protective clothing and barrier cream to the skin around the hair, start in the nape area using deep circular brush strokes in a horizontal pattern. This method is used to accommodate the cropped areas.

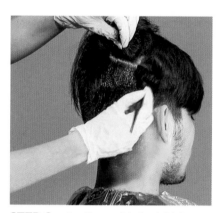

STEP 2 – Continue with the initial pattern up to the crown area.

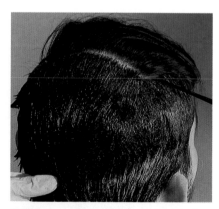

STEP 3 – Use the same method in both side areas, being mindful of the shorter cropped hair and ensuring even coverage.

STEP 4 – Now apply clear gloss to the remaining longer area through the top, starting in the crown and working horizontally through to the front hairline.

> **HANDY HINT**
>
> Quasi-permanent colours can also be applied on wet hair at the workstation by sectioning the hair and applying it like a full-head colour application. Apply the colour from root to point in medium-sized sections.

> **HANDY HINT**
>
> If quasi-permanent colours are used too regularly, a more permanent colour effect can occur and definite regrowth can be seen at the roots.

> **WHY DON'T YOU...**
>
> Watch a stylist carrying out colouring services.

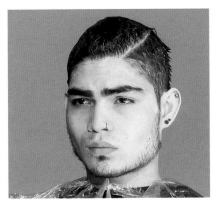

STEP 5 – Process and remove according to the manufacturer's instructions.

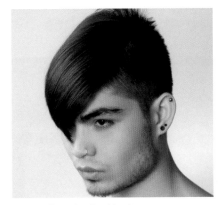

STEP 6 – The final look.

Applying permanent and high-lift products to the hair

Permanent and high-lift products can be used for regrowth and full-head colouring services.

Permanent regrowth service

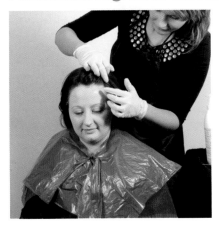

STEP 1 – Gown and protect your client, and apply barrier cream.

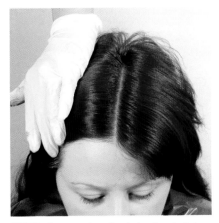

STEP 2 – Section the hair cleanly into four sections (hot-cross bun).

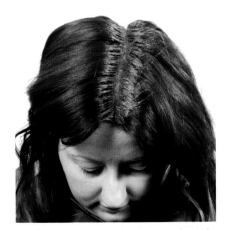

STEP 3 – Apply the colour evenly and cleanly to the root area.

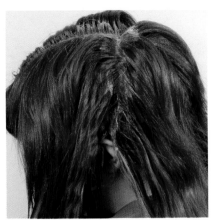

STEP 4 – Follow your section pattern for a thorough coverage.

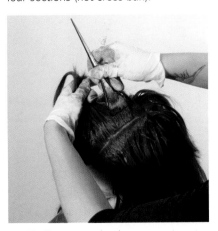

STEP 5 – Cross-check your sections to ensure even coverage.

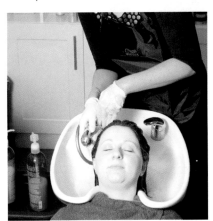

STEP 6 – After development and checking of the colour, rinse, emulsify, shampoo and condition.

Woven highlights

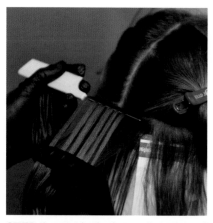

STEP 1 – Divide the hair to be coloured into manageable sections and weave your section.

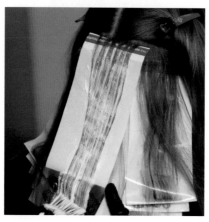

STEP 2 – Apply the product evenly without overloading the root area.

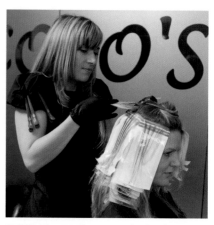

STEP 3 – Work in a methodical manner towards the top of the head.

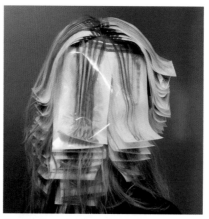

STEP 4 – When you have completed all the hair, leave it to develop.

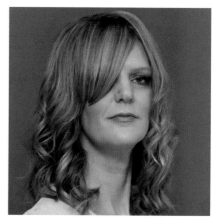

STEP 5 – The finished look.

Colour placement system, dip-dyed effect

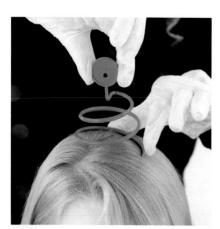

STEP 1 – Place the small twister (size 1) on the scalp and turn clockwise 360°.

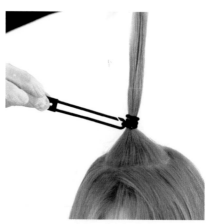

STEP 2 – Secure the sectioned hair with the soft band and attach the hook.

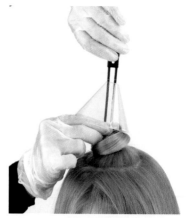

STEP 3 – Thread the hooked sectioned hair through the first shade and secure with the hook – this hair has not been coloured.

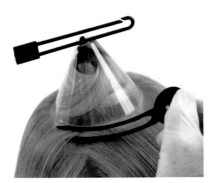

STEP 4 – Using the twin tail comb for accuracy, take the next section of hair.

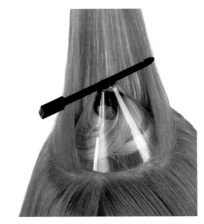

STEP 5 – Complete the section of hair around the shade.

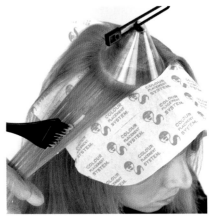

STEP 6 – Apply a colour guard over the first shade and lay the sectioned hair over the top.

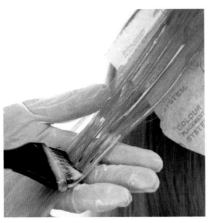

STEP 7 – Apply the colour to the hair using the colour guard to protect the root area.

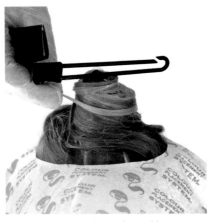

STEP 8 – Wrap the coloured hair around the shade securely.

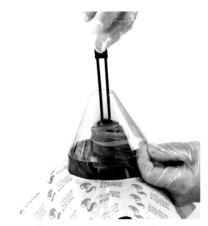

STEP 9 – Cover the coloured hair with the next-sized shade and secure with the hook.

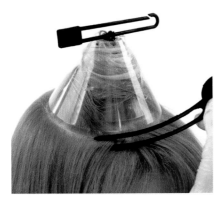

STEP 10 – Repeat the 360°-sectioning pattern and colour application as required.

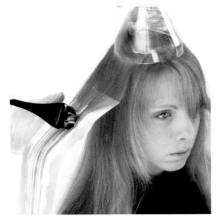

STEP 11 – Add a few woven highlights or slices of colour to the mid-lengths Leave colour to develop, following the manufacturers' instructions.

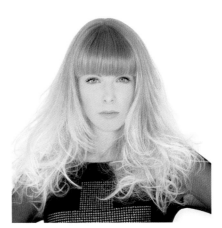

STEP 12 – The finished look.

Answers in the back of the book.

1 Which **one** of the following is the legislation that should be adhered to when using colour?

a The Trades Descriptions Act

b The Data Protection Act

c RIDDOR

d COSHH

2 **Statement one**

From November 2012, the use of HC orange No 2 is prohibited for use on under 16s.

Statement two

From November 2008, the use of 2-hydroxyethylamino-nitroanisole is restricted for use on under 18s.

Which **one** of the following is correct for the above statements?

a True   True

b True   False

c False   True

d False   False

3 Why is it important to use products economically?

a To minimise infection and ensure the best result

b To ensure the best outcome and prevent injury

c To maximise profits and minimise infection

d To minimise waste and maximise profits

4 Which **one** of the following is the recommended total service time for a full-head permanent colour?

a 50–70 minutes

b 80–110 minutes

c 120–140 minutes

d 150–170 minutes

5 Which **one** of the following is a hair classification that affects the colouring technique to be used?

a Very curly, frizzy hair

b Fine textured, white hair

c Naturally coloured, wavy hair

d Medium textured, straight hair

6 How long should a client wait after a relaxer before having a permanent colour?

a 2–3 days

b 7 days

c 2–3 weeks

d 7 weeks

7 **Statement one**

Depending on the natural depth of hair and the peroxide strength, high-lift tint will lift up to seven shades.

Statement two

Toners are used to remove unwanted tone left behind after lightening.

Which **one** of the following is correct for the above statements?

a True   True

b True   False

c False   True

d False   False

8 **Statement one**

One of the differences between quasi- and semi-permanent colour, is that a quasi- is mixed with a developer.

Statement two

Quasi-permanent colours act in the same way as semi-permanent colours; they just last longer.

Which **one** of the following is correct for the above statements?

a True   True

b True   False

c False   True

d False   False

9 Which **one** of the following is best used on the scalp for lifting up to six shades?

  a Gel bleach

  b Blue bleach powder

  c Permanent tint

  d White bleach powder

10 Which **one** of the following identify the chemical process and the most commonly used chemical for permanently colouring hair?

  a Reduction and hydrogen peroxide

  b Oxidation and hydrogen peroxide

  c Polymerisation and hydrogen

  d Polymerisation and oxygen

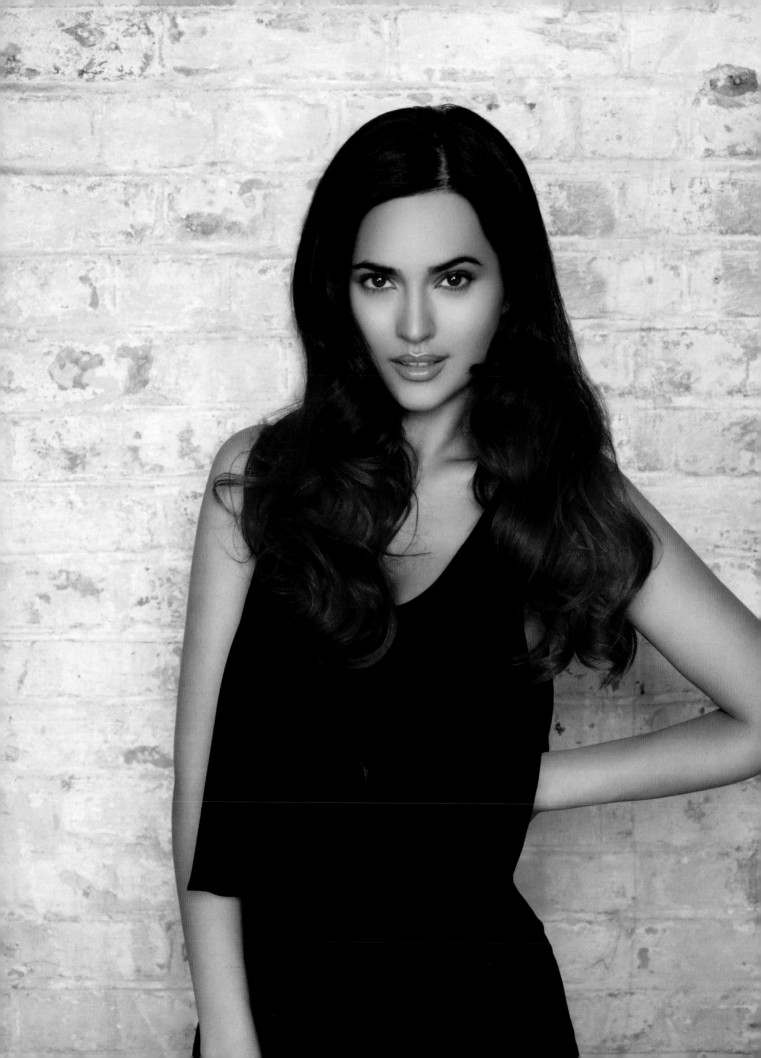

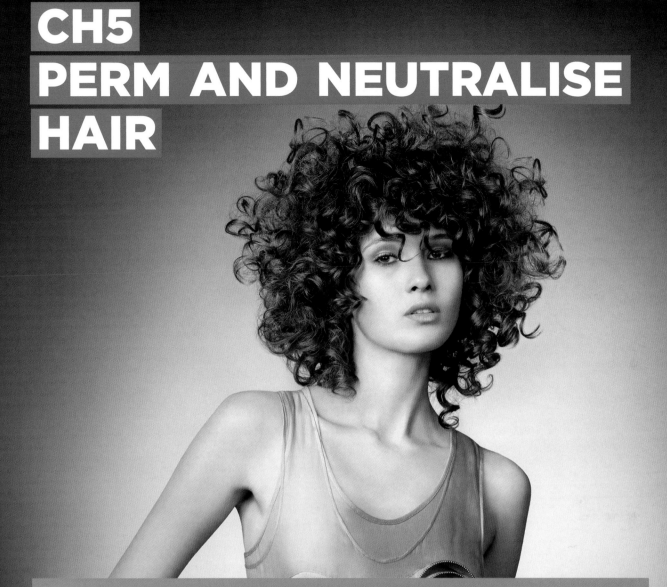

CH5
PERM AND NEUTRALISE HAIR

Perms are making a comeback, as curly hair is becoming more and more popular. Modern setting techniques are great, but they're high maintenance if your clients want to recreate the look themselves. Perming makes it possible for clients to recreate loose curls, spiral curls or a tousled look and, most importantly, maintain it at reasonable cost at home. Perm winding is creative and improves your dexterity, but understanding the science behind it is extremely important because you are working with strong chemicals and changing the hair's structure, and you don't want to damage your client's hair.

After reading this chapter you will:

- know how health and safety affects perming, neutralising and chemical rearranging services
- understand the factors that influence perming, neutralising and chemical rearranging services
- understand the science of the perming, neutralising and chemical rearranging services
- know the tools, equipment, products and techniques used for perming, neutralising and chemical rearranging services
- be able to perm and neutralise hair.

Health and safety

Your responsibilities under health and safety

HANDY HINT

When using chemicals, always follow SHUD, which is derived from COSHH: store, handle, use and dispose of substances correctly following the MFIs, your salon policy and local by-laws.

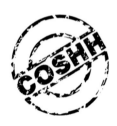

When perming, neutralising and chemically rearranging the hair you'll be using some very strong chemicals that can cause harm to yourself and your client. It is therefore important that you work safely throughout this service and ensure that both you and your client are effectively protected.

Activity

Refer to the health and safety and salon policies chapter and list your responsibilities under the health and safety legislation.

Protecting your client

You must protect your client's clothing with a gown, towel and a shoulder cape to ensure they remain dry and to avoid getting chemicals on their clothes. Before you apply the chemical rearranger or perm lotion or neutraliser, you should apply a barrier cream around your client's hairline to protect the skin from the chemicals. You must take particular care to avoid contact of the lotion with your client's eyes.

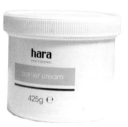
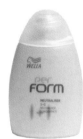

Barrier cream   Neutraliser

Personal protection, health and hygiene

You will be standing for long periods of time, so you must wear sensible, flat-soled, closed-in shoes and stand correctly. Always wear personal protective equipment (PPE) to protect your clothes and skin from the chemicals.

You must maintain your personal health and hygiene throughout the service by showering daily, wearing clean clothes, using deodorant, and carefully covering and protecting any cuts or open wounds. Always check that your body odour and your breath are fresh, as you'll be working in close **proximity** to your clients and colleagues.

Proximity

Closeness to, in terms of space.

HANDY HINT

Poor standards of hygiene can cause offence to your clients, give a poor salon image and cause cross-contamination.

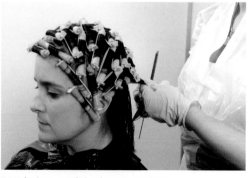

PPE being useful when perming

Salon waste

You must remove any used or wet soiled cotton wool after the perm or neutralising process. This will aid client comfort and prevent perm lotion coming into contact with the skin for long periods, which might cause chemical burns to the hairline area.

You must ensure that you dispose of all salon waste in the designated waste bin and rinse any excess products down the sink with plenty of cold water. This will ensure that chemicals are diluted and that you work within your salon policy, follow the MFIs and local by-laws.

If, during the service, you identify any stock shortages, you must report this to the relevant person who will add these products or resources to the stock order list.

Contra-indications that can affect the delivery of services

The following contra-indications may prevent or affect perming, neutralising and chemically rearranging services. We explore the implications of these contra-indications in the science section of this chapter:

- history of previous allergic reaction to perming products
- other known allergies
- skin disorders
- previous chemical treatments
- medical advice or instructions
- incompatible products
- recent removal of hair extensions or plaits.

> **HEALTH & SAFETY**
>
> Refer to the health and safety chapter to recap on environmental and sustainable working practices, such as:
> - reducing waste and safe disposal
> - using disposable items
> - reducing energy usage
> - preventing pollution.

> **VALUES & BEHAVIOURS**
>
> Refer to the values and behaviours chapter for more information on personal hygiene and protection, maintaining effective and safe methods for working and meeting your salon standards of behaviour.

Hazards and risks

Along with the hazards and risks identified in previous chapters and previous learning, you must be aware of the potential dangers in the perming, neutralising and chemically rearranging service.

HANDY HINT

If towels get damp from the shampoo or neutralising service, you must remove them from your client and replace them immediately with clean, dry ones.

HANDY HINT

A supply of clean towels and fresh shoulder capes should be available throughout the perming and neutralising process for your client's comfort.

Activity

Look at the hazard and risk diagram below and identify at least three more potential hazards and risks.

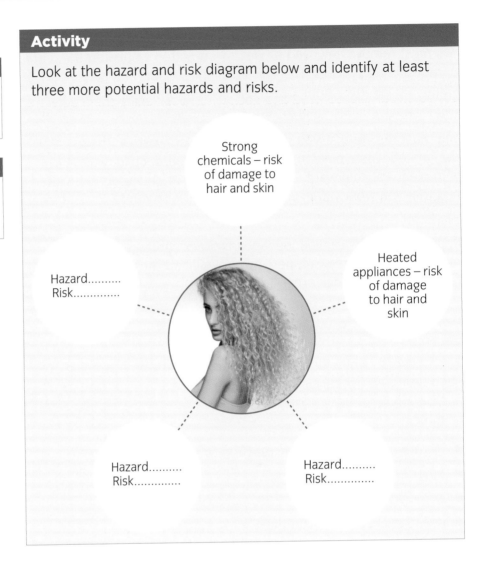

Strong chemicals – risk of damage to hair and skin

Heated appliances – risk of damage to hair and skin

Hazard..........
Risk..............

Hazard..........
Risk..............

Hazard..........
Risk..............

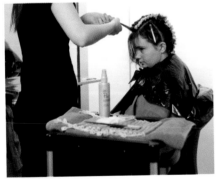

Prepare your trolley in advance of the service

Periodically

Sometimes or occasionally.

Safe and hygienic working practices

Before your client arrives, ensure you're prepared to carry out the service. Keep your work area clean and tidy to avoid potential hazards and risk of injury, to ensure the salon looks professional, and to minimise the risk of infection, infestation and cross-contamination.

Position your tools and equipment for ease of use

Prepare your trolley with the tools and equipment required, and clean and sterilise your tools before and after use. Always make effective use of your time to ensure you work to the commercially viable time.

Client positioning and preparation

You must always ensure that your client is comfortable; **periodically** ask about their comfort and offer refreshments. Ask your client to sit upright, with their back against the back of the salon chair and their legs uncrossed.

When you shampoo and neutralise their hair, ensure that you support your client's head and neck when positioning them down to the basin and, again, lifting their head and neck after the shampoo and neutralising process too.

To prepare the hair for a perming or chemical rearranging service, you should shampoo the hair with a clarifying or deep cleansing shampoo (pH 6–7) to remove any residue or styling product from the hair. Surface conditioner should not be used before the service, as it coats the hair and creates a barrier to the lotions.

Safe use of equipment and products
Equipment

Your equipment should have a yearly portable appliance test (PAT) carried out by an electrician to ensure it's safe and fit for use. Every time you use a piece of electrical equipment, you must check it visually by looking at the power cable, plug and main body to ensure that it's in good working order. This will prevent harm and risk of injury to you and others.

> **Activity**
>
> What visual checks must you carry out before using any electrical equipment? If you identify a faulty electrical appliance, what are your responsibilities under the Electricity at Work Regulations? Can you list three responsibilities?

Products

During these services you may use shampoo, pre- and post-perm conditioner, perm lotion, neutraliser, chemical rearrangers and styling products. All of these are substances which could be hazardous to your health, through **absorption**, inhalation or ingestion. Always follow the Control of Substances Hazardous to Health (COSHH) guidelines as well as the manufacturers' instructions (MFIs) and your salon policy. Wear PPE, for example gloves, aprons, eye protection and masks (particularly if you're asthmatic), and prepare the chemicals in a well-ventilated area.

> **Activity**
>
> Research contact dermatitis and write down three ways in which you can help prevent it.

> **HANDY HINT**
>
> Stand with your feet apart and your body weight evenly distributed. Avoid overstretching or bending too much to prevent fatigue and back problems.

> **HEALTH & SAFETY**
>
> Refer to the health and safety and salon policies chapter to recap on environmental and sustainable working practices.

> **HANDY HINT**
>
> Avoid wastage by turning off taps between shampoos and using the correct amount of product to avoid overloading the hair. This will help the environment and keep the salon profitable.

> **Absorption**
>
> The passage of a substance through the skin.

> **VALUES & BEHAVIOURS**
>
> Refer to the values and behaviours chapter for more information on maintaining effective, hygienic and safe working methods.

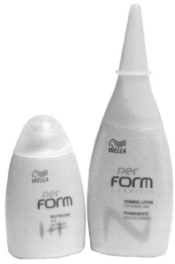

Neutraliser and perming lotion

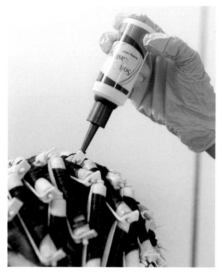

Wear gloves to protect your hands from dermatitis

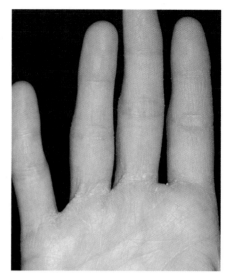

Dermatitis

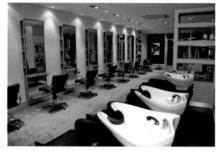

Clean and tidy salon

Preventing cross-infection and infestation

Work areas must be kept clean and tidy to promote a professional environment, maintain the image of the salon and prevent cross-contamination. Ensure your working methods are safe and hygienic, and minimise the risk of cross-infection and cross-infestation, by cleaning and sterilising tools, equipment and client protective clothing.

Activity

Which tools should be disinfected or sterilised using the following methods?

- autoclave
- UV light cabinet
- chemicals.

Preparing clients for the service

You'll need to prepare your client's hair for perming/chemical rearranging, and carry out a thorough consultation to ensure the desired result can be achieved. This will include:

- asking appropriate questions and listening to your client's responses
- analysing your client's hair
- identifying any contra-indications
- conducting relevant tests
- choosing the correct tools, equipment and products to use.

Questioning and listening

To identify the service that is best suited to your client's requirements and to achieve the desired result, you should ask a series of questions. Whether your client is new to perming/chemical rearranging or not, you'll need to ask them the same questions. Regular clients may want a change of curl, but even if a repeat service is required, you need to check whether anything has changed with the condition of the hair, their lifestyle or their health.

The types of question you should ask are:

- What do they want the service to achieve?
- What is their vision of the end result?
- What type of curl would they like?
- What size curl would they like?
- How much time do they have available to spend on their hair?
- Have they had this service before?
- When was their last perm?
- Have they had any previous problems with a chemical service?
- What chemicals (including relaxer) do they currently have on their hair, if any?
- Do they have any colour on their hair and, if so, what type of colour service did they have?
- Do they have any contra-indications such as allergies?

Record cards

If you are going to carry out a chemical service on a regular client, refer to their previous record card to check the service details and make sure that the last chemical service was to their satisfaction. Whether you are repeating the same service or changing it, you will need to add the details to the record card. For every client, regular or new, always ensure that their details are correct: check their name, address and contact details. Record the date, type of service, products used and the result, ensuring that the card is completed accurately and that it is easy to read. You must also record any relevant questions that you asked and the client's responses. This will ensure that:

- the correct service is carried out
- the records are available for future services
- you maintain a professional image
- you have documented evidence, in case of **litigation**.

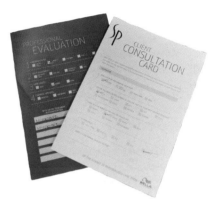

Check what products are on your client's hair and record your client's responses to questions asked

HANDY HINT

When completing record cards ensure you record the information and details accurately and write clearly and legibly.

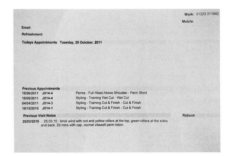

Completed record card

Litigation

Legal action.

WHY DON'T YOU...

Ask your manager if you can look at a client's service record card so you can see what details are recorded for future use.

HANDY HINT

Diversity

You will work on many different hair types to cover the range required. Some of the hair types you may perm or chemically rearrange could be European hair, Asian hair or African type hair. Clients will come from different ethnic groups, have different cultures and have different religions (or no religion). Make sure you respect other people's cultures and religions, even if they differ from your own personal views. See the values and behaviours chapter for more information on personal ethics.

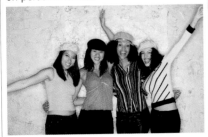

Factors that may influence services

To help you decide on the best rod/roller size and lotion choice and strength, you need to analyse your client's hair. By analysing the hair you can identify any potential problems that could occur. You should feel the hair and visually check it to identify the following factors:

- hair characteristics
- hair classifications
- temperature
- direction and degree of movement required
- hair length
- length of regrowth
- colour-treated hair.

How hair classifications might affect the service

Hair classification	Description	Impact on service
Type 1 – Straight hair Alkaline perm lotion	Fine/thin – hair tends to be very soft, shiny and oily and it can be difficult to hold a curl.	Although this type of hair is fine/thin it can be difficult to perm as it has tightly packed cuticles and is often shiny and oily. A slightly stronger perm lotion may be required to help lift the cuticle scales, or a smaller perm rod for a firmer curl.
	Medium – hair has lots of volume and body.	This hair type is likely to take well to perming and a lotion should be chosen to suit the hair condition and desired curl.
	Coarse – hair is normally extremely straight and difficult to curl.	A stronger perm product is likely to be required, it will need to be developed for the full development time and smaller rods may be required for the curl to be achieved.

Hair classification	Description	Impact on service
Type 2 – **Wavy hair** *Acid perm lotion*	Fine/thin – hair has a definite 'S' pattern. Normally can accomplish various styles.	This hair type is likely to take well to perming and a lotion should be chosen to suit the hair condition and desired curl.
	Medium – hair tends to be frizzy and a little resistant to styling.	This hair type is likely to take well to perming and a lotion should be chosen to suit the hair condition and desired curl, but care is needed to ensure the hair does not become any frizzier. A pre-perm treatment may be required to help even out porosity.
	Coarse – normally very frizzy; tends to have thicker waves.	This hair type is likely to take well to perming and a lotion should be chosen to suit the hair condition and desired curl. However, additional care is needed to ensure the hair does not become any frizzier and you need to use a pre-perm treatment to even out porosity. Consideration should be given to the rod size as the hair may curl very easily. A post-perm conditioner should be applied at the end of the service to help prevent the hair from drying out any more.
Type 3 – **Curly hair** *Curl boost perm (after rearranger perm lotion)*	Loose curls – it can be thick and full with lots of body, with a definite 'S' pattern. It also tends to be frizzy.	If perming loose curly hair to create smaller or tighter curls, you would need to consider the rod size and use of pre- and post-perm treatments, the lotion strength and choice, as the hair is likely to curl quickly and tightly. Otherwise the result could be frizzier hair. A larger perm rod could be used on this hair type to soften the curls.
	Tight curls – with a medium amount of curl.	Tight curly hair may need to be chemically rearranged to pre-soften the curls prior to winding a perm on larger rods to achieve the desired result.
Type 4 – **Very curly hair** *Chemical rearranger*	Soft – tightly coiled and has a more defined curly pattern.	Very curly hair will need to be chemically rearranged to pre-soften the curls prior to winding a perm on larger rods to achieve the desired result.
	Wiry – tightly coiled; however, with a less defined curly pattern – has more of a 'Z' pattern shape. This hair texture tends to be the most porous of all hair types.	

HANDY HINT

For more on hair classifications and characteristics, see chapter CHB9.

How hair characteristics might affect the service

There are a number of hair characteristics which may affect the service you provide:

- density
- texture
- elasticity
- porosity
- condition
- hair growth pattern.

Hair characteristic	Impact on service
Hair density 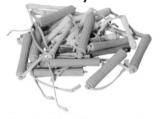 Choose the right size curlers for the hair's density	When checking the density of the hair, you are identifying whether the hair is sparse, medium or abundant. For sparse hair, a brick wind is the most suitable technique to use, as this prevents too many roller marks or partings being seen that would expose the scalp. Avoid too much tension, avoid winds that create roller section marks, use less lotion than normal and use a product that is milder on the hair. For abundant hair, you'll need more rods, more lotion and smaller sections when winding, so allow yourself sufficient time to wind the hair. Use larger rods on thick, abundant hair, as smaller rods may result in frizzy curls.
Hair texture 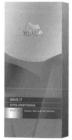 Choose the right perm lotion for the hair's texture	When checking the hair's texture, you are identifying whether the hair is fine, average or coarse. Services on fine soft hair may develop quicker than on coarse hair, and will require a softer lotion. However, if the hair is fine and resistant then it will take longer to develop and you're likely to need a stronger lotion. Coarse hair will take longer to develop, depending on its condition, and larger rods may be required. More lotion is likely to be required for coarse hair.

Hair characteristic	Impact on service
Elasticity 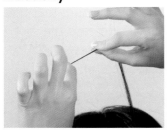 Elasticity test	An elasticity test must also be carried out to test the strength of the cortex layer. If the hair is weak, alternative services must be recommended instead of a perm/chemical rearranger, or you could suggest a series of conditioning or penetrating treatments for a few weeks before retesting the hair's strength. If the hair has weak elasticity it is unlikely to withstand a chemical rearranger and then a perming service. If the hair is normal or strong, then consider the lotion strength required.
Porosity 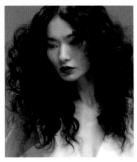 Pre-perm treatment	You must always carry out a porosity test to identify if the cuticle layers are open or closed and if the hair is porous, non-porous or even resistant. Porous hair will absorb the chemicals quickly so the ingredients will be active immediately. This hair will therefore need protecting from the chemicals and you may need to use a **pre-perm conditioner**, which is designed to even out the porosity of the hair. If the hair is very porous it is unlikely to withstand a chemical rearranger and then a perming service. Resistant hair is likely to require more lotion, longer development time and smaller rods, and sometimes you may benefit from **pre-damping** the hair with lotion prior to winding. Different hair types vary immensely in porosity – see the chart above on classifications and their varying characteristics. **Pre-perm conditioner** A spray-in conditioner that evens out the porosity of the hair. **Pre-damping** Winding with lotion already applied to the hair.
Condition 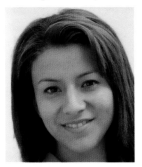 Long hair perm	The hair's condition will affect the porosity and elasticity of the hair (see the 'Elasticity' and 'Porosity' rows above). Longer hair, however, may have areas of weaker condition and pre-perm lotions may be required to level out the porosity and condition of the hair. A strand test is required during a service using a chemical rearranger to establish the effect the product has on the hair's condition.
Hair growth patterns Consider hair growth patterns like cowlicks	You should consider the growth patterns of the hair and wind accordingly. Consider a direction wind to work with strong double crowns or troublesome cowlicks.

Other factors that may affect the service	Impact on service
Temperature 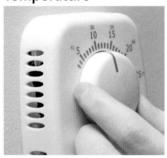	When you process a perm/chemical rearranger, you need to ensure that the environment is warm enough. If the salon is cold, this will increase the development time, as cool air slows down the development process. A warm salon or additional heat, such as an electronic accelerator, will decrease the development time. To decrease the development time, you may be able to use a rollerball, a climazone, a hood dryer or even just a disposable cap, as this will keep in natural heat generated from the head – always check whether your manufacturer's instructions state that heat can or can't be used.
Movement 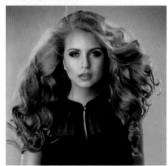	The client requirements for the direction of movement and how much movement and curl are required are key factors to consider. The more curl and movement that are required, the smaller the perm rod will need to be; the softer and looser the curl requirement, the larger the perm rod.
Hair length 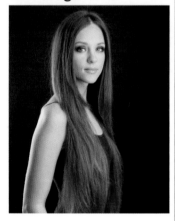	For longer hair you will need more time for the wind, more lotion to coat the hair and you may also need to consider your winding technique. If the hair is long and in good condition you may decide to wind with lotion – a technique called pre-damping. This ensures that all the hair is covered with lotion through to the ends, as the lotion might not penetrate to the ends if it is applied after winding. Longer hair will go around a rod more times than shorter hair and therefore create more movement. Although you may decide to use larger rods because of this, you must remember that the weight of long hair can pull the curls looser, so you must consider the density of the hair before making your final decision on rod size. When working with African type hair remember that the natural compact curl pattern will disguise the length of the hair and the hair will be elongated after chemical rearrangement.

Other factors that may affect the service	Impact on service
Length of regrowth 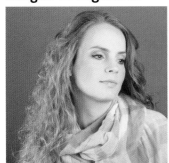	If the hair has previous perm on the hair you need to check how long ago the service took place. You'll need to find out if the hair needs to be cut before it's permed, if it needs a pre-perm conditioner on the mid-lengths and ends and if it is in good enough condition to take another chemical service.
Colour-treated hair 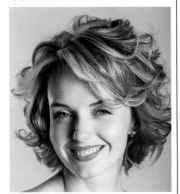	Hair that has been highlighted and tinted can often be permed with a perm lotion especially designed for highlighted hair, but a course of penetrating treatments may still be required before perming. Hair that has been bleached must not be permed or chemically rearranged. Before deciding on your perm choice you'll need to find the answer to these questions: Is there colour on the hair? Is it even and over the whole head or are there highlights, which may give an uneven porosity? Is there bleach on the hair? You should carry out an incompatibility test or a pre-perm test curl, if you are unsure as to what is on the client's hair.

Products, tools and equipment

Products

Pre-perm treatments

Pre-perm treatments generally refer to conditioners rather than the shampoo process. However, using a pre-perm shampoo prior to a perm is advisable. Chemical rearrangement is carried out on dry hair, for instance a relaxing service (using thioglycolate).

Pre-perm shampoo

A pre-perm shampoo should be used prior to perming. This type of shampoo has a neutral pH (pH 7) and therefore slightly opens the cuticle layer to allow the perm lotion to penetrate the cortex layer, where the changes during the perming process take place. A pre-perm shampoo helps to remove any dirt, products and oil residue from the hair that may coat the cuticle layer and create a barrier to the perm lotion.

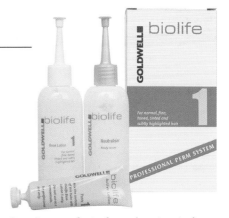

Perming products for colour-treated hair

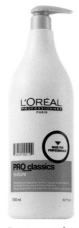

Pre-perm shampoo

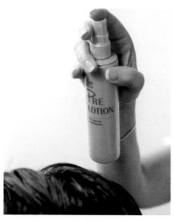

Pre-perm conditioner

Phial

Small bottle.

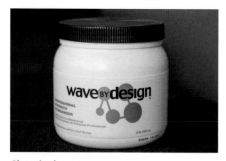

Chemical rearranger

Exothermic

Producing heat through a chemical reaction.

HANDY HINT

Use a pre-perm lotion on coloured hair to even out porosity.

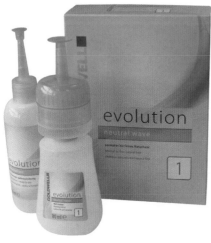

pH-neutral perm lotion

Pre-perm conditioner

A pre-perm conditioner should be used on the mid-lengths and ends of the hair if you have identified that the hair has an uneven porosity. A pre-perm conditioner can be sprayed (or sprinkled directly from a **phial**) on the hair before sectioning or winding the hair with the rods. It is important that you avoid spraying it on hair that has good porosity and aim it directly onto the porous and uneven areas of the hair. These conditioners even out the porosity and allow the perm lotion to penetrate evenly into the cortex layer.

Chemical rearranger

A chemical rearranger is generally used on African type hair to partially relax natural curls before a perm. Due to the natural shape of excessively curly hair with its many twists and turns along the hair, the surface is uneven. The product is often a cream emulsion rather than a lotion and it is applied to the hair in a four-section sequence to reduce the natural curl pattern. Once the hair is straighter, the rearranger is removed by rinsing thoroughly. This process will facilitate easy winding as the hair is now more easily adaptable to winding techniques. The hair is then permed with a perm lotion. Chemical rearrangers are alkaline and have a pH above 9.

Perming products

Perming products are available in varied forms, such as acidic, alkaline and **exothermic** perm lotions, and come in varied strengths to suit all hair types. When using a perm for African type hair use the perm lotion that comes from the same system as the rearranger as the pH and supporting ingredients will work effectively together. These are usually alkaline perms.

Perm lotion types may be written as:

- 0 or R – for resistant hair types, or hair that is difficult to perm (such as coarse hair)
- 1 or N – for normal hair types
- 2 or T – for tinted or coloured hair that is porous.

When deciding whether to use an acidic or an alkaline perm lotion, you should consider all of the following:

- what movement the client would like
- the hair's condition of the hair and what products are already on the hair
- the hair's texture, density and length
- whether the client wants a soft or long-lasting curl result.

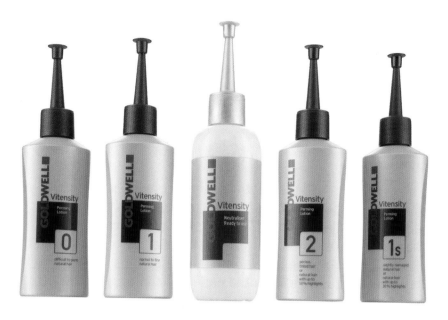

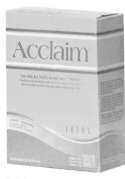

Acid perm

Acid perms

Acid perms are pH 6–7 and are therefore less damaging to the hair than alkaline perms. Acidic perms require a heat activator to help open the cuticle layer of the hair. This activator either comes in a separate bottle or can be 'hidden' in the screw cap of the perm lotion bottle. When the cap is twisted, it pierces the seal and the activator mixes with the perm lotion, activating it. Whether you add a separate activator or activate the product from the cap, when the two products mix, mild heat is generated. This heat helps to open the cuticle layer to allow the perm lotion into the cortex layer. You must only activate this product when the hair is wound and ready to be damped. If you activate it too early, the product strength will weaken. Therefore, acid perms can be used only for **post-damp** applications.

Acid perms are most suitable for sensitive hair, fine hair and softer curl requirements but they are available in varying strengths for resistant, normal and tinted hair.

Alkaline perms

Most alkaline perms are pH 8.5–9.5 but some can be much lower, around pH 7.1. The lower the pH, the milder the lotion and therefore the less damaging it is to the hair. Alkaline perms give firmer curls and are most suited to resistant, strong hair, oily hair and white hair.

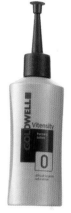

Product for difficult-to-perm natural hair

Post-damp

Applying the lotion after the wind.

Activity

Take two test cuttings of white hair and compare how well they perm with an acid perm lotion and an alkaline perm lotion.

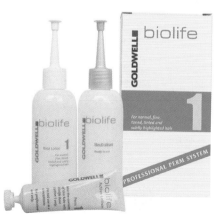

Alkaline perm

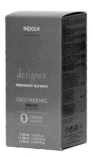

Exothermic perm product

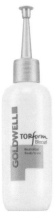

Neutraliser

Creeping oxidation

Where chemicals are left in the hair and they carry on working and cause damage.

Exothermic perms

Exothermic perms can be acid or alkaline, as the pH value varies. Exothermic perms produce their own heat when two separate chemicals are mixed together and the neutralising lotions also create heat when mixed together. These provide similar benefits to the acid perm lotions and are available for all hair types.

Neutralisers

You should always use the neutraliser that comes with your chosen perm lotion, as the manufacturer will have designed the two products to work together. Neutralisers are pH 3–5 and can be applied in different ways; refer to the MFIs. Some products must be applied directly from the bottle onto the rinsed rods; others may be diluted in a large applicator bottle and sprinkled over the rinsed rods. Another way to apply neutraliser is to pour the contents into a bowl and 'foam' it with a sponge. The neutraliser is then applied to the rods with the sponge and left to develop.

Post-perm treatment

After every perm service, a pH balancing conditioner should be used. We refer to these as post-perm treatments or conditioners. A post-perm treatment has the following special properties:

- it stops the chemical processing from continuing
- it stops **creeping oxidation**
- it returns the hair back to its natural pH of 4.5–5.5
- it closes the cuticle layer and stops the hair from losing moisture and becoming brittle.

Tools and equipment

Your trolley should be prepared with the items in the table below before your client arrives.

Tools and equipment	Purpose
Apron and gloves	To protect your clothes and skin from the chemicals.
Pintail comb	To section the hair during the winding process. A metal pintail comb cannot be used when winding with lotion (pre-damp technique) as the metal may react with the chemicals in the perm lotion.

Tools and equipment	Purpose
Section clips	To hold longer hair in sections in order to aid methodical working.
Detangling comb	To detangle the hair. This wide-toothed comb will prevent damaging the hair and minimise discomfort for the client.
End papers	To be used on the ends of the client's hair when winding the hair down the rod, enabling you to control the ends of the hair and wind without causing **fish hooks**.
Barrier cream	To be applied around the hairline before the damp cotton wool is applied. This prevents the perm lotion coming into contact with the scalp and skin, thereby avoiding discomfort or chemical burns.
Cotton wool	To be placed around the client's hairline when the perm lotion or neutraliser is being applied. Make sure the cotton wool is replaced if it becomes saturated or it might hold the chemicals against the client's skin.

Fish hooks

Buckled ends from poor winding technique.

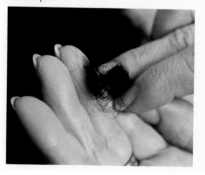

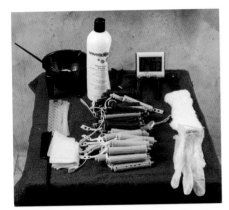

Trolley prepared for perming service

Tools and equipment	Purpose
Water spray	To be used during winding. Wound hair should be misted all over with the water spray to maintain an even moisture balance.
Plastic cap	To be placed over the wound head of hair once the perm lotion has been applied in order to keep in the natural heat from the head and aid development.
Timer	To time the development of the chemical process.

Once you have completed your consultation, relevant hair tests and decided which rod sizes are required to achieve the desired result, you can add the following items to your prepared trolley.

Tools and equipment	Purpose
Perm rods, small to medium	These are generally used when a client requests tighter curls but can also be used to achieve medium curls on dense hair. Longer hair may also require a slightly smaller rod, as the weight of the hair may pull the curls down, making them a little looser.
Perm rods, medium to large	Provide a looser curl for softer-looking curls.

Tools and equipment	Purpose
Bendy rods 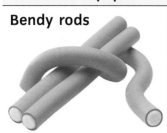	Bendy rods come in different sizes and can be used to produce spiral curls, tight curls and loose curls. The curl type will depend on the hair length, density, chosen wind and size of roller.
Accelerator 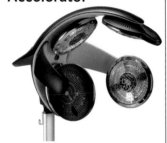	An accelerator can be used to speed up the development process of the perm (check the MFIs).

HANDY HINT

If you are using a hood dryer to develop the perm process, you must take care to prevent the dryer from drying out the perm lotion. Always ensure you use a plastic cap to contain the moisture.

When the perm has been completed and the neutralising process needs to take place, you will need two more items at the basin area.

Tools and equipment	Purpose
Bowl 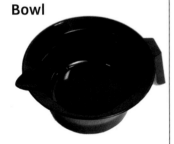	To contain the neutralising product (if you are applying the neutraliser with the bowl-and-sponge technique).
Sponge 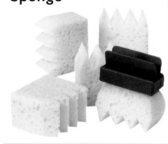	To froth/foam the neutraliser in the bowl before applying the neutralising product.

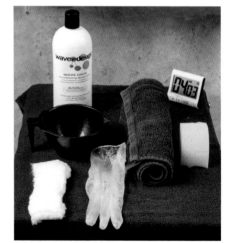

Trolley prepared for neutralising stage

Activity

After reading the previous lists, go and prepare your trolley for a perm service.

Write down anything you missed and discuss this with your tutor/manager.

HANDY HINT

Skin tests are only needed if the MFI states this. Perm lotions and rearrangers are irritants so usually there is no way of carrying out a skin test. Never carry out a perming service if the client has had an allergic reaction to perming products before.

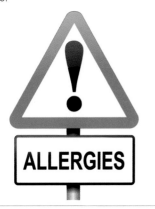

Science of perming, neutralising and chemical rearranging services

Test the hair and scalp

Recognising contra-indications

You'll need to ask appropriate questions to check whether your client has ever had any of the following problems:

- previous allergic reaction to perming products
- other known allergies
- skin disorders
- imcompatible products
- medical advice or instructions
- previous chemical treatments
- recent removal of hair extensions or plaits.

Contra-indication	Things to consider	Effect on the service
Previous allergic reaction to perming products	The client is more likely to suffer an allergic reaction to your perm product or a chemical rearranger if they have previously had an allergic reaction to perm products or relaxers.	If your client has had an allergic reaction to perming or relaxing products before, you must carry out a skin test using your chosen perm lotion or chemical rearranger prior to starting the service, but only where this is permitted in the MFIs (some products are too harsh to be used on the skin at all). If you are unsure, do not carry out the service, but recommend an alternative service and ask the client to seek medical advice before continuing with the service.
Other known allergies	The client is more prone to suffer an allergic reaction to your perming type products if they have a history of allergic reactions and allergies to other products.	Ask your client what their allergies are, check the ingredients in the chemical rearranger, perm lotion and neutraliser and carry out a skin test with the chosen product. If you are unsure, do not perm and recommend an alternative service.
Skin disorders	The disorder may cause discomfort to your client if open or sore. It may also be contagious and infectious.	If your client has a skin disorder on their head, check whether it is open or weeping. If it is, do not carry out the service. If it is not open, sore or weeping and you can protect it, proceed with care. Check that the disorder is not infectious or an infestation. If it is, do not carry out the service.

Contra-indication	Things to consider	Effect on the service
Incompatible products	Incompatible products may react with your perm products or chemical rearrangers and cause a chemical reaction or damage to the hair, skin or scalp.	Check with your client which products have already been used on the hair. If you have concerns that these products are not compatible with the perm lotion, carry out an incompatibility test on the hair. If the result is positive, do not carry out the service.
Medical advice or instructions	The hair may not be suitable to a chemical service if the client is on certain medications or in ill health.	Ask your client whether they are on any medication. If you are unsure as to the likely reaction of the hair while on this medication or the client's health as a result of perming the hair, do not carry out the service but refer your client to their GP for further advice.
Previous chemical treatments	The hair may have too many chemicals present on the hair and the condition may not be good enough to sustain another chemical service, or the chemicals on the hair may not be compatible – see 'Incompatible products' above.	Check with your client which products have already been used on the hair. Carry out porosity and elasticity tests and if you have concerns, carry out an incompatibility test. If the result is positive, do not carry out the service. If a client with African type hair has previously had a relaxing service to straighten the hair and hydroxides have been used it is also not possible to carry out a perm – thioglycolate and hydroxide are not compatible and if the two chemicals are overlapped the hair will break.
Recent removal of hair extensions or plaits	The scalp may be tender and the hair follicles inflamed after the removal of hair extensions or plaits. This could lead to hair loss if excessive tension is applied when perm winding or an infection of the follicles if perm lotion and/or chemical rearranger is then applied.	Check the scalp area for hair loss and inflamed follicles. Ask your client whether they have any discomfort. Do not carry out the service if there is evidence of hair loss, inflamed follicles or if extensions or plaits have been removed within seven days. It is important that the client has a course of strengthening treatments prior to a perm and after the removal of extensions or braids.

HANDY HINT

Remember: thioglycolate and hydroxide are not compatible and if the two chemicals are overlapped the hair will break!

HANDY HINT

Always seek guidance from your manager if you are unsure what to do about a contra-indication.

HANDY HINT

For each question you ask your client about contra-indications, you must record the answer on the client's record card and ask them to sign it for confirmation of what has been said and recorded. This will provide accurate information for future services and, in the event of an adverse reaction, you have documented proof of your client's responses in case of litigation.

Conducting relevant tests

Instructions from manufacturers will always vary, so make sure you always follow your MFIs in relation to these tests.

Test	When to carry out the test	How to carry out the test	Purpose	Action
Strand test Chemical rearranger strand test	This test is carried out prior to the rearranging process.	Apply the chemical rearranger to a discrete section of the hair and carry out the full development. If the test is on scalp, monitor every five minutes to determine whether the hair has been sufficiently 'smoothed' prior to the winding perm. If the test is off scalp, take small samples of hair from various areas of the head, secure them together and apply the rearranger – the results will determine if the condition of the hair is suitable to proceed with the service.	To establish the effect of the product on the hair and its condition, such as whether the degree of straightness/ smoothness has been achieved before winding	If condition of hair is good and outcome confirms the service can go ahead. Development time is confirmed and degree of straightness achieved. Do not proceed with the service if the degree of straightness is not achieved or the condition of the hair is weak.

HANDY HINT

It is important to confirm that straightening has been achieved by taking strand tests on different areas of the head and at suitable times in the chemical rearranging process to ensure the desired result has been achieved and that it is even throughout.

Test	When to carry out the test	How to carry out the test	Purpose	Action
Development test	This test is carried out during the perm development process	Partially unwind a perm roller and push the hair back towards the root. Do this in three to four areas around the head. A positive result shows an adequate S-bend in a similar size to the roller. A negative result can be either a weak S-bend, meaning the development time is insufficient or, if the hair has been overdeveloped, this test will identify that too many bonds have been broken within the hair and the S-bend will be much tighter than required.	To check whether the perm development time has been sufficient.	If the curl result is not achieved, re-wind the perm rod and develop for a longer period of time, following the MFIs. Later retest the same rod and an additional area. If the curl result has been achieved, then the hair is ready to be rinsed and neutralised. If the perm or chemical rearranger is overdeveloped then damage to and/or disintegration of the client's hair or skin may occur. The hair will need to be treated with a penetrating conditioner. Legal action may be taken by the client if their hair or skin is damaged, in which case your manager should inform their insurance company.

Test	When to carry out the test	How to carry out the test	Purpose	Action
Elasticity	This test is carried out before the perm service or chemical rearranger.	On wet hair, stretch a few hairs. See whether the hair stretches and returns to its original length	To test the strength of the cortex layer	If the hair stretches and returns then the elasticity is good – proceed with perm or chemical rearranger service. If the hair stretches and stays stretched or snaps, the hair is in weak condition and has poor elasticity. Offer alternative services and courses of conditioning treatments.
Porosity	This test is carried out before the perm service or chemical rearranger.	On dry hair, run your finger and thumb along the cuticle layer of the hair shaft towards the scalp. Feel whether your finger and thumb run along the hair smoothly or whether there is resistance and the hair feels bumpy.	To identify whether the cuticle layers are porous or non-porous	Good porosity results will mean you can proceed with the service. Porous hair will either need a pre-perm treatment or, if very porous, do not proceed with the service.

Test	When to carry out the test	How to carry out the test	Purpose	Action
Incompatibility 	This test is carried out before the perm service or chemical rearranger.	Take a test cutting and place hair in a solution of 20:1 liquid peroxide and ammonium hydroxide and leave for up to 30 minutes. If the hair bubbles, gets warm and/or causes hair discolouration then there are metallic salts present on the hair.	To test whether the hair has products on it that are incompatible with your salon products.	No reaction – proceed with service. Do not perm if the hair reacts in the solution. Offer treatments and retest in four to six weeks' time.

Potential consequences of failing to test hair

The results of these hair tests help you decide on the rod size, lotion strength, development time and most suitable service.

The results from these tests could prevent the service from taking place. Do not perm if a client has a positive reaction or if breakage occurs during a test as the hair and scalp may be damaged and the client may take legal action.

Offer advice for penetrating conditioning treatments and suggest alternative services. Always seek guidance from your manager if you are unsure what to do about a result of a hair test. You must record every test carried out and its result on the client's record card for future reference and in case of legal action.

VALUES & BEHAVIOURS

If a perm or chemical rearranger service cannot be carried out, refer to the values and behaviours chapter for more information on explaining clearly to clients any reasons why their needs or expectations cannot be met.

Activity

Feel the different textures and densities of the hair of the people in your salon. Look at their hair lengths and natural movement and identify which perm lotion would be most suitable. Don't forget to consider the hair's condition and what products have already been used. Ask each person to give you an indication of what sort of curl result they would like, so you can also choose the rod size.

Present your findings in an interesting way.

The effects of perming, chemical rearranging and neutralising on the hair structure

The perm/chemical rearranger and neutralising process goes through three stages: softening, moulding and fixing. The perm lotion/ chemical rearranger starts the softening stage, the development process is the moulding stage and the neutraliser fixes the hair in its new shape. Perm lotions and neutralisers are generally in a liquid form and chemical rearrangers are in a cream form.

The science

Recall that in chapter CH1 we covered that hair is made up of amino acids and peptide bonds, which originate in the hair follicle. The many amino acids and peptide bonds form the polypeptide chains (coils), which are held together by permanent and temporary bonds inside the cortex layer of the hair.

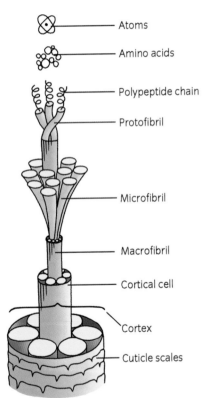

Detailed hair structure

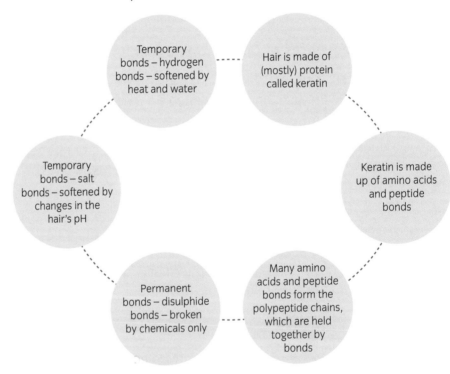

The diagram shows a single hair from the cuticle layer to the cortex layer. The polypeptide chains (coils) are found inside the cortex.

When you are blow drying, setting or styling with heated equipment, the temporary bonds are softened by the water and heat, and temporarily set into their new shape. When hair is permed, we are permanently changing the bonds with the use of chemicals. These bonds are called **disulphide bonds** (permanent bonds).

Disulphide bonds

Two sulphur atoms bonded together.

The temporary bonds hold the polypeptide chains in place along the length of the coils.

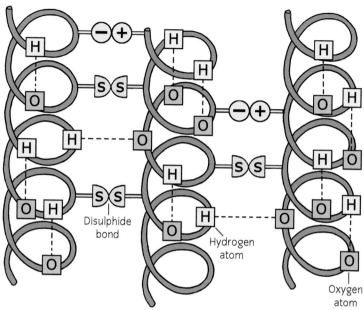

Temporary bonds of the hair

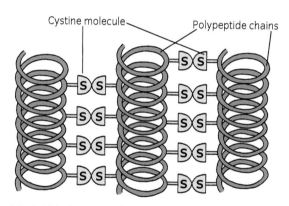

Disulphide bonds before perming process

The bonds that we change during perming are the disulphide bonds that hold the polypeptide chains in position across the coils from left to right.

A disulphide bond is also known as a cystine molecule, and is shown in the diagram.

The softening stage

When perm lotion/chemical rearranger is added to the hair, it uses either the heat generated from the acidic perm lotion to open the cuticle layer, or the pH of an alkaline lotion causes the cuticle layer to open. As the cuticle layer opens, the perm lotion penetrates the cortex layer and begins to soften the disulphide bonds that hold the polypeptide chains together.

When the perm lotion/chemical rearranger is applied, it adds hydrogen to the hair and the hydrogen breaks down some of the disulphide bonds, as shown.

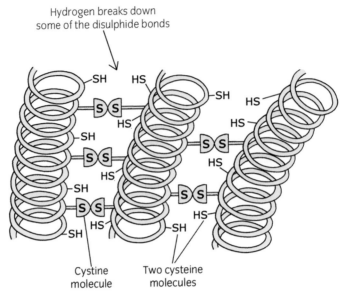

Hydrogen breaks down some of the disulphide bonds

Cystine molecule

Two cysteine molecules

Hair during the perming process

The moulding stage

As the disulphide bond is broken by the hydrogen, the cystine molecule is reduced into two cysteine molecules, as shown in the previous diagram.

When perming, the softened hair then starts to take on the shape of the perm rod, and begins to mould into its new shape.

When chemically rearranging, the hair is softened by the cream and combed straight to mould into its new position. This is to ensure that the hair is smoothly wrapped around the perming tool and will adapt to its new shape in a smooth and even curl formation. The hair is then permed and re-moulded around a perm rod to create a soft curl before being fixed by a neutraliser.

The fixing stage

The neutraliser stabilises the hair and permanently fixes it in its new shape.

The neutraliser is an oxidising agent and therefore contains oxygen. When the neutraliser is added, the oxygen combines with the hydrogen in the cysteine molecules, so there are now two hydrogen molecules and one oxygen molecule on the hair, which have reacted to form H_2O, the chemical formula for water, as shown.

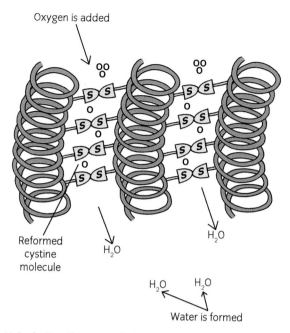

Hair during the neutralising process

The oxygen bonds with the hydrogen which leaves the cysteine molecules. This allows the recreation of one cystine molecule. The hair is now in its newly formed permanently bonded shape.

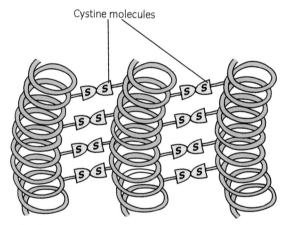

Hair after the neutralising process

HANDY HINT

During the development process, about 20–25% of the disulphide bonds should be broken. Any more than that and the hair could become frizzy and the hair structure will be permanently damaged. The development process can take 5–20 minutes, depending on the hair's condition.

This diagram summarises what you have just learnt.

As the water/H_2O leaves the hair, this allows the sulphur atoms to rebond, **fixing** the hair in its new shape, shown as **S–S**, a permanent disulphide bond (cystine)

When perming the hair, the permanent bonds that are broken are the disulphide bonds (cystine), shown as **S–S**

Neutraliser adds oxygen to the hair, which attaches to the hydrogen to form water, shown as

O
H   H

or **H_2O** – water

When perm lotion is added, we introduce hydrogen; this softens and breaks the disulphide bonds to form cysteine, shown as

H–H
S   S

During development the softened bonds are **moulded** around the rod and take on their new shape

S–S

H–H
S   S

O
H   H

S–S

Chemical rearranging

To partially relax naturally curly hair, a chemical rearranger is used on African type hair before a perm. This cream product is applied onto the hair which is then combed and smoothed into a straighter form. The rearranger softens the hair, swelling the cuticle and allowing penetration into the cortex. After it is developed it is rinsed off and the hair is then permed with a perm lotion.

Application methods of chemical rearrangers for regrowth and virgin hair

Depending on the length of the hair and whether or not it is a regrowth or virgin head application, the method of applying the chemical rearranger will vary.

For virgin application on longer hair lengths, the cream-based rearranger should be applied to the mid-lengths and ends first, and then the root area because of the heat produced from the head and the new growth of hair is freshly keratinised and is more sensitive to chemicals.

For short hair lengths, the product can be applied from root to tips, and for hair that has been previously permed, only the new growth towards the roots should be treated with the chemical rearranger.

How temperature affects the perm process

As previously mentioned, acid perms need an activating ingredient which produces heat to enable the cuticle layer to open and the perm to penetrate into the cortex layer. Alkaline perms and chemical rearrangers naturally open the cuticle layer because of their higher pH value.

When you process the perm, you need to ensure that the environment is warm enough. Cold salons will increase the development time, as cool air slows down the chemical process. A warm salon or additional heat, such as an accelerator, will decrease the development time. It is not recommended to use an accelerator on a chemical rearranger – a plastic cap can be used to regulate temperature.

To decrease the perm development time, you may be able to use a rollerball, a climazone, a hood dryer or even just a disposable cap, as this will keep in natural heat generated from the head – always check whether the MFIs allow additional heat to be applied.

> **HANDY HINT**
>
> It is important to restore the hair's pH balance after the perming and neutralising process to ensure that the cuticles are closed, that the hair is returned to a pH of 4.5 to 5.5 and the moisture is locked into the hair preventing it from drying out and becoming brittle.

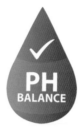

Techniques

To decide which technique to use, you need to complete the following:

1 consult with your client and confirm the curl result required
2 analyse your client's hair
3 identify any contra-indications and factors that could affect the desired result
4 carry out the relevant hair tests.

Choosing your technique

Post-damp or pre-damp?

Post-damping is winding the hair around the rods and then applying the perm lotion to each rod, one after the other. Pre-damping is applying a weak perm lotion to the hair prior to winding. For pre-damping, you'll need to wind the hair quickly to avoid over processing the hair. Remember to wear PPE to avoid allergic reactions or contact dermatitis from the chemicals used.

Pre-damping is not recommended on hair that has already been treated with a rearranger.

When deciding whether to use post-damping or pre-damping, you need to consider:

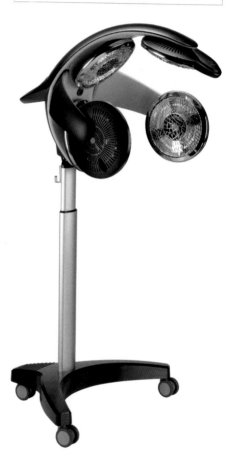

> **HANDY HINT**
>
> Not all perm manufacturers allow pre-damping techniques, so always read your MFIs.

- the sequence of the winding technique – particularly for pre-damping
- MFIs – post-damping is the only option for some perms
- the hair length – you might decide that pre-damping is the best option to ensure that you thoroughly cover the hair
- the hair texture and condition – never pre-damp fine or porous hair types, but consider the benefits to coarse, resistant hair or hair that is difficult to wind.

The main ingredient of acid perms is glycerol monothioglycolate and although acid perms are kinder to the hair, more clients suffer from allergic reactions to acid perms than alkaline perms. Remember to carry out skin tests on all clients with sensitive skin or those with a history of allergies (where the MFIs permit this).

Basic wind

Basic sectioning technique includes a six-section or nine-section perm wind.

Winding a nine-section perm helps you to control longer hair lengths and work in a methodical manner.

- Sections 1 and 2 go from the crown to the back of the nape, about the width of a rod.
- Sections 3 and 4, and 5 and 6 are on either side of sections 1 and 2, going from the top of the head to the back of the ear and down to the nape, splitting these sections in two – from the ear to the occipital bone.
- Sections 7 and 8 are the two front sections on either side.
- Section 9 is the top front section.

The benefits of a nine-section perm wind are that:

- it results in methodical winding
- it's easier to control the hair length.

For a six-section perm wind you would section the hair as follows:
- Sections 1 and 2 combined – crown to nape
- Sections 3 and 4 combined – left back section to nape
- Sections 5 and 6 combined – right back section to nape
- Section 7 – front left section
- Section 8 – front right section
- Section 9 – top section.

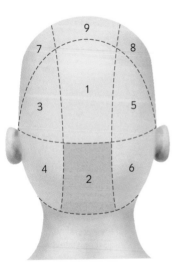

Nine-section wind sections

THE CITY & GUILDS TEXTBOOK

Directional wind

A directional wind is similar to a directional set; you wind the hair in a directed manner to suit the style requirements. The benefits of a directional wind are:

- the roots are wound in the direction that the style will be worn
- the hair is wound to suit the partings worn
- it is suitable for any hair length.

Brick wind

A brick wind perm has the same winding pattern as a brick wind setting technique. Wind the hair without any roller/rod sections, following the row pattern above.

The benefits of a brick wind perm are that:

- it avoids partings
- there are no rod/roller marks.

Winding on base or off base

When you are winding the hair, your rods should ideally be wound to sit on their own base. But, as with setting, you can wind on base to achieve maximum root lift or wind off base to prevent root lift.

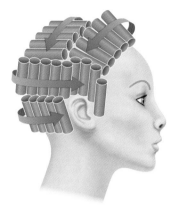

Directional wind

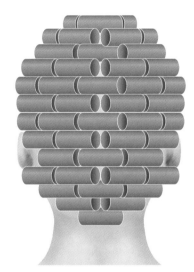

Brick wind sections

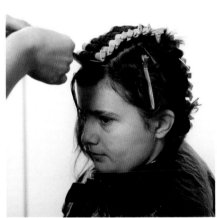

Wind on base

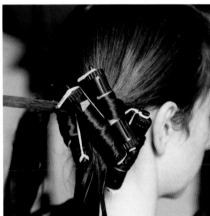

Off-base perm winding

Sectioning the hair

Once you have decided which winding technique and rod size to use, you can begin to wind. Each section of hair must be about the size of your rod choice. If you are using varied sizes, then your section sizes must vary too.

If the section size is too large for the rod, the curls may be uneven or too loose. If the section size is too small, you may struggle to get all the rods on the head and your resulting curls may be too tight.

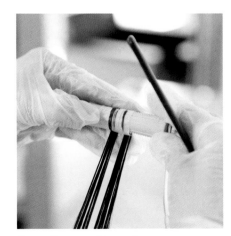

Correctly wound-in end paper

Securing the hair

To secure the hair in place as you wind, you must use an end paper. These are used on the ends of the hair to keep all the hairs in place and prevent buckled ends or fish hooks.

Once you have wound the hair around the rod, ensure that you secure it with a perm band. This band must go straight across the hair, without any twists. Bands that are twisted or secured too closely to the root area can break the hair.

The perm process

Once you have wound a full head of rods, you need to prepare the client fully for the perm lotion application.

Applying the lotion

1 Ensure your client is protected with a gown, towel and a waterproof cape.

2 Apply barrier cream around the hairline.

3 Attach misted/damp cotton wool around the hairline.

4 Mist the hair with water to ensure even porosity.

5 Activate and prepare the perm lotion of your choice.

6 Apply a few drops to each rod, starting from the back and working towards the front (the resistant areas to the weaker areas).

7 After the initial application, thoroughly coat each rod a second time, without flooding the scalp with lotion.

8 Change the cotton wool if the lotion drips.

9 Place a disposable cap on the client's head.

10 Use heat if suitable.

11 Offer your client refreshments and explain the development process and roughly how long it will take.

Accurate timing

You must always follow the MFIs in relation to the suggested development times. These will give you a guideline, but the timing will also depend on:

- hair texture
- hair density
- hair type – remember white hair can be misleading
- hair length
- temperature of the salon
- winding method – if you wind with lotion (pre-damped) then the development time will be decreased once all the rods are in place;

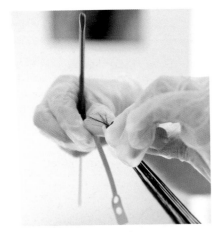
Incorrectly wound-in end paper

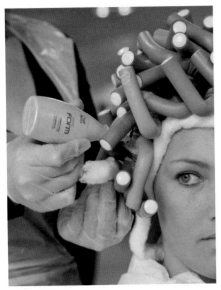
Applying the lotion

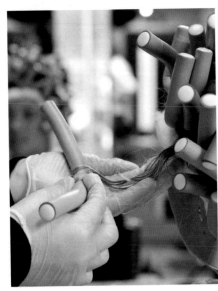
Development test curl

if you apply the lotion after the wind (post-damped) then the perm may take longer to develop.

If the perm lotion is underdeveloped, an insufficient number of bonds will break and the hair won't take on the new shape. If the neutraliser is underdeveloped, the curl will not be fixed in its new position. Either way, the curl is likely to drop and produce an unsatisfactory result.

If the perm lotion is overdeveloped, too many disulphide bonds are broken (over 25%) and the hair may become frizzy. If either the perm lotion or the neutraliser are overdeveloped, the hair condition can deteriorate and the hair's structure may be weakened.

You must always carry out a development test and check the S-bend to see if the perm has sufficiently developed.

Developing the perm

1 Leave the perm to develop without disturbing the hair for at least 5–10 minutes, depending on the MFIs.

2 Complete a development test.

3 If the hair requires further development, leave it for another 5 minutes and then check every 2–3 minutes until the development test curl produces an S-bend that resembles the size of the rod.

4 When the development test is positive, escort your client to the basin area.

The importance of water temperature

When you shampoo the hair in preparation for the perm, you should use warm water to help cleanse the hair, removing products, oil and dirt. Warm water will also aid the opening of the cuticle layer, ready for the lotion to be applied.

When you rinse the perm lotion from the hair, again use warm water to keep the cuticle layers open, ready for the neutraliser to fix the hair in its new shape. Remember that the scalp may be sensitive from the chemicals, so consider your client's comfort and ensure the water is not too hot.

Rinsing the hair

When the perm lotion is developed and the development test identifies that about 20% of the disulphide bonds are broken, the hair must be thoroughly rinsed to remove all traces of perm lotion. Perm lotion and neutraliser react together and can cause chemical burns to the hair and scalp, so you must rinse the hair, not only to stop the perm lotion from continuing to work, but to prevent chemical burns when the neutraliser is applied.

HANDY HINT

You must accurately time a perm's development to prevent overprocessing the perm and damaging the hair. Make sure you calculate this time correctly.

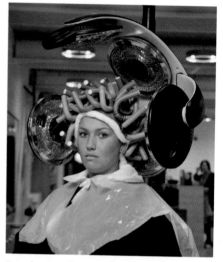

Developing the perm

HANDY HINT

If the water is too hot, then your client may suffer discomfort or scalp irritation, and the perm may process more quickly than expected. But if the water is not warm enough, the cuticle layer will not be sufficiently opened to allow the chemicals to penetrate the cortex layer, which could slow down the development process.

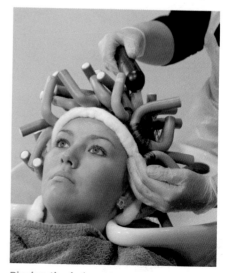

Rinsing the hair

Once the perm lotion has been thoroughly rinsed, blot dry the hair to avoid diluting the neutraliser and apply the fixing agent/neutraliser.

When developed, the neutraliser must also be thoroughly rinsed from the hair to prevent overdevelopment which damages the hair's structure.

Rinsing and neutralising

HANDY HINT

Remember to turn off taps in between use to save water.

HANDY HINT

Always rinse the perm lotion and neutraliser thoroughly from the hair to ensure the products are removed and to prevent the hair from overprocessing.

1 Ensure your client is adequately protected.

2 Rinse the hair for at least 5 minutes, depending on the MFIs and the hair length, taking care with the temperature, direction and pressure of the water.

3 Carefully blot the rods dry with hand towels, paper towels or cotton wool, so as not to disturb them and to prevent diluting the neutraliser, and reapply cotton wool to the hairline.

4 Apply the neutraliser either from the applicator bottle or foam it in a bowl and apply with a sponge.

5 Leave the hair to develop for about 5 minutes, depending on MFIs, and then either remove the rods and gently reapply the neutraliser to the unwound hair, or leave the rods in place and reapply the neutraliser.

6 Leave the hair for a further 5 minutes, depending on MFIs, and then remove the rods if you have not already done so.

7 Remove all the cotton wool from the hairline.

8 Thoroughly rinse the hair and apply a pH-balancing or post-perm conditioner.

9 Leave the conditioner on for a few minutes, depending on the MFIs, and thoroughly rinse the hair.

10 Towel dry the hair and comb through with a wide-toothed comb.

11 Escort your client back to the workstation for any further service.

12 Your desired look should have been achieved. Check that your client is happy with the result.

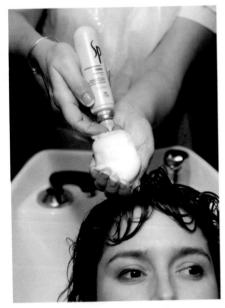

Applying post-perm treatment

Importance of following instructions

You must follow the instructions of your suppliers and the manufacturers when using your equipment to ensure it is used correctly and safely and to aid you achieving the best perm results for your client.

Instructions for perming and neutralising products vary immensely, so always read them carefully before applying the products to your client's hair to ensure you achieve the best result and do not cause damage to their hair, skin or scalp.

Factors can affect your choice of perming and neutralising products, such as:

- how straight or curly a client's hair is and their desired result
- the length, condition, density and texture of the hair
- any previous service on the hair
- any contra-indications.

Ensure you check all of the above and take these points into consideration when reading the MFIs.

Activity

If you have several different perm products in your salon or at college, compare the manufacturers' instructions and take notes any variations in application techniques, development times, rinsing of products, etc.

VALUES & BEHAVIOURS

Refer to the values and behaviours chapter for more information on adhering to workplace, supplier or manufacturer instructions.

Activity

What would happen if you did not rinse the perm lotion from the hair prior to adding the neutraliser? For the purpose of research, and under the supervision of your manager/tutor, mix a small amount of perm lotion with an equal amount of neutraliser in a measuring jug. Feel the container and note how hot the two products become when mixed together. Remember to wear PPE!

Now imagine how your client would feel if this was put on their head!

Perming problems – causes and remedies

As with all services, problems can occur. Problems with perming can often be overcome, once you know what has caused them.

The following tables show the types of problem that can occur, their likely causes and how they can be remedied.

HANDY HINT

Don't forget not to flood the scalp when you apply the perm lotion – you are perming the hair not the scalp!

Problems noticed during the perm or neutralising process

Problem	Likely cause	Resolution
Scalp irritation	■ Lotion on the scalp ■ Allergic reaction to the lotion ■ Tension or rods too tight	■ Rinse the hair and scalp with cool water. ■ Refer to GP if required.

Problem	Likely cause	Resolution
Rods fall out when rinsing the hair	■ Water pressure too high ■ Hair too short ■ Rods wound too loosely	■ Lower the water pressure. ■ Use a hair net to secure in place. ■ Rewind the rods.
The perm process is slow	■ The salon is too cold ■ Insufficient lotion used ■ Lotion too weak	■ Add heat and use an accelerator (check MFIs). ■ Add more lotion. ■ Add stronger lotion.

Problems noticed after the perm process

Problem	Likely cause	Resolution
Fish hooks 	■ Poor wind, the hair has been buckled or bent during the wind	■ Trim the ends of the hair.
Some straight pieces 	■ Sections too large ■ Rod size too large ■ Poor wind – too loose ■ Uneven application of lotion ■ Rods loosened during rinsing	■ Reperm the straight pieces if the hair condition allows.

Problem	Likely cause	Resolution
Frizzy hair	■ Rod size too small ■ Wind too tight ■ Lotion too strong ■ Overdeveloped ■ Overlapped product	■ Apply conditioning treatments. ■ Regular trims in order to remove the damaged hair gradually.

Hair breakage	■ Poor wind – bands are twisted or positioned too close to the root.
	■ Rods are too tightly wound.
	■ Incompatible products.
	■ Lotion too strong.
	■ Overdeveloped.
	■ Overlapped product.
		■ There is no remedy other than cutting to reduce the visible effects of breakage, but the following may help prevent further breakage:
		  ● conditioning treatments and restructurants
		  ● regular trims.

Discolouration of hair	■ Incompatible products ■ Neutraliser has faded recent colour service.	■ Use a semi-permanent or temporary colour to tone the hair colour.
The curl is too tight	■ Rods too small ■ Sections too small ■ Overdeveloped	■ Apply deep conditioning treatments. ■ If condition allows, you could reperm on larger rods or relax the hair.

Problem	Likely cause	Resolution
The hair is straight 	■ Barrier on the hair ■ Resistant hair ■ Incorrect perm choice – too weak ■ Underdeveloped ■ Faulty lotion	■ Reperm the hair if the condition allows.
The curl is uneven 	■ Sections too large ■ Poor wind – uneven ■ Incorrect rod size ■ Uneven product application ■ Rods loosened during rinsing stage	■ Reperm if condition allows.

Problems noticed a couple of days later causing client to return

Problem	Likely cause	Resolution
The curl has dropped 	■ Uneven tension when winding ■ Insufficient coverage of perm lotion or neutraliser ■ Uneven application of perm lotion or neutraliser ■ Underdeveloped perm lotion or neutraliser	Reperm if hair condition allows.

WHY DON'T YOU...
Find out from your salon manager which of these problems you can deal with yourself and which ones you should refer to your manager.

HANDY HINT

In some cases, the salon's insurance company may need to be notified if the client is dissatisfied or if there is damage or breakage to their hair or skin.

VALUES & BEHAVIOURS

If you encounter a problem, refer to the values and behaviours chapter for more information on explaining clearly to clients any reasons why their needs or expectations cannot be met, keeping the client informed and reassured and adapting your behaviour to respond effectively to different client behaviour.

Providing advice and recommendations

It is important that you provide your client with aftercare advice following a perm because of the strength of the chemicals used. They need to know how to maintain the curl and their hair condition.

You must provide your client with advice on:

- which retail products to use
- which tools and equipment they should use
- which additional services they would benefit from
- when to return to the salon for future services.

Always give clear, accurate and constructive advice, and consider your client's time constraints in relation to maintaining their hairstyle. If your client has an active lifestyle and/or enjoys swimming, make sure that you consider this and recommend suitable products.

Explain to your clients that they should not wash their hair for 24–48 hours after a perm, and avoid excessive tension on the hair, as this can cause the curls to loosen.

Recommending products

You must advise your clients which shampoos and conditioners they should use to maintain moisture levels and the condition of the hair. Suggest regular deep-penetrating conditioning treatments, which can either be used at home or carried out in the salon.

You should make recommendations to your clients about the use of styling and finishing products. Advise them which styling products to use when the hair is wet, to avoid the hair looking frizzy, and which finishing products to use to hold the curls in place. Show your clients how much of the product to use, depending on their hair length, and how to use it with their styling tools.

When making your recommendations, use your English communication skills, maintain eye contact and use positive, open body language to promote trust and a good client–stylist relationship.

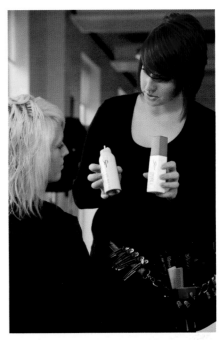

Recommend products suitable for permed hair

Recommending tools and equipment

Always clearly explain to your client which tools, such as brushes and combs, they should use, and which to avoid. Inform your clients that they should always use a wide-toothed comb on wet hair. Promote the use of a diffuser to maintain the curls without disturbing or separating the curls or causing the hair to look fluffy or frizzy. Explain that excessive use of heated styling equipment will increase the porosity and reduce elasticity, causing damage to the hair.

Recommending further services

Future colouring services may need to be suggested or avoided, depending on the condition of the client's hair. If a colour has faded slightly during the perming process, you may need to recommend a semi-permanent or a temporary colour to brighten the faded colour. The perm service carried out may, however, restrict your client to certain colour services in the future, and you must make your client aware of this.

Recommending when to return

Recommend to your clients when to return to the salon for a trim, and make them aware of the signs that indicate that their hair needs to be cut and styled again.

Make suggestions for future colouring services and conditioning treatments, and tell your clients how long the perm should be expected to last.

It is ideal if your clients book their next appointment while they are still in the salon, when your advice is clear in their mind.

Dry permed hair with a diffuser

HANDY HINT

When using your consultation skills you are also developing and maintaining your speaking and listening skills. These skills are vital in hairdressing.

WHY DON'T YOU...
Practise perm winding on a training head and time yourself.

Activity

Find out how long you are allocated in your salon for a perm service. How long are you booked out for the perm wind?

Step by steps

Chemical rearranging

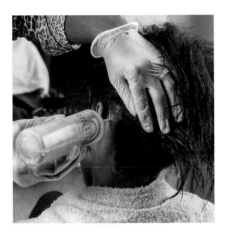

STEP 1 – Apply the scalp protector around the nape of the neck and the hairline. Detangle the hair first using your hands, then a wide-toothed/afro comb. Check the scalp thoroughly for any cuts or abrasions.

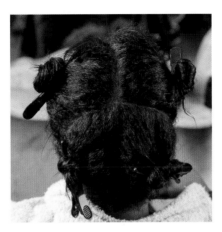

STEP 2 – Divide the hair into four neat sections from hairline to nape and ear to ear. Use plastic clips to secure the hair.

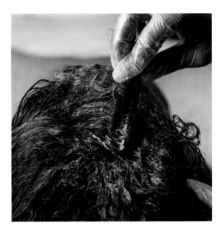

STEP 3 – Take ½cm (¼in) sections and using a spatula or tint brush, apply the rearranger solution starting on the ends and then the mid-lengths of the hair. Once the ends and mid-lengths are covered, begin applying the rearranger solution to any new growth area, being careful to avoid contact with the skin as the rearranger solution can cause damage and burning to the scalp and skin.

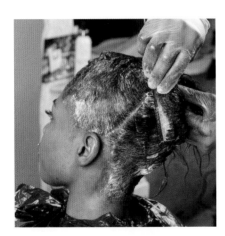

STEP 4 – Repeat application of the rearranger until the entire head is covered. Once the application is complete, smooth the rearranger into place with gloved hands or the back of a comb. Set timer according to MFIs.

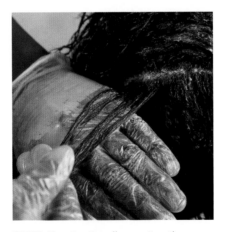

STEP 5 – Continually monitor the development of the rearranger, carrying out a curl reduction test to evaluate curl reduction after 10 minutes. Do not over-straighten the hair as this will cause the hair to become weak and increases the potential for breakage. Ensure you check client comfort throughout the process. Always follow the MFIs for maximum development time. Check for curl reduction every 5 minutes.

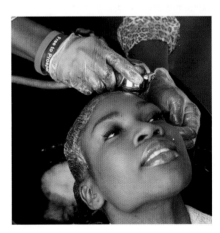

STEP 6 – Thoroughly rinse out the chemical rearranger from the hair with tepid water, avoiding excess water pressure or rough handling of the hair. Proceed to winding phase.

Directional perm wind

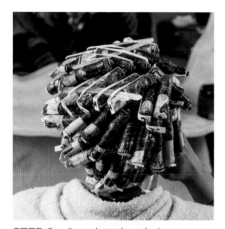

STEP 1 – Complete the whole area to be wound. Follow MFIs for the application of perm lotion.

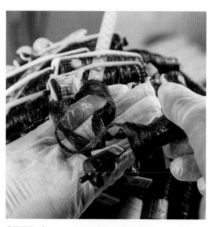

STEP 2 – Carry out a development test curl.

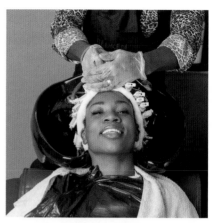

STEP 3 – Once the correct level of curl has been achieved, rinse the hair thoroughly at the basin to remove all traces of perm lotion.

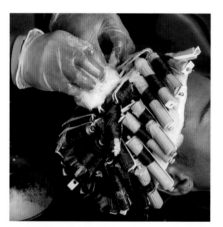

STEP 4 – **Blot dry** the hair with a towel, so that you do not dilute the neutraliser. Apply neutraliser following MFIs.

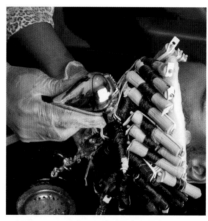

STEP 5 – Develop for 5 minutes, or according to MFIs, then rinse on the rods.

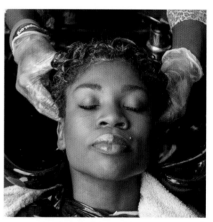

STEP 6 – Gently remove the rods and rinse the hair thoroughly.

Blot dry

To soak up excess water using cotton wool, hand towels or paper towels, without rubbing the hair.

HANDY HINT

Keeping the hair misted with water while winding makes it easier to control.

HANDY HINT

Ensure that the completed wind is not too tight, as this can cause scalp irritation and damage the hair.

WHY DON'T YOU...

Watch the stylists in your salon wind a directional perm and then practise on a mannequin.

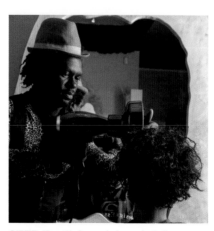

STEP 7 – Style and dress hair to complete the look.

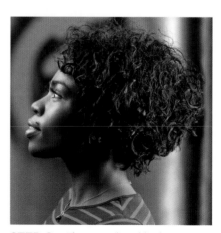

STEP 8 – The completed look – chemical rearranger on African type hair with directional perm wind.

Basic nine-section perm wind

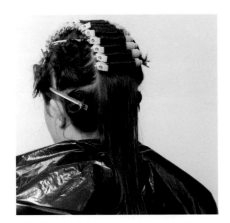

STEP 1 – Divide the hair into nine sections. Start to wind from the top front section, or the crown, towards the back.

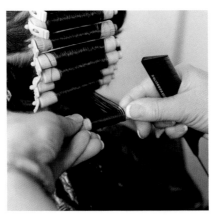

STEP 2 – Continue the winding process down towards the nape section.

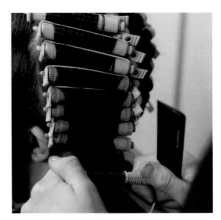

STEP 3 – Complete the nape section and start on the side sections.

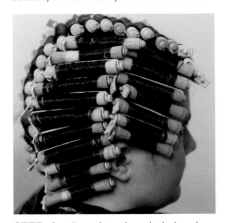

STEP 4 – Complete the whole head wind, maintaining tension throughout.

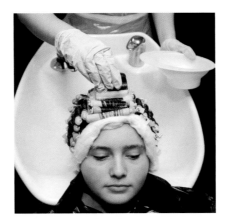

STEP 5 – Develop the perm, then rinse the hair. Neutralise using a bowl-and-sponge technique.

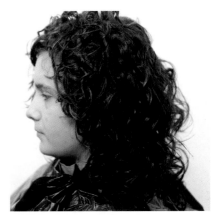

STEP 6 – The completed perm and desired result.

HANDY HINT

You must ensure that you maintain the tension from root to point when winding the hair, otherwise the end result may be uneven.

Partial-head brick wind

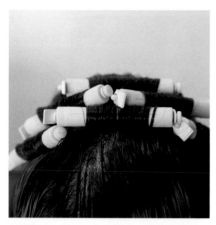

STEP 1 – Start at the top of the head using a brick winding technique.

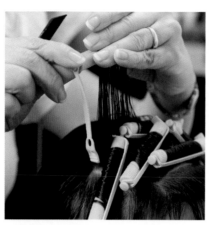

STEP 2 – Wind the crown area, maintaining even tension throughout.

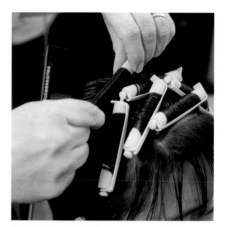

STEP 3 – Complete the rest of the crown in a brick wind.

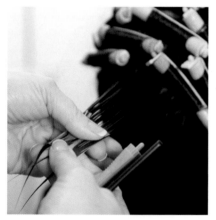

STEP 4 – Work down towards the nape area.

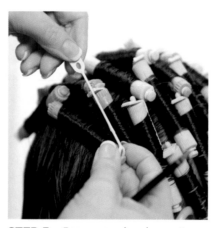

STEP 5 – Ensure your bands aren't twisted or too tight.

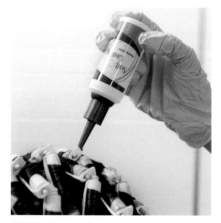

STEP 6 – Apply perm lotion, being careful not to flood the scalp.

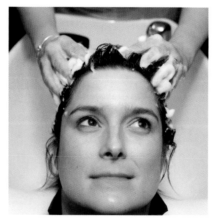

STEP 7 – Apply a post-perm treatment after neutralising.

> **HANDY HINT**
>
> Make sure you decide whether you are winding on base or off base before you begin. If your aim is to wind on base and you create root drag as you wind, the resulting curl will be similar to that of off-base winding, and no root lift will be achieved.

Answers in the back of the book.

1 Statement one

COSHH controls the use, storage and disposal of substances that can be inhaled, absorbed or ingested.

Statement two

Chemical burns is a risk involved with perming hair.

Which **one** of the following is correct for the above statements?

a True   True

b True   False

c False   True

d False   False

2. Which one of the following is the most difficult hair to curl?

a Type 1 coarse hair

b Type 2 fine hair

c Type 3 medium hair

d Type 4 soft hair

3 A client has very abundant hair. Which one of the following is the most likely impact on the perming service?

a A weaker lotion is used which may result in the curl being loose

b A stronger lotion is used which may result in hair damage

c Longer development time and larger rods are required

d More rods are required and smaller sections are taken

4 Statement one

Porous hair will absorb perm lotion quickly; a pre-perm conditioner will protect the hair by slowing the process.

Statement two

When using chemical rearranger, a strand test is used to establish the effect on the hair's condition.

Which **one** of the following is correct for the above statements?

a True   True

b True   False

c False   True

d False   False

5 Which **one** of the following is a technique used on long hair to ensure the lotion has even coverage?

a Pre-damping

b Post-damping

c Pre-conditioning

d Post-conditioning

6 Which one of the following lotions is best used on sensitive hair?

a Exothermic perm 0

b Alkaline perm 1

c Acid perm 2

d Acid perm 0

7 **Statement one**

Creeping oxidation describes when a chemical has been left in the hair and carries on developing.

Statement two

A post-perm conditioner is used to close the cuticle and stop creeping oxidation.

Which **one** of the following is correct for the above statements?

a True   True

b True   False

c False   True

d False   False

8 Which **one** of the following describes the reduction and oxidation stages of perming and chemical rearranging?

a Softening and moulding

b Fixing and moulding

c Softening and fixing

d Fixing and softening

9 Which **one** of the following describes the effect of perm lotion and chemical rearranger on the structure of hair?

a The cortex is chemically changed which fixes the curl pattern

b The cuticle is opened and hydrogen changes cystine to cysteine

c The cuticle is opened and oxygen breaks the disulphide bonds

d The cortex is chemically changed from cysteine to cystine

10 **Statement one**

During neutralising, oxygen combines with hydrogen and re-forms the disulphide bonds.

Statement two

When chemically rearranging long virgin hair, it is best applied from roots to tips.

Which **one** of the following is correct for the above statements?

a True   True

b True   False

c False   True

d False   False

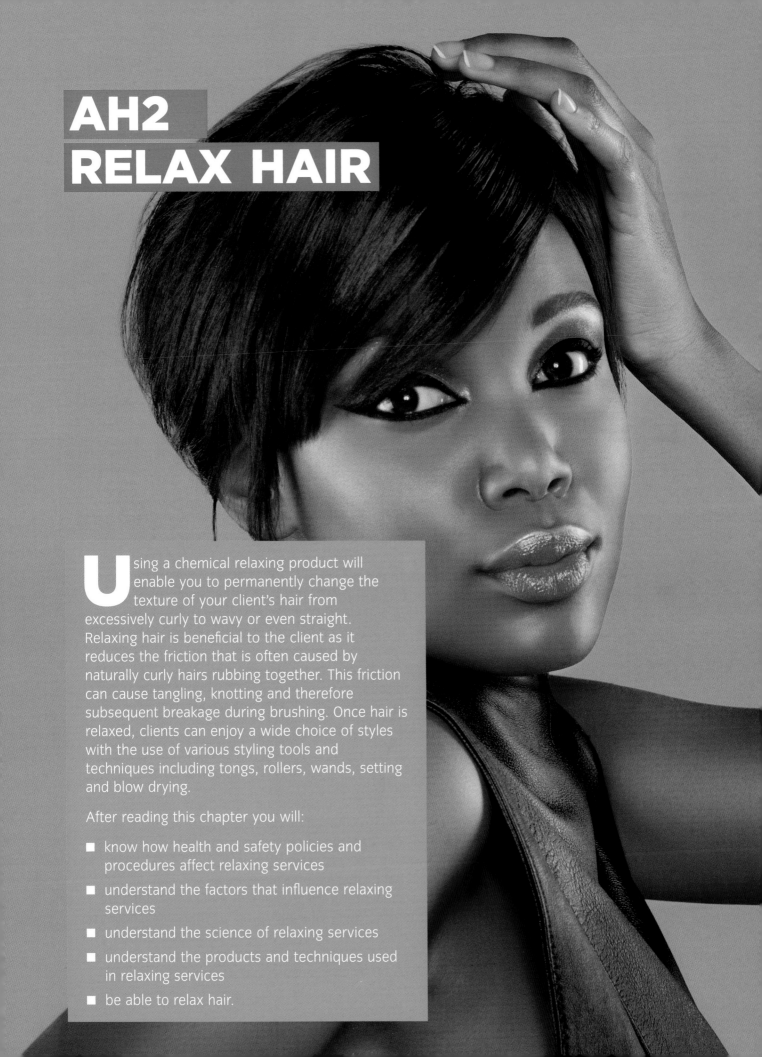

AH2
RELAX HAIR

Using a chemical relaxing product will enable you to permanently change the texture of your client's hair from excessively curly to wavy or even straight. Relaxing hair is beneficial to the client as it reduces the friction that is often caused by naturally curly hairs rubbing together. This friction can cause tangling, knotting and therefore subsequent breakage during brushing. Once hair is relaxed, clients can enjoy a wide choice of styles with the use of various styling tools and techniques including tongs, rollers, wands, setting and blow drying.

After reading this chapter you will:

■ know how health and safety policies and procedures affect relaxing services

■ understand the factors that influence relaxing services

■ understand the science of relaxing services

■ understand the products and techniques used in relaxing services

■ be able to relax hair.

Benefits of relaxing hair

WHY DON'T YOU...
Find out about manufacturers' training for relaxing services?

Carrying out a relaxing service on a client is a great opportunity to transform your client's appearance with a total change of hair texture. The option to give your client the flexibility of having straight hair and wearing their hair in many different styles will allow you to be very creative. You will develop skills such as dexterity, precision and speed.

Having clients who visit your salon for a relaxer will help you build a profitable clientele as the service will need to be maintained with future appointments and regular treatments. Understanding the new technology and techniques that are frequently updated by manufacturers to make this service better and better will enable you to continue your learning process throughout your career.

Health and safety

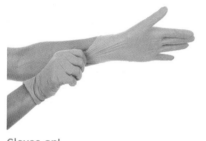

Gloves on!

Prepare for relaxing services

Your own hair and grooming should reflect the salon image and create a professional impression. Pay attention to oral and personal hygiene, wear clean clothes daily and use deodorant to keep fresh and odour-free. Ensure that your hands are clean and that your nails are free from dirt. Your nails should also be maintained so that they are free from splits that can catch on the client's hair and scalp during application and service. Use hand cream to keep your hands from becoming dry and to prevent dermatitis. Make sure to use the correct personal protective equipment (PPE) such as protective gowns, aprons and gloves. Always dispose of gloves in a closed bin once you have finished using them. Ensure that your tools and equipment are clean and sterilised before each use.

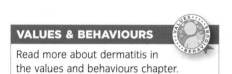

VALUES & BEHAVIOURS

Read more about dermatitis in the values and behaviours chapter.

Prepare yourself and your client

WHY DON'T YOU...
Compare the manufacturers' instructions and make notes on the differences for lye and no-lye relaxer products?

When carrying out a relaxing service on your client, the chemicals used can be harmful to yourself or your client. If used incorrectly, these chemicals can damage the skin, scalp and hair. Paying close attention to working safely is essential to safeguard yourself and your client. It is vital that protective measures are always carried out. You should wear personal protective equipment (PPE) when applying products in order to protect your hands and clothes. Tools must be cleaned and sterilised after each client, and you should always use fresh, clean towels. Wipe and clean around basins before and after removing a relaxer, as this will ensure that no product that could cause damage to the skin and hair will be transferred onto your clients and cause harm. Always follow the manufacturers' instructions (MFIs) when preparing your products, tools and appliances for use throughout the service.

The workstation and safe working methods

Preparing your workstation before a client arrives for a relaxing service helps to convey a professional impression to your client and enables you to work cleanly and safely. In a well-prepared and tidy environment you can avoid potential hazards and risk of injury, and minimise the risk of infection, infestation and cross-contamination. It is important that your tools are cleaned and sterilised after each use.

Activity

Make a list of all the tools and products that you will need to carry out a relaxing service and describe their uses. Be sure to spell and punctuate accurately!

As a relaxer requires a fast and precise application technique, it is important to have your tools close to hand. To avoid adopting bad postures ensure the trolley is within easy reach on the side that you work (depending on whether you are left- or right-handed) and that it is free from unnecessary tools or products. Posture is important, as standing correctly can help you avoid fatigue, and leg and back pains. Make sure the styling chair is positioned at the correct height to enable you to work comfortably. Stand with your feet slightly apart and your weight distributed evenly; work around your client as you apply the relaxer to the hair.

The position of your client is also important. Your client needs to be sitting straight in the chair and in the centre of the workstation and the mirror. You need to be able to see the balance of your application and the outline of your client's head clearly with no obstructions. Make sure the client is relaxed with their back against the chair with their legs uncrossed.

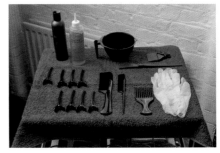

A trolley ready for service

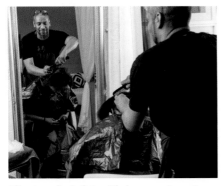

Client and stylist with incorrect posture

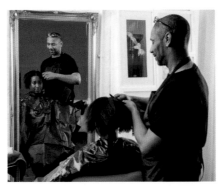

Client and stylist with correct posture

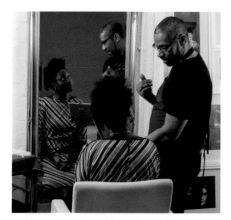
Consultation for relaxing service

Hazards and risks

Hazards can frequently occur in a busy salon environment and everyone should be aware of the safety implications. As part of personal responsibility, you will need to be able to recognise when the hazard needs to be dealt with immediately, or when help may be needed, and whether it needs to be reported to a supervisor, lecturer, technician or manager.

It is important to be able to identify hazards before they become risks. Should they become risks it is essential to know how to deal with them.

Client consultation and tests

A thorough consultation will help you to identify your client's requirements, choose the most suitable product to carry out the service and identify any influencing factors. During the consultation you will also be able to discuss the results achievable.

Follow these steps to deliver an appropriate consultation for relaxing services:

- ask appropriate questions and listen to your client's responses
- make a detailed analysis of your client's hair
- identify contra-indications
- conduct relevant tests
- choose the correct tools and equipment and products to use.

Activity

Research and make a 'look book' of celebrities with hair styles where a relaxing service has been used to create the style. You can use this as a consultation tool.

Activity

Create a list of open and closed questions that help you identify your client's wishes. Try to use words that will help you confirm your client's expectations.

Whether your client has a relaxing service carried out regularly or it is the first time, it is essential to understand the client's expectations, styling habits, lifestyle, the condition of their hair and their general health. Even if they are a returning client, these things may have changed since their last visit.

Always make a record of the discussions that you have had during your consultation. This information is extremely important for future reference and should include:

- dates of services
- test results
- allergies
- skin and scalp conditions.

This will also help you decide on your technique and application methods.

Questions to ask before carrying out a relaxing service

Ensuring that the hairstyle is suitable for the client's lifestyle and face shape and that they are able to maintain the style that you have created are significant. It is also important to be aware of their curl and natural growth patterns, and to consider whether the style agreed is achievable. The guidance that you give your client in choosing the correct hairstyle for them will demonstrate your professional skills and will help build trust between yourself and your client.

Ask the following questions:

- When did you last have a relaxing service carried out?
- What type of relaxer was used?
- Have you ever experienced irritation, burning or skin sensitivity whilst having a relaxing service?
- When did you last shampoo your hair?
- When did you last colour your hair?
- Have you ever used a lightening product on your hair?
- Have you recently had braids or extensions removed from your hair?
- Do you suffer from soreness of the scalp? Is your scalp free from cuts and abrasions?
- Is the hair very dry or brittle?

Factors that may influence the service

So that you are able to choose the correct relaxer and technique you first need to analyse the hair and scalp. This will enable you to determine whether the procedure is suitable for the client. You will also be able to identify any potential problems that may occur. It is important to visually check and handle the hair to determine the factors during the analysis of the hair.

Natural curl pattern

Curl patterns can range from curly, coily and excessively curly to Z-shaped patterns. The classification of curl patterns refers to the tightness of the curl:

- Curly hair tends to have an open S-shaped bend and can be styled between curly and straight with relative ease.
- Coiled hair will have a tighter spiral shape to the hair.
- Excessively curly hair has a combination of coils and curls, and can compress by up to half of its length.
- Z-shaped pattern hair will curl, coil and double back on itself. This hair type tends to be very fragile as the many directional changes along the hair create many points of weakness.

Hair growth pattern

Excessively curly hair does not usually have any natural partings. However, there can be differences in hairline shapes which need to be considered when carrying out relaxing services.

Face shape

You will also need consider how the shape of the face will influence the finished look. A perfect style to complement a relaxer service is a feminine pixie crop or a funky graduated bob. If your client has a very round face then a relaxer will be very flattering as it will reduce the overall rounded look of the face.

Client lifestyle

Will the client be able to maintain the style you have created? Factors include:

- the time they can spend on styling their hair
- the client's working environment (is this casual or corporate?)
- the client's ability to attend regular salon visits.

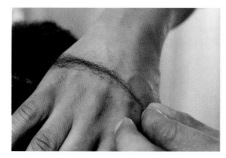

Z-shaped pattern hair

> **HANDY HINT**
>
> For more on hair types and curl patterns, see chapter CHB9.

> **HANDY HINT**
>
> It is often considered that all African type hair is thick but this is a misrepresentation. There are many different textures of hair within the hair category and therefore identifying the texture during a consultation is vital.

> **WHY DON'T YOU...**
>
> Research different textures of African type hair in magazines and on the internet, and make a note of their curl patterns and texture?

Length of the hair

The natural curl pattern of African type hair disguises the length of the hair. You must determine if you can achieve the style required and whether the hairstyle will be affected by the length.

Texture of the hair

The texture of the hair also influences the relaxing service and end texture your client can expect. When checking the texture of the hair we are identifying whether the hair is fine, medium or thick. We can determine this by the diameter of each hair. Is it narrow (fine), wide (thick) or in between the two (medium)? Fine hair can absorb less moisture and therefore can process more quickly so will need a more gentle formula. Thick hair can absorb more moisture and may take a longer processing time so may need a slightly stronger formula.

Density of the hair

Identifying the density of the hair helps us understand if the hair is sparse, regular or abundant. For hair that is sparse we need to ensure that we avoid too much tension or pulling on the hair. The density of hair will have an impact on the relaxer formula chosen. For abundant hair the application process will take a little longer and therefore we must be mindful of the processing time to ensure it does not exceed the manufacturer's instructions.

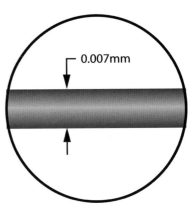

Determine the diameter of the hair

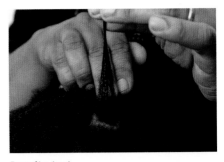

Density test

HANDY HINT

To identify the density of the hair take a 2.5cm² (1in²) section and evaluate how many hairs are growing from the scalp and how close the hairs are growing next to each other. If the section is very full of hair then this can be identified as abundant. If there are fewer hairs in the section then the hair is sparse. If it falls between the two it is regular.

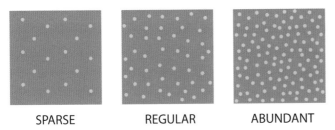

| SPARSE | REGULAR | ABUNDANT |

Density of the hair when looking at a cross-section of the scalp

Curl pattern

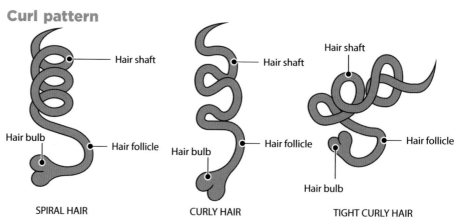

SPIRAL HAIR   CURLY HAIR   TIGHT CURLY HAIR

Curl patterns

WHY DON'T YOU...
Make a ponytail on your own hair and then make one on someone else and measure the thickness of each one?

The natural curl patterns of African type hair are variable. The tightness of the curl disguises the length of the hair which is often quite long when straightened. The direction of hair growth varies and the hair does not fall into regular patterns or natural partings like Caucasian or Asian hair, which tends to be uniform in thickness from the root to the ends. African type hair will twist, turn, bend, kink and forms into coil shapes and the diameter can differ along the hair shaft creating some narrower segments which can cause points of weakness in the hair, leaving it prone to breakage. Even once a relaxing service has been carried out, these original weaknesses are still present and must be considered during styling and maintaining the hair's condition.

Porosity

A porosity test should be carried out to evaluate the status of the surface of the hair. Porosity refers to the hair's ability to absorb liquids into the cortex. Porosity is determined by whether the cuticle layers are open or closed. Porous hair absorbs lotion more quickly so care is therefore required to choose the correct lotion strength and a precise development time. Open cuticles are revealed by the sensation of bumps along the surface of the hair. Run your finger and thumb along the hair shaft towards the root – if the surface is smooth it means the cuticles are closed (not porous); if the surface is rough it means the cuticles are open and the hair is porous. As previously covered in the curl pattern section above, excessively curly hair has twists, turns and bends along its surface. This uneven exterior will result in the hair generating a variable uptake of liquids and will result in inconsistent processing. It is therefore advisable to use a treatment to even out the porosity of the hair prior to a relaxing service being carried out.

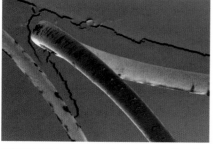

Microscope view: curl and porosity of West African natural hair

Some of the methods used during the styling of African type hair can also be much harsher than those used on Caucasian hair, for example excessive heat and continued stretching, and this can also lead to the cuticles remaining open and the hair being porous.

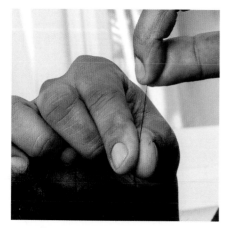

Porosity test

Elasticity

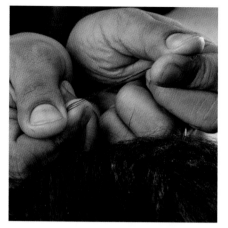

Elasticity test

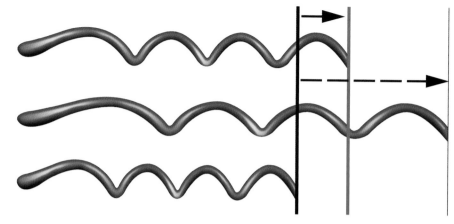

Elasticity

An elasticity test must be carried out to determine whether the condition of the hair is good enough to withstand processing. When hair is healthy it is able to stretch and return to its original length while resisting breakage. Elasticity is what allows the hair to change its shape, for instance from curly to straight or vice versa, during styling, setting or blow drying. The elasticity in the hair is determined by the bonds in the hair. Strong **polypeptide chains** make strong hair and vice versa. It is preferable to carry out an elasticity test on African type hair when it is damp, as it is possible to **manipulate** the hair over a greater range of movement when wet. When dry, African type hair is much more prone to snap when stretched due to the **inherent** parched nature of the hair.

To test elasticity, a single hair or small group of hairs should be held at two points some distance apart along the hair shaft. Whilst keeping the heels of the hands together, pull the hair gently in opposing directions. If the hair stretches significantly without springing back or breaks easily, any further processing should be avoided because this indicates damage within the cortex. Treatments should be carried out in order to improve the condition of the hair.

Polypeptide chains

These are the chains that coil and fold to form a spiral.

Manipulate

Handle or control in a skilful manner

Inherent

Existing in something as a permanent characteristic.

Scalp health

In order to have healthy hair it is essential for the scalp to be clean, pliable and nourished. Before carrying out a relaxer service it is important to check that there are no cuts, abrasions, infections or infestations. If you discover any skin disorders on the head during your inspection and the scalp has any areas that are open or weeping, do not proceed with a relaxing service. As African type hair has no natural partings and can grow in abundance, it is extremely important that your scalp check is carried out thoroughly as it can be easy to miss any smaller areas. While you are checking the health of the scalp it would be a good time to question your client regarding

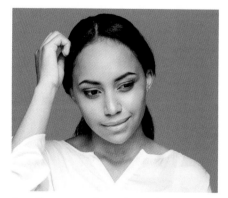

Question your client about their scalp health

previous relaxing services and ask them if they have ever experienced scalp sensitivity or have any known allergies.

Degree of straightness

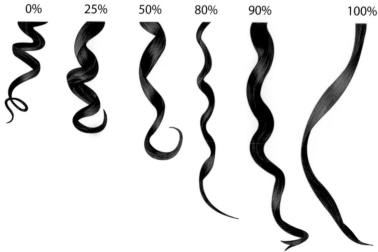

0%   25%   50%   80%   90%   100%

If you relax the hair until it is dead straight you are essentially overprocessing the hair, and it will not have the elasticity that it needs to be strong and withstand the general styling whims of your client. It is not advised to reduce the curl further than 65% of its natural curl pattern. Over a period of time of continuous overrelaxation, blow drying and thermal styling, the hair will become damaged and prone to breakage. If you encounter a client whose hair has experienced damage due to previous relaxing services, it is important to stress the need for regular conditioning treatments to restore the condition of the hair.

Contra-indications

Contra-indications are factors that could prevent you from carrying out a relaxing service on your client. It is important to ask your client questions that will help you establish if there are any contra-indications. The responses that your client gives must be recorded on a client record card and will enable you to establish whether to proceed with the relaxing service, continue with further testing, or stop and not proceed with the service.

The consultation is an ideal time to look for evidence of infestations such as head lice. If you notice any signs of infestation do not proceed with the relaxing service. You may require the assistance of a senior member of your salon team as you will need to inform your client of the infestation. Once the client has left the salon, ensure that you sterilise all gowns, towels and equipment that have been used.

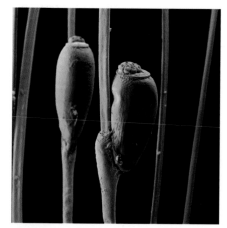

Microscope view: head lice eggs (nits)

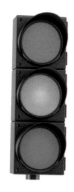

Stop and do not proceed with the service.

Continue with further testing.

Proceed with the relaxing service.

Contra-indication	Outcome
Skin sensitivities	
	If your client has previously experienced skin sensitivity during the application of a sodium (lye) relaxer do not proceed with a sodium (lye) formula.
	It may be possible to proceed with the service if your client has previously had a no-lye relaxer without experiencing sensitivity. No-lye relaxers are known to be more gentle on the scalp.
Previous allergic reactions	
	As relaxer cream is not designed to be applied directly to the skin, it is not suitable to carry out a skin allergy test. If the client has had a previous reaction during the application of a relaxer, do not proceed.
Other known allergies	
	Ask your client if they know what may trigger an allergy. Check the ingredients within the products including oils and fragrances.
	If the client is unsure of what may trigger allergies but has experienced allergic reactions to hair products in the past, do not proceed.
	If there is a formula that contains an ingredient to which your client is allergic, choose an alternative product.
Skin disorders	
	If your client has a skin disorder on their scalp and there are signs of open or weeping areas, do not proceed.
	If the skin is not broken and there are no signs of weeping and you can protect the area sufficiently, you may proceed with care.
Incompatible products	
	Check with your client which products have already been used in the past on their hair. If you have any concerns about previous treatments, carry out an incompatibility test.

Contra-indication	Outcome
	If the results show incompatibility, do not proceed. Remember that **thioglycolate** used in perming is never compatible with **hydroxide** and will cause breakage.
	Thioglycolate In hairdressing, this refers to the compound ammonium thioglycolate, also known as perm salt.	**Hydroxide** In hairdressing, this refers to strong alkaline compounds such as sodium hydroxide.
Medical history	Ask your client if they are taking any medication. If you are unsure as to the likely reaction of the hair, carry out an incompatibility test. If the incompatibility test is positive, do not proceed.
Time interval	Retouch relaxer applications should be measured by the amount of new hair growth. This can vary from client to client, depending on their rate of hair growth. It is advisable to wet a small section of the hair, approximately 2.5cm^2 (1in^2), to see if there is any curl pattern close to the root area. Remember to apply relaxer 0.5cm/⅛in away from the scalp and without overlapping onto the previously relaxed hair. Anything more frequent can lead to breakage and overprocessing. If you can't see a visible regrowth, do not proceed with the relaxing service. Be aware the client may have used thermal styling tools and therefore new growth may not be visible. If there is ¾–1in/2–2.5cm of new growth, you can proceed with the relaxing service.
Recent removal of extensions or braids	Check with your client when their hair was last in a braid or extensions. If your client has removed either braids or extensions within the past two weeks, do not proceed with the relaxing service. It is important to leave at least two weeks between the removal of braids or extensions as the hair is very fragile during this time. Advise your client to have a deep conditioning treatment before rebooking them for their relaxer after an appropriate period of time.
Interval of time from colour	If the client has not had a permanent colour service within two weeks, proceed with relaxing service. If your client is unsure which type of colour has been applied to the hair, carry out a strand test to identify the condition of the hair.

Once you have identified a contra-indication or have a problem test result, you need to know whom to ask for assistance in your salon. It is important that this person knows how to assess both contra-indications and hair test results, and will normally be a more senior member of your salon team. If you are unsure what to do when you have one of the listed problems, you can ask this colleague to help you decide what action to take.

Previous chemical treatments

Retouch relaxer applications should be measured by the amount of new hair growth. This can vary from client to client, depending on their rate of hair growth. The guidelines for a safe regrowth are 2–2.5cm/¾–1in of new growth. It is essential not to overlap the relaxer cream during application as this will cause a reduction of the remaining bonds within the cortex and this will lead to breakage. The client may have thermally straightened their hair prior to the consultation and therefore the hair will appear straight at the regrowth area. To ensure that you are conducting an accurate analysis follow the steps below:

- Dampen a small section of the hair approximately 5cm²/2in² near the root area. (Do not oversaturate the scalp as this may cause sensitivity if you proceed with the application.)

- Review the hair's return to its original curl pattern: if the curl springs back to a curl and is at least 2–2.5cm/¾–1in from the scalp, then it is safe to proceed with the relaxing service.

- Make sure you check with your client whether they have had any other straightening services carried out on the hair.

- If the client has previously had a thioglycolate lotion applied to the hair (ie if they have had a perm) and it is possible that the effects of this service still remain in the hair, then do not proceed with a relaxer service.

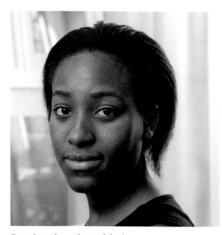
Previously relaxed hair

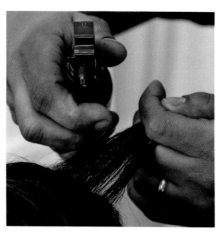
Dampen hair to check the original curl pattern

HANDY HINT

Curly perms and relaxer services are usually not compatible as they use different chemicals and the combination of the two chemicals will cause the hair to break.

HANDY HINT

If you are unsure about previous chemicals always do a strand test. Take a few strands of hair from various areas if the client's head. Place this sample in some relaxer cream, monitor the processing and ensure that the hair remains in optimum condition.

HANDY HINT

If your client has used straightening irons to style their hair at home before the consultation, remember that this may disguise the amount of new growth. Therefore, dampen a small section of the hair to see the natural curl pattern of the hair – do not wet the scalp as this may cause sensitivity if you choose to proceed with the relaxing service.

HEALTH & SAFETY

Remember thioglycolate and hydroxide chemicals are not compatible and will cause the hair to break.

Activity

A client's straightened hair is 4cm (1½in) long when dry but when it is wet it is 2cm (¾in) long. What is the percentage of 'shrinkage'? What does this tell you about how the hair was straightened?

Activity

If a client's hair grows 1.25cm (½in) per month, how many centimetres of regrowth would the client have after three months?

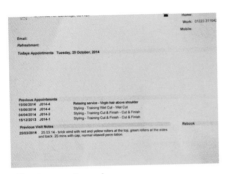

Client record card

HANDY HINT

More information about the Data Protection Act can be found in chapter CHB9.

Client history

For every client either regular or new, it is always essential that you have a detailed record card with their correct details outlined. The information on the record card should include their name, address and contact details. Record the dates of services, types of service, products used and the result, ensuring that the card is completed accurately and easy to read. You must always record the outcome of any tests carried out and your client's verbal responses to any questions asked. This will be very helpful in case you need to refer back to the information in future. If any problems occur, you will need evidence of your client's comments.

Always follow the Data Protection Act to ensure only authorised personnel have access to your client's data, that the record cards are kept in a secure location, that they are used for professional use only and that they are kept up to date.

Basic science

When carrying out a relaxing service on the hair it is important to understand the science of the hair and what happens during the relaxing process.

Characteristics of African type hair

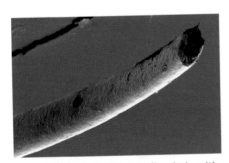

Microscope view: West Indian hair with a flattened surface

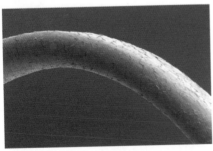

Microscope view: African type hair in its natural curved shape

Due to the distinct shape and formation of African type hair in its natural state, the features of the hair are unique. It is rare that there is any uniformity in the distribution of curls, twists and bends throughout the hair strand. Even during the early growth phases from the scalp, the hair grows at a variety of angles. This is why there are no distinct partings, as opposed to Caucasian or Asian hair which grows more directly upwards from the scalp. Excessively curly hair has a more oval shape and when viewed under a microscope looks more ribbon-like than other hair types. While other hair types tend to have more uniformity in thickness from the root to the end of the hair, the diameter of African type hair tends to differ along the shaft. Even when African type hair is chemically altered or straightened, this thinning of the hair fibre at points where the natural bends were positioned are still present and therefore form points of weakness along the hair shaft. The points of weakness along the strand of hair mean that the force required to break a strand of African type hair is much less than required to break Caucasian or Asian hair. This means that the hair is very fragile.

The nature of curly hair means that it contracts tightly and makes the hair appear much shorter than it actually is. Coily hair can shrink to half its actual length and this must be considered when carrying out relaxing services and styling.

It is considered that African type hair is naturally drier than other hair types. This happens when the sebum, which is produced to protect the surface of the hair, and gives flexibility and shine, is obstructed by the uneven surface of the hair and therefore rarely makes it beyond the mid-lengths of the hair to the ends. This lack of natural moisturiser to the surface of the hair can cause 'shedding', which is when the tips of the hair become extremely dehydrated and break off.

There are many different curl types that fall within the African type hair classification. However, these characteristics can be found throughout many different ethnicities. Therefore, it is important when analysing the hair to focus on the type of hair that you are working with rather than the **ethnic group** of the client. Excessively curly hair types share a common characteristic of dryness. It is the tightness of the curls that produce a more undulating surface. These twists and turns cause the hair to have two differing cortex components, the **ortho**-cortex and **para**-cortex. The ortho-cortex has a thinner and therefore weaker structure because this side of the hair bends outwards and is stretched. The para-cortex is the opposite side of the hair and bends inwards, so is less stretched and thicker. The fact that one side of a stand of hair can be weaker means that care must be taken during the processing time of a relaxer.

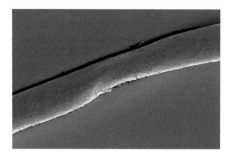

Microscope view: trichorrhexis nodosa – nodes that thicken and can cause breakage

Ethnic group

People with shared physical appearance based on genetic origins.

Ortho

Refers to the surface of the curl bending outwards (convex).

Para

Refers to the surface of the curl bending inwards (concave).

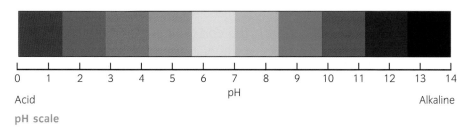

pH scale

Hair is subject to the laws of chemistry even in its natural state. When you are changing the shape and texture of the hair with a chemical relaxer it is important to understand the pH of the product that you are working with. The pH of a relaxer is highly alkaline and usually falls between 12 and 14 on the pH scale. The relaxer products usually come in the form of a cream emulsion and are prepared with the support of proteins, moisturisers and vitamins. The reduction phase of a relaxing service is followed by a normalising/neutralising shampoo and conditioner. These are both acid-balanced to restore the hair back to its natural acidity of 4.5–5.5.

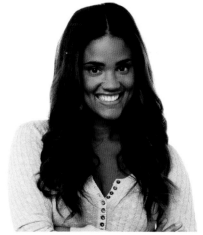

African type hair, Brazilian client

Activity

A pH of 3 is ten times more acidic than a pH of 4 and 100 times (10 times 10) more acidic than a pH value of 5. What is the difference in value of a pH of 3 and 6?

The structure of the hair – layers within the hair

Each hair is made up of three layers:

- cuticle
- cortex
- medulla.

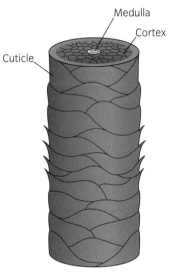

Structure of the hair

Tattered

Torn or frayed.

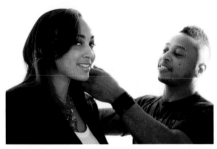

If sebum cannot reach the ends, hair becomes dry

Cuticle

The cuticle is made up of colourless overlapping layers of hardened keratin. The number of cuticle layers varies depending on the ethnic background of the client. Typical African type hair has between five and eleven layers whereas Caucasian hair has four to seven and Asian hair has up to eleven. The hair colour that we see is actually the pigmentation found within the cortex. The healthy appearance of hair depends almost entirely upon the condition of the cuticle. **Tattered** cuticles reflect the light much less and therefore cause the hair to have less ability to shine. In its natural state the curls, coils and bends in excessively curly hair cause the cuticle scales to be slightly lifted and, as a result, chemicals can enter the hair more rapidly. A relaxer is an alkaline and is designed to open the cuticle scales allowing the chemicals to work within the cortex.

Cortex

Immediately under the cuticle is the cortex. It is within the cortex that the strength and elasticity of the hair are determined. The cortex comprises long, fibrous, cable-like chains of keratin which run parallel with each other, down the length of each hair. The cortex makes up the greatest percentage of the hair strand, responsible for 80–90% of the hair's weight. This is also where we find hair's bonds: hydrogen bonds, salt bonds and disulphide bonds. It is the change in the disulphide bonds that enables a reduction of curls when a relaxer is applied.

Medulla

The medulla can be found at the innermost layer of the hair shaft. However, the medulla is not always present and has not been demonstrated to have any significance in hair's condition. The medulla when present simply makes the hair shafts naturally thicker than those without it.

The structure of the cortex

It is the cortex that is most affected by our client's various styling impulses and chemical processes to the hair. It is the keratin in the cortex that gives hair its physical characteristics (colour, curl, strength, etc).

The cortex consists mainly of keratin, which looks like a rope or cable when looked at under a very strong microscope. It consists of a series of cable-like chains. Within these chains are even finer chains:

- these finer chains are called polypeptide chains, which are made up of a combination of 18 **amino acids**
- polypeptide chains form a spiral shape which is known as an alpha-helix
- these alpha-helices twist together to form a protofibril
- these protofibrils are joined together by several different cross-linkages or bonds which form a ladder-like structure
- the protofibrils twist together to form a stranded cable-like structure which is called a microfibril
- microfibrils fall into irregular bundles called macrofibrils
- these macrofibril bundles make up the main bulk of the cortex.

Amino acids

Compounds found in living cells that contain carbon, oxygen, hydrogen and nitrogen.

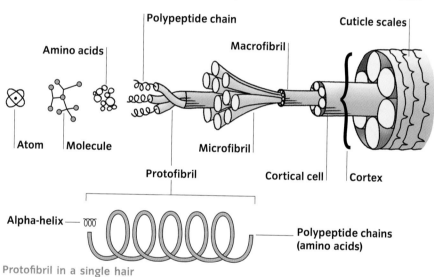

Protofibril in a single hair

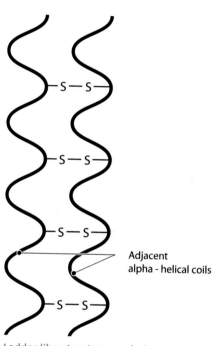

Ladder-like structure made by cross-linkages in the microfibril

So to simplify this:

Amino acids ➡ polypeptide chain (keratin/alpha-helix) ➡ protofibril (three twisted alpha-helices ➡ microfibril ➡ macrofibril (hundreds of bundles) ➡ cortex (joined-up macrofibrils)

It is the cross-linkages between the protofibrils in the microfibril that are affected during the chemical action of a relaxing service. Cysteine linkages are the strongest of the cross-linkages in keratin. Each molecule of the amino acid cystine forms part of two adjacent polypeptide chains with the cysteine linkage making a bridge between the chains. The cysteine linkages each contain two sulphur atoms, also known as disulphide bonds. These disulphide bonds are broken during the reduction phase of a relaxing service.

HANDY HINT

The smell of 'burnt hair' is the sulphur atoms being released from within the cysteine.

HANDY HINT

During the reduction phase the hydroxide changes the *cysteine* to *cystine*.

The effects of relaxer on the hair structure

The high alkalinity of the relaxer opens up the cuticle scales, allowing the chemicals to enter the cortex.

When active in the cortex the hydroxides within the relaxer cream break one of the two disulphide bonds – this is known as **hydrolysis**. It is the cross-linkages that are affected during the chemical action of a relaxing service.

Cystine linkages are the strongest of the cross-linkages in keratin. Each molecule of amino acid cysteine forms part of two adjacent polypeptide chains with the cystine linkage making a bridge between the chains. The cystine linkages each contain two sulphur atoms which are held together, also known as disulphide bonds.

During a relaxer service, the disuphide bonds (cross-linkages) are broken by the chemical action in the cortex. A new bond, called a **lanthionine linkage**, is formed. These lanthionine linkages are permanent bonds containing only one sulphur atom instead of the two sulphur atoms in a cystine linkage. This process is shown in the following illustration.

Hydrolysis

Chemical breakdown in which a compound is split into other compounds by reacting with water.

Cystine

Amino acid formed by the oxidation of two cysteine molecules that link via a disulphide bond.

Lanthionine linkages

Bond formed when the double bonds of a disulphide are reduced by a hydroxide.

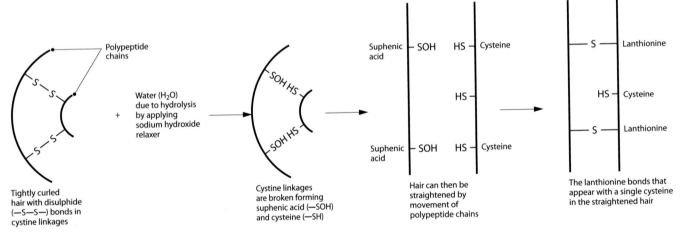

Chemical processes occurring during hair relaxing treatment

Activity

Discuss the differences between the permanent changes in the disulphide bonds in perming and relaxing procedures, and the temporary changes in the hydrogen bonds using heat (see chapter CH1).

If you relax the hair until it is very straight, you are essentially overrelaxing the hair. This removes any degree of elasticity, thus weakening the hair. Over time, continuous overrelaxation, blow drying and hot curling will cause the hair to become damaged and prone to breakage.

To avoid irreparable damage and maintain the integrity of the hair it is recommended straightening the hair 65–70%. It is important to understand that the chemical reaction of a hydroxide relaxer is a permanent change and the bonds can never return to their original formation.

Prepare for the service

Tests

Test	When to carry out the test	How to carry out the test	Purpose	Action
Elasticity 	During the consultation and analysis of the hair before proceeding with the service	Holding a few wet hairs gently between the fingers, gently pull the hair no more than 2cm (¾in) and allow it to stretch.	To check the strength of the hair. Ensure there is no breakage due to the bonds being deteriorated	If the hair does not return to its original length when stretched then this means the elasticity is impaired and therefore the hair may be too weak to withstand the relaxing service.
Porosity 	During the consultation and analysis of the hair before proceeding with the service	Holding a small group of hairs upright at the tips of the hair, slide your fingers towards the root area feeling for a raised surface.	To evaluate how quickly the product will be absorbed and therefore which strength of relaxer cream to use	Applying a relaxer to hair that is very porous could lead to damage as the product will be absorbed very quickly, breaking too many bonds, leading to hair breakage.
Density 	During the consultation and analysis of the hair before proceeding with the service	Take a $2.5cm^2/1in^2$ cross-section of the scalp and see how many hairs are growing from this area.	You will need to establish if the hair is sparse (thin), regular (medium) or abundant (thick). This knowledge will help you to use the correct strength of relaxer cream to carry out the service.	If the hair is sparse, the relaxer may take rapid effect and overprocess – avoid pulling the hair during application and preparation. If the hair is abundant, then this will have an impact on the time taken to apply the relaxer cream.

HANDY HINT

Take careful notice not to exceed the development time given on the manufacturer's instructions.

Test	When to carry out the test	How to carry out the test	Purpose	Action
Texture	During the consultation and analysis of the hair before proceeding with the service	Isolate individual hairs from the head and compare the diameter to that of your own or a colleague's hair.	Assess the diameter of each hair to establish how much relaxer can be absorbed and which strength of product to use.	Thick (coarse) hair – process longer; may be more resistant to processing. Medium hair – does not pose any special problems or concerns. Fine hair – more fragile, easier to process, and more susceptible to damage from chemical services than coarse or medium hair.
Incompatibility test	During the consultation and analysis of the hair before proceeding with the service	Coat 2–3 hairs in the chosen relaxer cream in a plastic bowl and process for the manufacturer's recommended development time.	To determine whether there are any residues or incompatible product within the cortex or cuticle of the hair. These could be metallic salts or some compound henna products.	If there is deterioration of the hair sample, do not proceed with the service. Carry out some conditioning treatments in the salon and suggest other hairstyle options to the client.

Tools and equipment

Each manufacturer may have some tools which are exclusive to their brands and it is important to follow the manufacturer's guidelines throughout the process of the relaxing service.

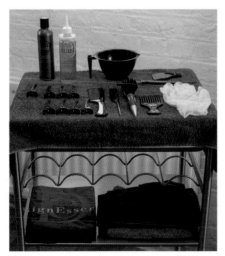

Trolley prepared for protective stage of relaxing service

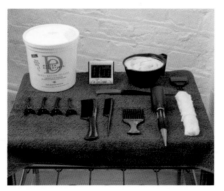

Trolley prepared for relaxing stage of service

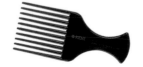

Tools and equipment	Function
Cape/towels	To ensure your client is suitably protected from the chemicals that you will be using during the relaxing service. Always ensure that your client is wearing a protective gown and has a towel placed around their neck. You can also use a disposable plastic cape.
Personal protective equipment/PPE (stylist apron, gloves)	Used to protect your own clothing and skin from the harsh chemicals used during a relaxing service.
Detangling comb	It is important to detangle the hair prior to the relaxing service. Make sure you have detangled with your hands before trying to comb the hair. Always comb the hair in small sections, each time starting the stroke further towards the roots than the previous stroke.
Tail comb	Used to section the hair during application of the scalp protector, mid-length and ends protector and relaxer cream. Ensure that your comb is free from product build-up throughout the application – this will help to prevent product transferring onto areas that you do not wish the product to contact.
Tint brush/spatula and non-metallic bowl	Use either a spatula or tint brush to apply the relaxer. Using a spatula is very gentle on the scalp and will not disturb the surface of the scalp or placement of the scalp protector. Dispense your relaxer into a non-metallic bowl. This will allow you to avoid cross-contamination and avoid using excessive amounts of product.
Timer	It is important to have a timer in order to continually monitor the processing time of your relaxer. Ensure that you follow the manufacturer's instructions and do not exceed the processing time. The processing time will include the time it takes to apply the product.
Plastic clips	Use non-metallic clips to keep hair in neat sections during application of the relaxer. Clips that are coated with metals may cause a reaction with the relaxer.
Styling comb	Used during styling and dressing of the hair.
Paddle brush/vent brush	Use a paddle or vent brush to create a smooth blow dry. These brushes will help you achieve the desired result without excessive tension to the hair which can cause breakage.
Hair dryer	Used for styling the hair after the relaxer service. Keep heat low and avoid contact with the hair and nozzle during drying as this can cause extreme damage to the cuticle, especially immediately after a relaxer.

Products

Choose the correct relaxer based on the texture, density, porosity, elasticity and curl pattern of your client's hair. The records made during your conversation with your client will give you an understanding of the expected outcome, the client's lifestyle and their ability to maintain the style that you are going to create.

Lye and no-lye relaxers

A relaxing service on excessively curly hair is usually carried out using 1–4.5% sodium hydroxide (sometimes known as 'lye') in a cream emulsion. The cream emulsion will also be enhanced with vitamins, moisturisers and proteins to help protect the hair during processing. Sodium hydroxide is a **caustic** alkali and has a pH of 12–14. A sodium relaxer will break down the bonds more quickly and the hair is left with more shine. However, sodium hydroxide can be more irritating on the scalp. If used incorrectly it will burn the skin and if overprocessed, it will have a **depilatory** effect and destroy the hair.

The alternatives to a sodium hydroxide (lye) relaxer are lithium hydroxide, potassium hydroxide, calcium hydroxide and guanidine hydroxide. These are also known as no-lye relaxers. The most common active ingredient in a no-lye relaxer is calcium hydroxide or guanidine hydroxide with a liquid activator of guanidine carbonate, which is added to the relaxer cream just before use. Although the pH level of a no-lye relaxer is typically lower than a lye one, no-lye relaxers are often associated with dryer hair due to potential calcium build-up. One of the major reasons someone may prefer a no-lye relaxer is if the scalp is sensitive, as the chemicals in this type of relaxer can be milder on the scalp. This does not mean that no-lye relaxers can't burn – they can.

Caustic

Able to burn or corrode organic tissue by chemical action.

Depilatory

Capable of removing hair.

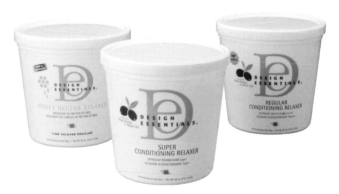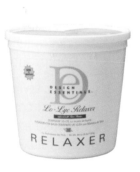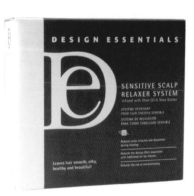

Regular sodium hydroxide (lye) and calcium hydroxide or guanidine hydroxide (no-lye) relaxers

THE CITY & GUILDS TEXTBOOK

Relaxer strengths

There are many different strengths of relaxer available. The percentage of hydroxide used in a relaxer determines its strength. For example, 'super strength' contains a higher concentration of sodium hydroxide than a 'regular strength' relaxer. Although the result from a relaxer, irrespective of strength, is straighter, more manageable hair, the strength of the relaxer used to achieve the result is very important. The goal is to avoid hair and scalp damage based on the texture of the hair, so you should only use the highest strength for the most resistant healthy hair. Always follow the manufacturer's instructions for the specific processing time for the relaxer you have chosen to use on your client, following a detailed consultation and analysis of the hair.

Products

Product	Function
Scalp protector	Applied before the relaxer cream, this is used to protect the client's skin and scalp during the processing period. A lightweight gel that provides a soothing barrier between chemical and scalp, it usually contains menthol, aloe, vitamin E and shea butter.
Lengths and ends protector	Applied before the relaxer cream, this is used to protect previously processed hair. Apply to the length and ends of the hair that has been treated with either colour or relaxer. Do not rinse. It contains a blend of conditioners, vitamins, minerals and proteins and provides conditioning protection before, during and after a chemical service.

Product	Function
Relaxer cream 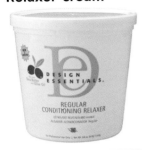	Hydroxide relaxer cream using either sodium hydroxide (lye) or lithium hydroxide, potassium hydroxide, calcium hydroxide or guanidine hydroxide (no lye). A relaxer cream's pH falls between 12 and 14 and it is used to transform the disulphide bonds into lanthionine bonds. It also contains moisturising and strengthening ingredients to retain the optimum condition of the hair during the process. Follow the manufacturer's instructions regarding optimum application and processing times.
Neutralising conditioning shampoo 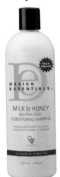	Neutralising conditioning shampoo is an acidic formula which removes all traces of chemical residue using a colour indicator and restores hair to its normal pH level of 4.5–5. Developed to neutralise and condition the hair after the curl reduction process with hydroxides, it contains protein and vitamin complexes which restore the balance of the hair.
Reconstructive treatment 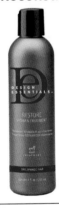	Vitamin and protein complexes prevent and protect against breakage. This type of treatment moisturises, softens, detangles and evens porosity. It seals the cuticles and restores hair to a normal pH level. Check the manufacturer's instructions for the appropriate after-service treatment.

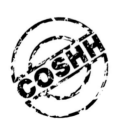

Product disposal

It is essential to store, use, handle and dispose of products in accordance with manufacturers' instructions, salon policy and local bye-laws. When dealing with resources in the salon, you will be expected to have a good working knowledge of the Control of Substances Hazardous to Health (COSHH) Regulations, thereby minimising the risk of harm or injury to yourself and others.

Apply relaxing treatment

Scalp protector

It is important that the client has not recently shampooed their hair prior to a relaxer application as a freshly cleansed scalp will contain very little natural oil and this will cause heightened sensitivity. Protection of the scalp and hair is essential during a relaxing service whether using lye or no-lye products – failure to protect the scalp, hairline and tops of the ears sufficiently can lead to chemical burns of the skin. Applying a scalp protector will help with this but minimum contact with the skin and the scalp should also be achieved through precision during application of the relaxer.

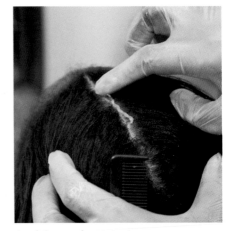

Applying scalp protector

Length and ends protector

Protective treatments for the hair are available from most manufacturers. These products will help to regulate the absorption of the relaxer cream and are enhanced with vitamins and strengthening ingredients which will fill and smooth the cuticle. However these products will not prevent overprocessing of the hair and if the recommended processing time is exceeded, the hair will become damaged and has the potential to break.

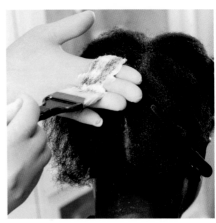

Applying lengths and ends protector

Categories of relaxer services

A relaxer service can be either a regrowth application or a virgin hair application.

Regrowth application

This technique is used on hair that has been previously relaxed. The product is applied to the new growth of hair only and should be carried out between 8 and 12 weeks after the original service.

Virgin hair application

This is where a relaxer has never been used on the hair before. The product is applied on the mid-lengths and ends where the hair is more resistant. Relaxer is then applied to the new growth of hair and processed – as the hair has just grown it is freshly keratinised and therefore softer. The natural heat from the scalp will also cause the hair in this area to process more quickly.

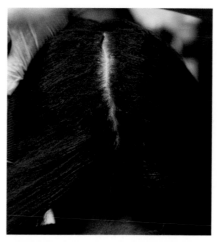

Regrowth area prior to relaxing application

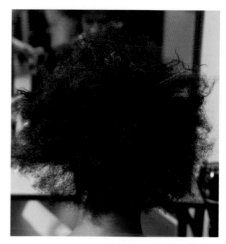

Virgin hair prior to relaxing application

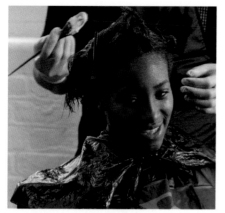

Processing time includes the time it takes to apply the product

Accurate timing

Processing times vary from client to client, depending on the density, texture and curl patterns. However, most processing times are a maximum of 20–25 minutes. Do not exceed the manufacturer's instructions for processing times for the variety of relaxer cream that you have chosen. The processing time will include the time it takes to apply the product. Carry out a curl reduction test to ensure that you have achieved the desired amount of curl reduction.

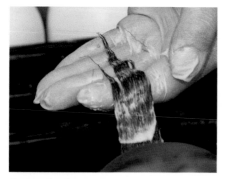

Curl reduction test

Curl reduction test

This test is to determine if the curls have been reduced enough during the relaxing service process. Wearing the recommended protective clothing and gloves (PPE), gently wipe the relaxer cream from a few strands of hair. If you have not reached the desired result, re-apply the relaxer cream to these strands and continue checks frequently.

If the curls spring back spontaneously then the relaxer has not been processed sufficiently. If the curls look smoother and loosened significantly, then the desired result has been achieved. Be careful not to overprocess the hair as this will cause breakage and damage.

The normalising phase

When the straightening is complete the hair must first be thoroughly rinsed with **tepid** water, taking care that all of the relaxer cream is removed.

The alkali must then be washed out of the hair, using a specialised neutralising shampoo with a pH of 4–5. This process is a true chemical neutralisation between acid and alkali.

This shampoo process will remove any alkali left on the hair, stop further reduction of the bonds, reduce the swelling of the hair shaft and return the hair to its normal slightly acidic state. The neutralizing shampoo usually contains a chemical indicator, which will cause a colour change to the lather if any alkali remains in the hair.

It is important to treat the hair with great care during this phase as the hair is extremely fragile and undergoing an extreme chemical change. Neutralising shampoos are not interchangeable and you should always use the neutralising shampoo that accompanies the relaxer cream.

Temperature

As a relaxer cream is a highly alkaline cream emulsion using hydroxides the formula is designed to work at the temperature of the scalp – it is not suitable to use any form of heat source to accelerate the processing time. If the salon is extremely warm, ensure that you continually monitor the progress of the reduction phase of your relaxing service.

Tepid
Moderately warm/lukewarm water.

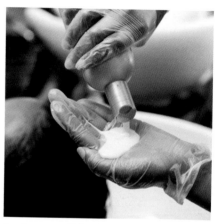

Apply neutralising shampoo at least twice to ensure all the relaxing cream has been removed

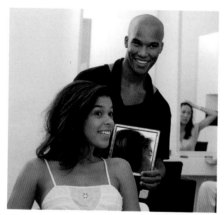

Check that the client is happy with the result

Combining relaxing and colouring

Care must be taken when using colouring products on hair that has been relaxed, as the combination of the two chemicals can cause the hair to become weak and fragile. It is recommended to leave an interval of at least two weeks between carrying out a relaxing service and a permanent colour service.

HEALTH & SAFETY

An oxidising agent or neutraliser for a perm lotion should never be used in replacement of this phase as it will cause breakage to the hair.

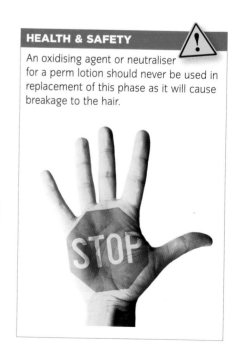

It can be possible to carry out a quasi-permanent or semi-permanent colour on the same day as a relaxer by reducing the development time of the colour. However, you must follow the manufacturer's instructions.

The safest colour procedure on the same day as a relaxing service would be the use of topical staining rinses only. These are colours that do not require any oxidation, they should contain no ammonia nor have the ability to make changes to the bonds within the cortex.

It is important to carry out a stand test to establish if it is possible to proceed with colouring.

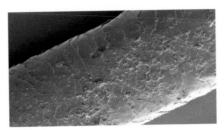

Microscope view: West Indian hair processed with a relaxer

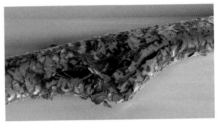

Microscope view: West Indian hair damaged by using both a relaxer and pre-lightener

Problems that may occur during a relaxing service

You may encounter some challenges whilst carrying out a relaxing service. It is essential that you know how to respond to any challenges. The table below will give you a summary of challenges that may occur and how to remedy them.

Challenge	Cause	Remedy
Scalp irritation	The scalp has become sensitised during the process due to the product strength. Recent shampooing – wait at least 48 hours between shampooing and the application of relaxer cream. Removal of extensions or braids can cause scalp sensitivity due the length of time that the hair has been lying directionally. Use of inappropriate tools can scratch the scalp. Hot drinks during the service.	Frequently check the client's comfort. If the client states scalp discomfort, remove the relaxer immediately. Use tepid water. If the discomfort is isolated to one small area, remove the relaxer cream from this area with dry cotton wool – avoid rubbing the skin. (Ensure you are wearing the correct PPE.)
Discolouration of white hair	White hair can become yellowish during the relaxing service when oxidation causes the melanin to lose its colour, leaving some residual red and gold colours. In addition, since the keratin is naturally yellow, this accentuates the appearance of the yellow tint of the hair after these treatments.	After the normalising phase is complete, use a silver-toned styling mousse, setting lotion or conditioner to counteract the yellow.

Challenge	Cause	Remedy
Signs of hair breakage/loss	The curl reduction could be too extreme. Application time could have been too long. Formula strength too strong.	Rinse directly in tepid water. Be very gentle with the hair. Apply an intense reconstructing treatment.
Curl pattern remains too strong	Not enough product applied or insufficient curl test. Underprocessed – not enough bonds reduced. Application was not thorough.	Carry out reconstructing treatments. Once the hair is in optimum condition reapply the relaxer. Always follow manufacturers' instructions.
Trichorrhexis nodosa	A defect in the hair shaft characterised by thickening or weak points (nodes) that cause the hair to break off easily.	Handle hair with care and avoid harsh brushing or excessive exposure to thermal styling tools. Carry out reconstructing treatments. Only proceed with relaxer once the hair is in optimum condition and breakage has stopped.

Advice and recommendations

Activity

Keep up to date! The hairdressing industry is extremely progressive with new technology and techniques under constant development. Research events, shows and exhibitions and read about the competitions held by different manufacturers. These can be found online or in trade magazines.

Time intervals between relaxing services

Your client will need to understand the importance of time intervals between their relaxing services. If you relax the hair too frequently then you can cause damage by overlapping the chemicals and this will cause extreme deterioration to the hair. However, if the interval is too long the hair will become difficult for the client to manage and become too full in the regrowth area making it difficult to maintain smooth styles.

Shampooing

This will vary from client to client but once a client has undergone a relaxing service, it will facilitate future cleansing and conditioning of the hair meaning the client can wash and condition the hair more frequently.

Suitable conditioning treatments

Having changed the physical shape of the hair during a relaxing service, it is important to maintain the condition of the hair. Advising your client about the importance of carrying out regular protein and moisture treatments will help them to preserve the condition of their hair.

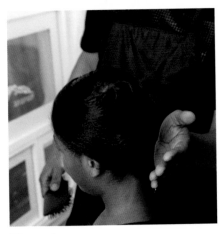

Client recommendations after service

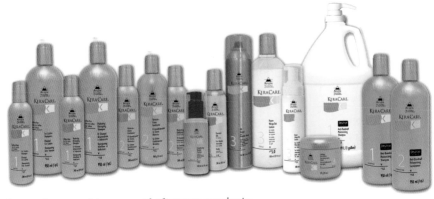

Choose from a wide range of aftercare products

Wrapping the hair

It is important that your client understands the importance of protecting the hair at night. Introducing a smooth and silky pillowcase or hair cover (satin is considered to be the best material) is a great way to reduce breakage due to friction. There are several ways the client can put up their hair before they go to sleep. In the morning, all they'll have to do is take it down and go, which means no heat-styling with flat irons. Relaxed hair will benefit from wrapping at night. It keeps the hair smooth and tangle-free.

Depending on the length of the hair, they can either begin at the nape of the neck and wrap in a clockwise or counter-clockwise direction, or they can part the hair into three sections and begin wrapping at the back. Your client should use a vent brush, boar bristle brush or wide-toothed comb along with the hands, to smooth the hair and mould it to their scalp as they work their way round. They can use long pins to hold hair in place if it has trouble staying on its own. However, there are lots of 'night-time treatments' available that will enhance the condition and make it easy to wrap the hair. Once the hair is wrapped, your client should tie a satin scarf around the hairline.

Wrap set

HANDY HINT

For more details on wrap setting, see chapter CH2.

Intervals between haircuts

Ensure that your client understands that trimming the hair regularly will help them achieve longer, healthier hair. Hair that is not trimmed regularly will become very dry and brittle on the ends and will begin to 'pop' or 'shed'. This will inhibit the ability for the hair to grow.

Styling tools

Brushes and combs should have teeth or bristles that are widely spaced apart to avoid snagging and tearing the hair. It is very important that your client understands that they need to be extremely gentle whilst brushing the hair when it is dry, as this can cause damage even though the hair is now in a straighter form.

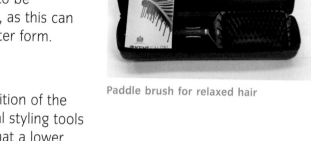

Paddle brush for relaxed hair

Thermal styling tools

The use of heat can have a negative effect on the condition of the hair and therefore it is important to explain that thermal styling tools and hairdryers should be temperature-controlled and that a lower heat and less contact with the hair are desirable.

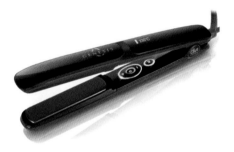
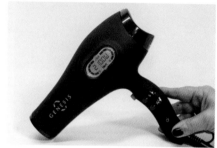

Thermal controlled styling tools

Step by steps

Regrowth application

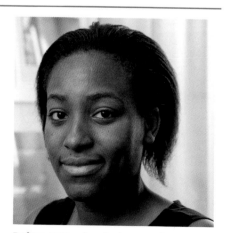

Before retouch relaxing service

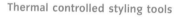
HEALTH & SAFETY

Ensure stylist and client are wearing suitable PPE throughout the service.

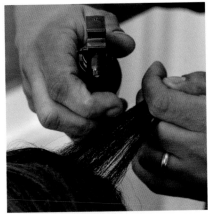

STEP 1 – As the client may have used irons to straighten the hair prior to an appointment, using a waterspray, dampen a small area of the hair to determine the natural curl pattern and regrowth.

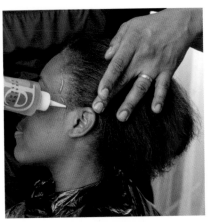

STEP 2 – Apply the scalp protector around the nape of the neck and all around the hairline.

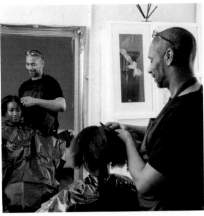

STEP 3 – Detangle the hair thoroughly first using your hands and then a wide-toothed comb. Neatly separate the hair into four sections.

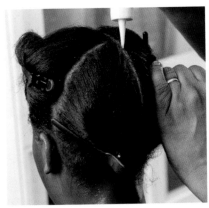

STEP 4 – Using an applicator bottle, apply the scalp protector to the scalp using 0.5cm (¼in) sections, parting throughout the head, being careful to cause as little disturbance to the scalp as possible. Rubbing the scalp or too much disturbance can cause scalp sensitivity.

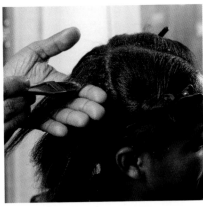

STEP 5 – Still working neatly in a four-section pattern, begin applying a protector to all of the lengths and ends of the hair that have previously been treated with relaxer or colour to prevent damage to the hair.

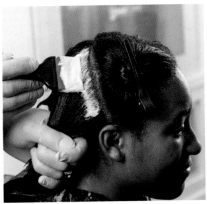

STEP 6 – Taking 0.5cm (¼in) sections, and using a spatula or tint brush, apply the appropriate relaxer cream 0.25cm (⅛in) from the scalp on new growth only, being careful to avoid contact with the skin as the relaxer cream can cause damage. For the same reason, make sure that you are wearing protective gloves.

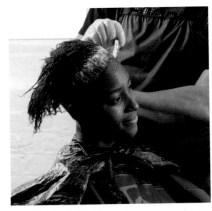

STEP 7 – Once the relaxer cream has been applied to the entire regrowth area, begin gently smoothing the hair with the back of a tail comb or spatula to ensure a smooth result.

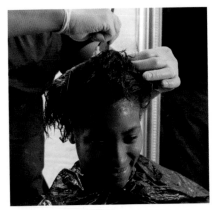

STEP 8 – Monitor the development time, carry out curl tests and ensure client comfort throughout the service.

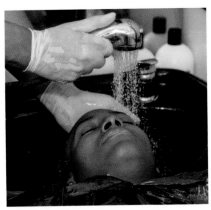

STEP 9 – Rinse the hair thoroughly to remove all traces of the relaxer cream.

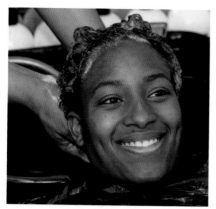

STEP 10 – Proceed with the neutralising shampoo up to three times. A colour indicator will help you decide when all the alkali has been removed from the hair and the hair has been restored to its acidic balance of 4.5–5.5.

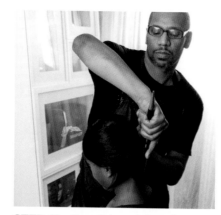

STEP 11 – Dry, style and dress hair to complete the look.

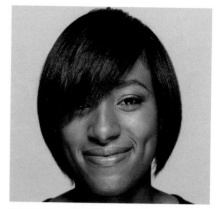

STEP 12 – Final look – retouch relaxer.

HANDY HINT

For more details on wrap setting, see chapter CH2.

Virgin hair application

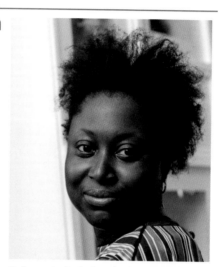

Before virgin hair relaxing service

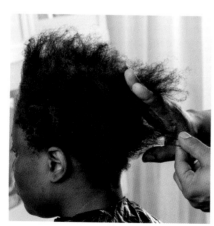

STEP 1 – Detangle the hair thoroughly first using your hands.

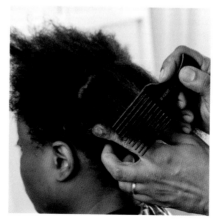

STEP 2 – Next detangle it with a wide-toothed comb.

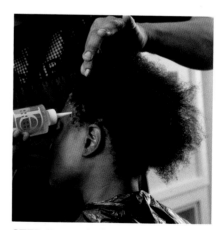

STEP 3 – Apply the scalp protector around the nape of the neck and the hairline.

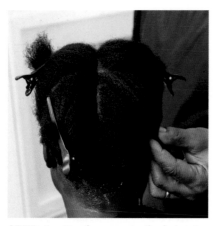

STEP 4 – Neatly separate the hair into four sections using the plastic clips to secure hair.

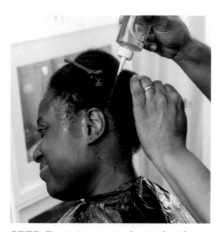

STEP 5 – Using an applicator bottle, apply the scalp protector to the scalp using 0.5cm (¼in) sections, parting throughout the head, being careful to cause as little disturbance to the scalp as possible. Rubbing the scalp or too much disturbance can cause scalp sensitivity. (If the hair is very dry due to mechanical damage, you can also protect the lengths and ends.)

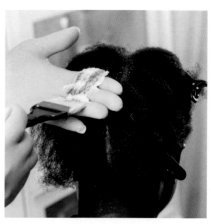

STEP 6 – Taking 0.5cm (¼in) sections, and using a spatula or tint brush, apply the appropriate relaxer cream starting on the ends and then the mid-lengths of the hair.

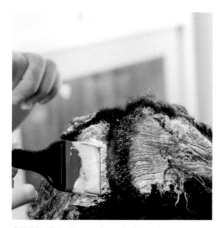

STEP 7 – Once the ends and mid-lengths are sufficiently infused with product, begin applying the relaxer cream to the new growth area, 0.25cm (⅛in) from the scalp, being careful to avoid contact with the skin as the relaxer cream can cause damage and burning to the skin and scalp.

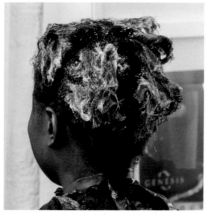

STEP 8 – Repeat the application of the relaxer cream until the entire head is covered, checking client comfort throughout.

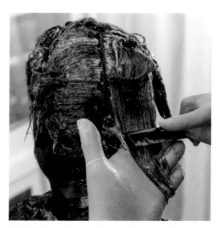

STEP 9 – Once the application is complete, begin smoothing with your hands or the flat back of a tail comb, working in the same direction as the initial application.

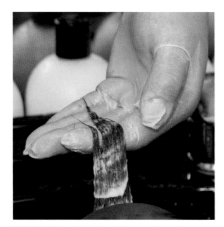

STEP 10 – Continually monitor the development of your relaxing service, carrying out a curl test to evaluate curl reduction. If a wavy or texturised look is required, ensure that you are allowing sufficient curl to remain in the hair. If you require a smoother look, continue to process. However, do not overstraighten the hair as this will cause the hair to become weak and potentially break. Check for client comfort throughout the service. Always follow the MFIs for maximum development time.

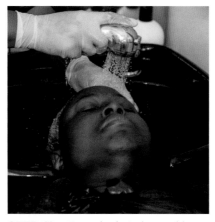

STEP 11 – Rinse the hair thoroughly with tepid water, avoiding excess water pressure or rough handling of the hair.

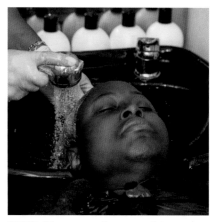

STEP 12 – Once all traces of the relaxer cream have been rinsed from the hair, continue to the normalising/ neutralising phase by shampooing the hair with the neutralising shampoo up to three times. A colour indicator will help you decide when all the alkali has been removed from the hair and the hair has been restored to its acidic balance of 4.5–5.

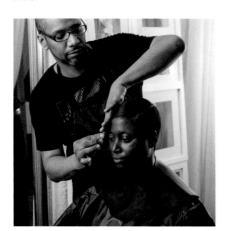

STEP 13 – Dry and trim the hair as required.

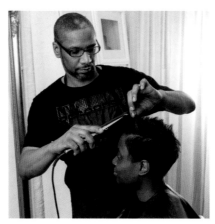

STEP 14 – Style the hair to complete the look.

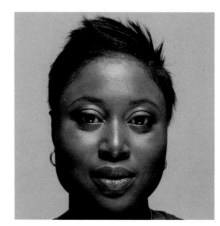

STEP 15 – Final look – virgin hair relaxer.

Answers in the back of the book.

1 A client has complained that their clothing has been stained during the service. Which one of the following should have been carried out?

 a Reading manufacturers' instructions

 b Wearing protective clothing

 c Following COSHH

 d Using PPE

2 Which one of the following is **not** a contra-indication to a relaxing service?

 a Poor elasticity

 b Cuts on the scalp

 c Head lice

 d Abundant hair

3 **Statement one**

 Due to the curl pattern of type 4 hair, it can appear much shorter when relaxed.

 Statement two

 Sparse, medium and abundant are the three categories of hair texture.

 Which **one** of the following is correct for the above statements?

 a True   True

 b True   False

 c False   True

 d False   False

4 Why is tightly curled hair often weaker than straight hair?

 a Because the keratin is very elastic

 b Because the keratin is very porous

 c Because of the narrow segments of keratin along the hair shaft

 d Because of the keratin being very thick at points along the shaft

5 The polypeptide chains in the cortex

 a Make the hair feel brittle

 b Establish the strength of hair

 c Make the hair feel dehydrated

 d Establish the curl pattern of hair

6 Why is it important to avoid 100% straightness when relaxing?

 a To avoid touching the skin with the product

 b To avoid hair becoming too curly

 c To avoid spending too long on the service

 d To avoid over-processing the hair

7 When should a client be recommended to return to the salon for a retouch relaxer?

 a After a minimum of four weeks

 b After a minimum of three months

 c When the hair has grown at least 2–2.5cm/¾–1in

 d When the hair has grown at least 1.25–2cm/½–¾in

8 Which one of the following identifies the pH of a sodium hydroxide relaxer and describes how it can affect the hair?

 a 3–5 which can break the hair

 b 8–10 which can make the hair brittle

 c 12–14 which can severely damage hair

 d 6–8 which can make the hair extremely porous

9 A relaxer can have a depilatory action on the hair. What does the term depilatory mean?

 a It is capable of removing hair

 b It will increase the pH of hair

 c It makes the scalp sensitive

 d It makes the hair brittle

10 Which two of the following describe how lanthionine is formed when relaxing hair?

 1 By the disulphide bonds breaking

 2 By the pH of hair changing to an acid

 3 By hydrogen bonds being broken

 4 By cysteine and supheric acid being formed

 a 1 and 2

 b 2 and 3

 c 3 and 4

 d 4 and 1

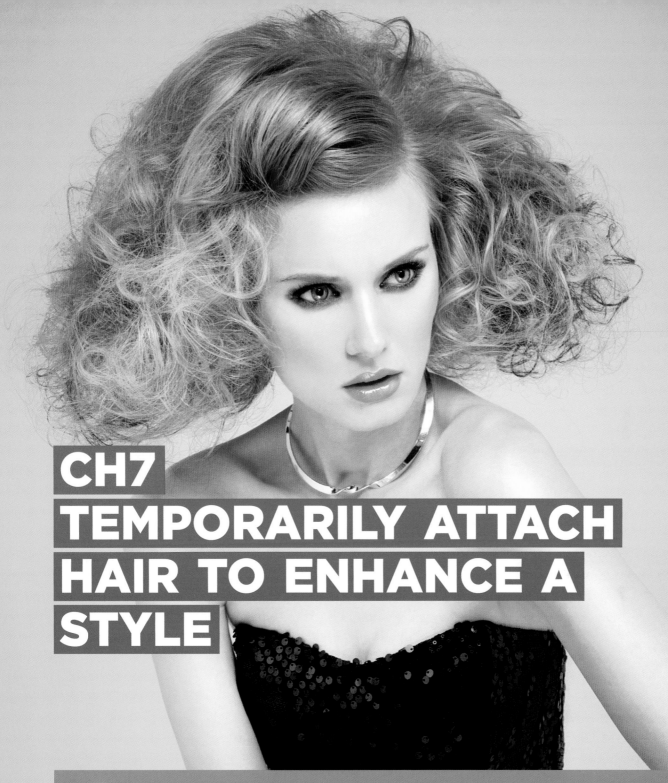

CH7
TEMPORARILY ATTACH HAIR TO ENHANCE A STYLE

Attaching hair to enhance a style can create a quick image change that adds colour, texture, volume and/or length. The result can be dramatic or subtle to suit your client's requirements, and can last from 24 hours to up to six weeks, depending on the method of attachment. Attaching hair has become a very popular service in many salons because of its flexibility, the immediate result and varied looks that can be achieved.

After reading this chapter you will:

- know how health and safety affects hair attachment services
- understand the factors that influence hair attachment services
- know the tools, equipment, products and techniques used to attach and remove added hair
- be able to attach hair to enhance the style.

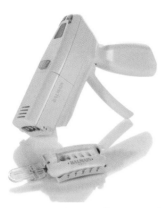

Hair extension applicator tool

HANDY HINT

Keep mints and deodorant in your locker or bag to enable you to freshen up when required, and avoid offending clients with unpleasant body odours. Don't bring your germs to work: stay at home if you have a contagious illness.

HEALTH & SAFETY

Refer to the health and safety and salon policies chapter to refresh yourself on the main health and safety legislation.

VALUES & BEHAVIOURS

Refer to the values and behaviours chapter for more information on maintaining effective, hygienic and safe working practices, ensuring standards of personal hygiene and protection meet accepted industry and organisational requirements (values), and maintaining salon standards of behaviour (behaviours).

HANDY HINT

Always cover any open wounds and avoid going to work if you have a contagious illness or disease. Maintain a healthy, balanced diet and exercise regularly.

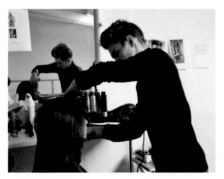

Maintain a good posture whilst working

Health and safety

Throughout this service it is vital that you maintain safe methods of working to prevent hazards and accidents, and work effectively to achieve a suitable end result. You may use a variety of methods to secure the hair, which can involve glue or needles and thread. These are quite different from your day-to-day tools, so you must always take care and follow the manufacturers' instructions (MFIs).

Responsibilities under health and safety

As with all services it is important to maintain health and safety to ensure that you, your client and others are not put at risk of harm or injury.

Your own personal hygiene is important. Salons can become hot and humid with all the hairdryers, steamers and warm water used, so it is essential that you start your day showered and wearing fresh, clean clothes suitable for work. Use deodorant and freshen your breath after your lunch. If you have long hair, you should tie it back during these services, to avoid it getting in the way and sticking in the glue.

Ensure you use your tools and equipment safely. If you are using an electrical glue gun, you must take extra care not to burn yourself, your client or those around you. Use your tools only for the purpose for which they are intended, to minimise the risks to you and others, and to avoid damage to the tools. Always follow the Electricity at Work Regulations and remember visually to check the plug, power cable and body of the glue gun for any signs of damage prior to use. If the electrical glue gun is faulty, you must label it, remove it from the salon area and inform the relevant person.

You must make sure that your tools, equipment and resources are all cleaned, sterilised and prepared for the service to avoid cross-infection and infestation, and to ensure that the salon's reputation is maintained.

As you prepare for the service, ensure that your trolley is arranged and on the correct side for your convenience. Check that your client is comfortable, with their back supported by the chair, legs uncrossed and feet on the floor or supported with a footrest.

As you will be standing throughout the service, try to avoid bending and twisting your back unnecessarily. Stand with your body weight evenly distributed and your back straight. Some hair attachment services require you to stand for long periods of time, and you'll risk back injury or fatigue if you do not stand correctly.

Hazards and risks

Hazards and risks in this chapter include all the usual ones, such as slippery services, faulty electrical equipment, use of chemicals or substances, risks of injury and skin conditions, but also include the use of glue for hair attachments and needles for sewing hair to plaits.

When using glue, always follow the Control of Substances Hazardous to Health (COSHH) regulations, local by-laws and your salon policy. These will tell you how to correctly use and store the product and dispose of empty containers.

Safe working practices

Always follow your salon's requirements for client preparation and when using products to secure hair attachments, for example glue, you must ensure that you wear gloves, wash and dry your hands properly and use a moisturising hand cream. Always follow the MFIs for these products and glues, as they will outline how to use them, the precautions to take and tests to complete. Your salon will have a policy on where to store products and glues, and this must be followed at all times.

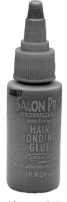

Always follow the MFIs when using bonding glue

Environmental and sustainable working practices

As part of your working practice, you should always try to maintain environmental and sustainable working practices:

- reduce energy usage – switch off lights and electrical items after use
- reduce water wastage – turn off taps
- reduce waste and use the correct quantities of products
- recycle, re-use and dispose of waste safely.

HEALTH & SAFETY

Refer to the health and safety and salon policies chapter for more information on environmental and sustainable working practices.

Preventing dermatitis

Remember to protect yourself by wearing personal protective equipment (PPE) to protect your clothes from damage and your skin from dermatitis. Contact dermatitis can be recognised by red itchy skin that might become cracked and inflamed.

Preventing cross-infection and infestation

Keeping a clean and tidy workstation helps you to prevent cross-infection and infestations. Always ensure that your tools and equipment are cleaned with warm, soapy water and then disinfected or sterilised before being used on any client.

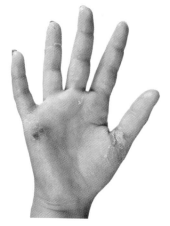

Dermatitis

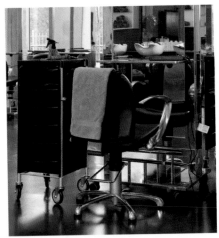

Maintain a clean and tidy work area throughout the service

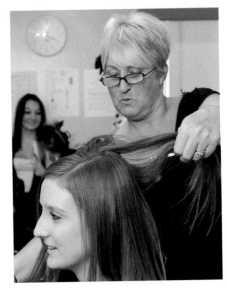

Visually check the hair to ensure suitability of the service

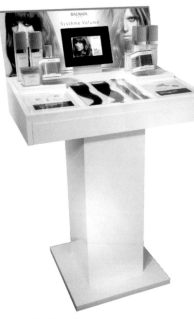

Consultation desk

You can use disinfectant sprays, solutions and wipes for cleaning, a UV light cabinet to keep tools sterile, or an autoclave to sterilise. Disinfecting and sterilising your tools and equipment will ensure you do not cross-contaminate.

> ### Activity
>
> In the salon you may come across a client whose personal hygiene is not good and they may smell of body odour. This may upset staff and other clients. Discuss how you would deal with this situation. Ask your salon managers what you should do in this situation.

Importance of questioning clients

First, you will need to find out your client's vision of the end result; this will help you to establish their requirements. For this part of the consultation you should ask your client how long the style is needed to last. Hair attachments can last from 24 hours when you use a clip-in method, to up to six weeks for plaited, blended or fused methods.

Ask your client whether they want the attachment to include additional colours, or blend with the natural colour. Attachments can be added in any colour, from vibrant fashion shades to neutral or natural tones.

You should ask your client if they would like to add texture with the hair additions to make it curly or straight, or work with the natural texture of their own hair. Finally, ask if they would like to add length, volume, or both.

> ### Activity
>
> List three open questions and three closed questions you should ask your client to gain relevant information on your client requirements for adding hair services.

> ### Activity
>
> In pairs carry out the following role-plays on client diversity:
> - a consultation with a client who is not fluent in English
> - a consultation with a client who is hard of hearing
> - a consultation with a client who is partially sighted.

Record cards

For every hair attachment service you must keep a client record card. Prepare the card before the service; check the client's details are up to date and correct, and completed accurately and clearly. Always follow the Data Protection Act with your client's personal information and ensure that you:

- keep and store client records confidentially
- give client record access only to authorised staff
- use client records for professional salon use only
- keep client records up to date and accurate
- dispose of client records after a year if the client no longer visits the salon
- dispose of client records by shredding the cards or securely deleting the computer records
- register with the Data Protection Registrar if client information is stored on a computer.

Activity

Write down all the details that should be listed on your client's record card – ensure your writing is neat and accurate, and check your spellings.

Planning

During the consultation, you need to examine the hair physically and visually to identify any factors that might affect the service. You will need to ask your client appropriate questions to identify any contra-indications that could prevent the service from taking place or cause problems. You'll also need to carry out the relevant hair tests to ensure the hair and scalp are suitable for the service required.

Factors that may influence services

Salons will allow quite varied time frames for attaching hair services, as the service itself is very variable. You should follow your salon's guide for service times. The salon will need to consider the attachment method, the quantity of hair that is being added and the blending required. You will need to consider your section sizes and the desired finished style.

As a guide, the clip-in attachments may be quickly and easily applied in 10–20 minutes, but grip-in techniques can take between 20–60 minutes, depending on the quantity of grip-in hair being added. Bonding **wefts** can take one to two hours, and fusing and sewn-in techniques are likely to take at least two hours.

Weft

A section of prepared hair.

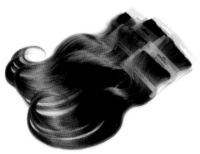

Wefts of hair

Activity

Find out the different time frames your salon allows for attaching hair services. If you carried out these services all day, how many of each service could you carry out in a 7.5-hour working day?

Life expectancy of the style

First, clarify with your clients how long they require the style to last. Hair attachments can last up to six weeks, and the desired time will affect the method you use to apply them.

The table below shows how to attach the hair and the expected life of the style produced.

Method	How to attach the hair	Life expectancy of the style
Clipped in 	Using clips that are attached to the added hair – these are secured to the client's own hair for a one-off look.	24 hours
Clipped-in rings Micro rings	Using small rings of added hair, each ring of hair is clipped to the client's own hair.	Up to 6 weeks
Plaited 	The added hair is entwined with the client's hair and plaited together to secure it in place.	Up to 6 weeks

Method	How to attach the hair	Life expectancy of the style
Sewn in 	The hair attachment is sewn onto cornrow plaits and stitched in place using a needle and thread.	Up to 6 weeks
Bonded/cold bonding (latex) 	Using a glue applicator bottle, the weft of hair is glued to the root of the client's hair.	Guide: 4–6 weeks
Fused 	Using a glue gun, the melted glue is applied to the hair to be added which is then attached to client's hair.	Guide: 4–6 weeks

Activity

If a client had a sewn-in added hair service every six weeks, how many times would she visit in one year?

If this service were charged at £85, how much money would she generate for the salon?

If each service costs the salon £28 in products, what is the total year's profit for the salon?

Other factors

There are many factors that could affect the outcome of this service and you will need to consider all of them.

As with all styles, you'll need to consider the hair characteristics and classifications, the shape of the face and head, the scalp condition and the client's lifestyle to be able to confirm that the desired look can be achieved.

Always carry out a thorough consultation with your client to determine how long the style needs to last, what the client's expectations of the finished image are, and to ensure you have time to consider all the factors.

Hair characteristics

Characteristic	Impact on service
Density and texture 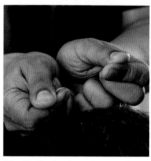 Traction alopecia	The amount of hair your client has will help you to decide on the best method of applying the added hair. For fine hair that is sparse, you would benefit from plaiting the hair and stitching the wefts to the plaits, as this would make the hair look and feel thicker. However, you will also need to avoid too much additional weight and length, as this would put too much tension on the root area and could cause **traction alopecia**. Clients with abundant hair are less likely to request hair extensions unless they wish to gain length, but of course this will add volume and thickness too. Clients may add a clip-in hairpiece to add curls for a look that will last up to 24 hours. **Traction alopecia** Hair loss caused by excessive tension.
Elasticity, porosity and hair condition Elasticity test	You must not add hair attachments to hair that is weak in elasticity, as it will not be able to withstand the additional weight or tension. Clients with porous hair should also avoid hair extensions unless using clip-in techniques that are due to last 24 hours. This service should also be avoided if there is evidence of hair damage at the roots. Clients with hair in good condition or with good elasticity and porosity are free to have any type of hair attachment.

Characteristic	Impact on service
Hair growth patterns 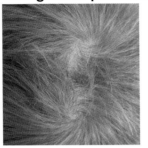 Double crown	As with most services, you are best to work with growth patterns. Always consider the growth patterns and avoid attaching hair in areas where the hair has a tendency to stick up or out, such as the crown area. In this area you will need to consider the best place and type of hair attachment service.

Hair classifications

Classification	Impact on service
Straight hair 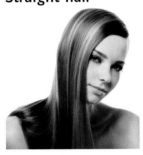	Fine or thin straight hair has a tendency to be very soft, shiny and oily, and therefore some types of hair attachments may not attach securely. Take care with fine hair and make sure the added hair is not too heavy, as this will cause the added hair to be less secure and will put tension on the scalp and hair. Medium straight hair has lots of volume and body and can be great hair to work with and create good results. Coarse straight hair can be extremely straight but attachments should grip well to it. As this hair type is difficult to curl, you'll need to make sure the attaching hair is of similar texture, so that it blends in well.
Wavy hair 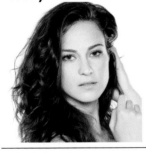	Fine/thin wavy hair can accomplish various styles and the wave can be enhanced or made to look straighter. Take care with fine hair and make sure the added hair is not too heavy and does not put tension on the hair or scalp. Medium wavy hair can sometimes be frizzy, so take care to create a suitable match with the added hair texture. Coarse hair tends to have thicker waves and needs to be matched carefully.
Curly hair 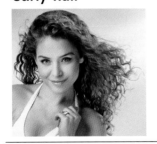	Loose curls are often of combination texture; the hair can be thick with lots of body too, so be careful not to 'overfill' the hair with more added hair. Tight curls will need to be controlled carefully and the hair handled gently. Curly and very curly hair can be weak and porous. Be careful not to overload the hair and additional hair, or create damage with glue and the weight of the wefts.

Classification	Impact on service
Very curly hair 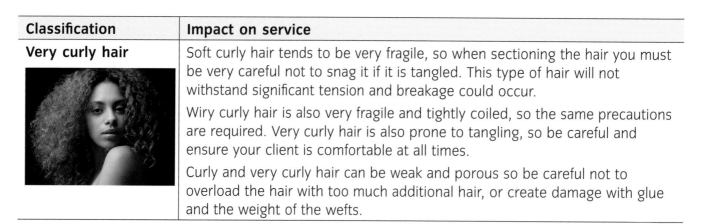	Soft curly hair tends to be very fragile, so when sectioning the hair you must be very careful not to snag it if it is tangled. This type of hair will not withstand significant tension and breakage could occur. Wiry curly hair is also very fragile and tightly coiled, so the same precautions are required. Very curly hair is also prone to tangling, so be careful and ensure your client is comfortable at all times. Curly and very curly hair can be weak and porous so be careful not to overload the hair with too much additional hair, or create damage with glue and the weight of the wefts.

HANDY HINT

For more on hair characteristics and classifications, including curl types, see chapter CHB9.

Testing the hair and scalp

You must carry out the relevant tests before beginning the service. You will need to carry out an elasticity test, a pull test, and, if using glue, a skin test.

Test	When and why you do the test	How to do the test	Possible results	Consequences of not carrying out the test
Pull	Before the service. To evaluate if there is excessive or abnormal hair loss.	Gently pull a small section of hair at the root area.	One to two hairs may be lost at the root area. If 12 or more hairs are lost from the root area, then there is evidence of excessive or abnormal hair loss.	Could cause damage to the hair, further hair loss or traction alopecia. Client would be unhappy. Result might not be achievable and the added hair might fall out. Client might take legal action.

Test	When and why you do the test	How to do the test	Possible results	Consequences of not carrying out the test
Skin	Before the service. To test for an allergic reaction to the glue products.	Clean an area behind the ear or on the inner elbow. Apply a small amount of the glue that will be used to the skin, and leave for 24–48 hours. Always follow the MFIs and your salon's procedures as skin test instructions vary.	A negative result means there is no allergic reaction. A positive result means there is an allergic reaction, for example skin irritation, redness soreness, weeping pustules, itching and/or swelling.	The client could suffer an allergic reaction. Client might take legal action.
Elasticity	Before the service. To test the strength of the cortex and inner structure of the hair.	Take one to two hairs, mist with water and stretch between both hands.	Hair stretches and then springs back, returning to its original length. A poor or weakly conditioned cortex will cause the hair to stretch and stay stretched or break.	Could cause damage to the hair. Client would be unhappy. Result might not be achievable and the added hair might fall out. Client might take legal action.
Porosity	Before the service. To test the condition of the cuticle layer.	Take a few strands of dry hair and run your finger and thumb along the hair shaft towards the roots.	On porous hair the cuticles will feel raised and open. On non-porous hair the cuticles will feel smooth and closed.	Could cause damage to the hair. Client would be unhappy. Result might not be achievable and the added hair might fall out. Client might take legal action.

HANDY HINT

You must always follow the manufacturers' instructions when carrying out tests, to ensure they are carried out correctly. Record the outcomes of every test on the client record card, in case you need to refer back to the information at a later date or if it is needed in the case of legal action.

Activity

Practise and carry out a pull test and skin test on a colleague.

Adverse reactions to tests

Test	Effect of adverse reaction
Pull test	Do not add additional hair to a style if 12 or more hairs are lost from the head after a pull test.
Skin test	If your client has an allergic reaction to the glue, do not carry out the service, consider alternative methods of adding hair. You should suggest that your client visits their GP for medical advice if they suffer from allergies.
Elasticity test	If the cortex is weak, it will not withstand the weight of additional hair. A 24-hour added hair service may still be a viable option but not a service that will last for up to six weeks.
Porosity test	If the hair is porous and the cuticles are raised the hair will tangle easily. If the strength of the hair (cortex) is good, the service may still be suitable, but ensure the client is advised on how to maintain the strength of the cortex and does not make the hair more porous.

HANDY HINT

When using glue for bonding or fusing it should not touch the scalp. A skin test is carried out in case it does touch the scalp and causes an allergic reaction.

HANDY HINT

You must accurately note the questions you asked and the client's responses on the client's record card. This will be useful in case there are problems after the service, and if the client decides to take any legal action.

Identifying contra-indications

You will need to ask your client appropriate questions in order to identify any contra-indications that might limit or prohibit a service. Identifying contra-indications will help you to recognise any potential problems that might occur and to choose the most suitable products to use and services to carry out.

Contra-indication	Effect on the service
Skin sensitivities 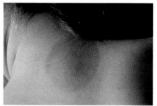	Carry out a skin test for glue products. Avoid methods of attaching hair that require tension.
History of previous allergic reactions Redness – reaction to skin test for glue	Ask your client to obtain medical advice prior to the service, carry out a skin test for glue products, recommend alternative services if necessary or do not carry out the service.

Contra-indication	Effect on the service
Hair, skin and scalp disorders 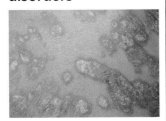	Ask your client to obtain medical advice prior to the service. Check if the scalp or skin disorder is contagious and, if it is, do not carry out the service. Added hair may not be suitable for clients with eczema or psoriasis on the scalp because the scalp might be difficult to access for applying treatments, frequent washing of the hair is not always possible and the products required may cause further irritation.
Medical advice or instructions 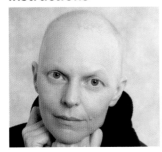 Chemotherapy	Always follow the advice given by medical experts, and do not offer the service if you are unsure. If your client has recently had chemotherapy, you must avoid adding hair, but suggest instead a full wig that will not put any tension on the weak hair recovering from treatment.

Consequences of excessive tension

Traction alopecia is caused by excessive tension on the hair's follicle. Hair becomes sparse or dull, the hairline can begin to recede and the scalp feels sensitive. Raised follicles may also be evidence of traction alopecia.

Traction alopecia can be identified by hair loss or thinning. Further symptoms of traction alopecia are a receding hairline and a sensitive scalp.

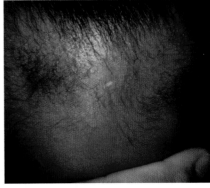

Traction alopecia

Attachment method

You will need to consider which of the following attachment methods is most suited to the client's needs and hair condition:

- sewn
- plaited
- rings
- tapes
- clip-in hairpieces and additions
- taped weft
- cold bonding (latex)
- wefted hair-tracks/rows
- plaited cornrows.

HANDY HINT

You must carefully prepare the added hair and products, following the MFIs. This will enable you to achieve the best possible results.

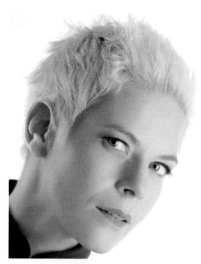

Hair too short for extensions

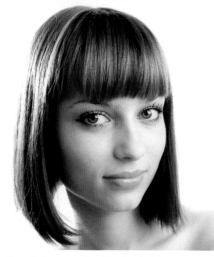

Fine hair cannot withstand thick or heavy extensions

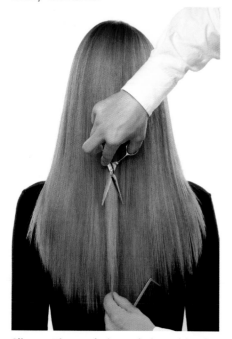

Slice cutting techniques help to blend in the added hair

Direction and fall of added hair

You will need to take into consideration how your client wears their hair and any partings. Visually check the natural fall of the hair and any hair growth patterns – remember to work with them, not against them.

Client's own hair length

The client's natural hairstyle and cut both need to be considered in order for the attachments to blend effectively. Hairstyles with layers and texture will blend better with added hair than those with blunt looks. Some styles may be too short to add hairpieces.

Quantity of added hair

To help you to decide how much hair to add, you will need to feel the density and texture of the client's hair. If the hair is very dense, you may need to add double thicknesses of wefts to help them to blend, but this will also make the hair feel thicker.

Although fine hair will need less added hair, it will not be able to withstand too much extra weight. If you are attaching clip-in hair, make sure it is not too thick or heavy.

Head and face shape

When considering the volume required for the finished style, you will need to look at your client's head and face shape. Big volume styles will not suit round faces as they will accentuate the roundness, whereas flat head shapes benefit from additional volume at the occipital bone area. Long face shapes do not benefit from additional length, but added volume might be suitable. Clients might wish to soften strong features, such as sharp noses or chins, so consider the partings and direction of the hair fall to choose a flattering style.

Blending the hair

For blending you will need to consider the colour and length of the hair. Discuss with your clients the length that they require and inform them that you may need to cut the natural and added hair in order to blend it effectively.

Lifestyle factors

Having a style with added hair will not suit everyone's lifestyle. Although some styles are quick and easy to achieve and maintain, others are limiting and time-consuming. Clients with busy lifestyles may find these styles hard to maintain. Those with an active sports life might find that the results do not last and the style is quickly lost. Chlorine and salt water do not mix well with added hair as the hair may become tangled and matted. Clients who often wear crash helmets may find that glue-based hairpieces quickly become loose because of heat from the head and the friction of the helmet.

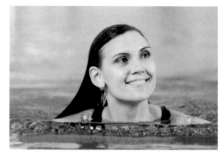

Chlorine and salt water may make extensions matted

Activity

Ask a colleague to visualise an end result for added hair. Ask them relevant questions to identify the service required and whether it would be achievable on their hair.

Activity

Hair that is used for hair extensions can come from all over the world and there are some very sad stories about Indian girls selling their hair for money just to be able to eat. In some cultures hair is sacred. Research where hair extension hair comes from and how you can donate hair to charities for wig-making for cancer patients. Present your findings in an interesting way.

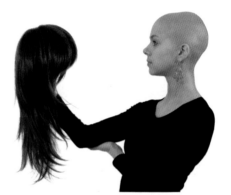

Hair can be donated to charity for wig-making for cancer patients

Tools, equipment and products

Once you have identified any limiting factors, contra-indications and have the results from the hair tests, you can consider which type of added hair service to carry out. Then you will be able to identify which tools and equipment you will need and the most suitable products to use.

Where possible, you should prepare your trolley and the hair attachment in advance of the service. You must ensure that the tools and equipment required are well maintained. Always check that they are clean before use and that you clean and sterilise them afterwards. If you use a glue gun, put it somewhere safe while it cools down and remove any glue from the nozzle once it has sufficiently cooled. Dried glue can block the nozzle and prevent future use.

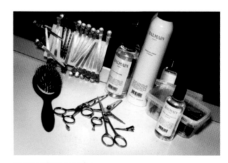

Extension tools

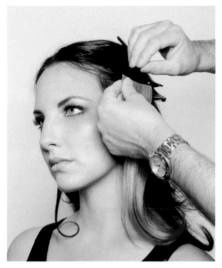

Select the length, colour and texture of the added hair to suit the client's requirements

HANDY HINT

When cutting hair wefts to size, use household scissors. Haircutting scissors will be damaged and become blunt if you use them to cut the edge of the weft.

HANDY HINT

You should compare a colour swatch to the client's natural hair colour. Avoid comparing it to the root colour and aim for mid-lengths and ends for a suitable match.

WHY DON'T YOU...
Practise colour matching with swatches on your colleagues.

HANDY HINT

Always ensure that your workstation is clean, tidy and presentable to the client.

Selecting the hair

Whether you are using a hair clip attachment or a weft, you will need to consider the texture, colour, length and width required.

■ Texture – choose a texture that will work with the style to be worn. Your client may have curly hair, but if a straight style is required, your hair attachments will need to be straight.

■ Colour – if you are aiming for a colour match, rather than adding a new colour to the hair, then you should match the colour to the mid-lengths and ends, and not the root area.

■ Length – when choosing the length of the added hair, you will need to consider the weight of the hair. Ideally, you should not go longer than double the client's natural hair length for long periods of time, as this can cause traction alopecia. For example, if the client's hair is 15cm (6 inches) long, the extensions should be no longer than 30cm (12 inches). If you are using a hair clip attachment for a one-off event, then adding long hair to well-conditioned, strong hair for a short period of time should not be a problem. You must not add long attachments to weak hair for any period of time.

■ Width – when you are adding wefts to the hair, you need to cut them to size.

Preparing the hair prior to attaching hair

You need to make the best use of your time by working methodically and effectively. Once your client is gowned and ready for the service, you should:

■ prepare your client's hair and brush it through to remove any tangles

■ section the hair to suit the desired outcome

■ prepare the wefts to be attached, and measure and cut them to size, if relevant, or

■ prepare any other types of hair attachment and position them on the trolley to avoid them becoming tangled

■ keep the lid on the glue, if using, until you are ready to use it in order to prevent accidents and spillages – glue will also go hard if left with the lid off for long periods of time.

Preparing tools and equipment for use

You must ensure that your tools and equipment are used for their intended purpose only and that they are fit for use. Keep them clean and sterilised and carry them safely. When carrying out added hair services, you are likely to use the following items.

Tool	Use
Brushes	To use on dry hair before you section the hair ready to attach the wefts. You should brush the hair in downwards strokes starting each stroke further towards the root of the hair to avoid tangles and damaging the cuticle layer. Use a dressing-out brush to smooth, detangle and brush the added hair.
Combs Wide-toothed comb Pintail comb	A specialist comb or wide-toothed comb can be used on wet hair after shampooing and conditioning. Section the hair and comb the hair in downwards strokes starting each stroke further towards the root of the hair to avoid damaging the cuticle layer. A backcomb can be used to backcomb the hair if you are attaching clip-in attachments. A pintail or tail comb can be used to section the hair.
Scissors or razors	Use to blend the added hair into the natural hair. Remember to use only household scissors to cut the wefts to the correct size.
Section clips	To use when sectioning the hair to aid control and keep the hair you are working on visible to you.
Applicator	A hot glue gun is used when applying glue to wefts or the hair.

Tool	Use
Professional hair bands 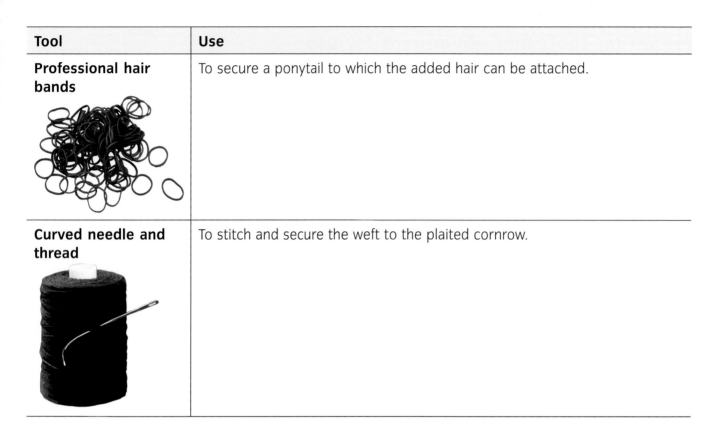	To secure a ponytail to which the added hair can be attached.
Curved needle and thread	To stitch and secure the weft to the plaited cornrow.

Activity

Describe how you would maintain and sterilise your tools and equipment.

Activity

Give yourself five minutes and list all the items you'll need to prepare your trolley for a hair attachment service. Discuss and compare your list with a colleague. Did you forget anything? From this activity you can identify how long it takes to be prepared for this service.

If a salon of five stylists each ran 18 minutes late in a day because they were unprepared for their clients and services, how much time would have been wasted in this salon?

Products

Always follow the MFIs when using products, to ensure you use them correctly and achieve the best possible results.

Product	Use
Shampoo and conditioner	Prepares the hair for the service.
Lotion	Styles and smooth the hair prior to adding the attachments.
Serums	Smoothes the cuticle layers and add shine.
Sprays	Holds the hairstyle in place.
Glue or adhesive	Adds to the hair ready for attaching the weft, or to add to the hairpieces to attach to the natural hair.

HANDY HINT

Overloading the hair with products can make it feel heavy, oily or crispy, which will spoil the end result and the hair will need shampooing more quickly, which could also ruin the result.

HANDY HINT

Oils must not be applied to attachments requiring glue, as this will prevent the glue from bonding to the hair.

Always follow manufacturers' MFIs when adding hair

Activity

Can you identify any other suitable products from your salon's product range that could be used after a service adding hair?

Methods of attaching, maintaining and removing hair attachments

You will need to know which techniques are available, how to section the hair effectively and how to secure the attachments in place.

At the end of the consultation you should be able to confirm with your client that the desired result will be suitable and adaptable enough for them, their hair and their lifestyle. You are now ready to commence the service.

Depending on the technique, the added hair can last between 24 hours, as a one-off look, or up to six weeks for a longer-lasting style.

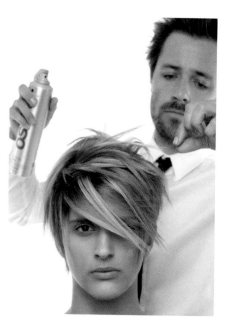

Choose suitable products to define the end result

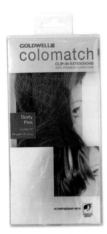

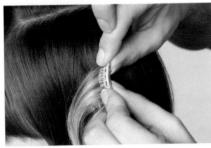

Clip-in attachments

Stylist adding clip-in extensions

Short-term effects – 24 hours

Clip-on techniques

The benefits of clip-in techniques are that they are:

- perfect for quick transformations
- easy to attach
- no commitment.

The disadvantages of clip-in techniques are that:

- the style does not last long
- limited looks are achievable
- sometimes clips and attachments can be seen through the natural hair.

Grip-in techniques

The benefits of grip-in techniques are that:

- they are perfect for quick transformations
- they are easy to attach
- there is no commitment.

The disadvantages of grip-in techniques are that:

- the style does not last long
- limited looks are achievable
- sometimes grips and attachments can be seen through the natural hair.

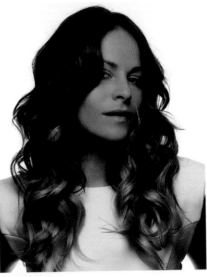

Grip-in extensions used to create an ombre effect

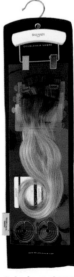

Grip-in extensions

Longer-lasting effects – up to six weeks
Plaited techniques including plaited cornrows

The benefits of plaited techniques are that:

- there is flexible movement in the style
- there is an extended range of possible looks
- they can look natural
- they are good for increasing the density of fine hair.

The disadvantages of plaited techniques are that:

- they can cause traction alopecia
- they can reduce the hair's natural moisture levels
- you might need an assistant to help you apply the added hair
- the finished result is not very adaptable.

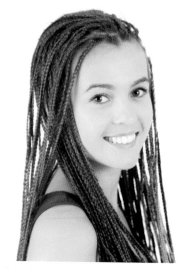

Plaited extensions

Sewn-in techniques

The benefits of sewn-in techniques are that:

- there is access to the scalp to aid cleansing or applying products
- there is minimal damage to the hair and scalp
- they are easy to remove.

The disadvantages of sewn-in techniques are that:

- the attached hair can look lumpy
- movement of the hair is reduced
- the planning of the style takes longer
- after a few days the attached hair can begin to cause discomfort to the client.

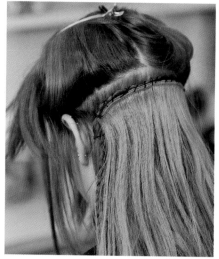

Sewn-in extension

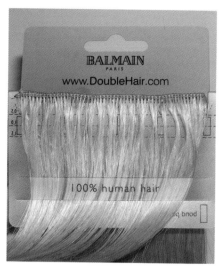

Extension for sewing in

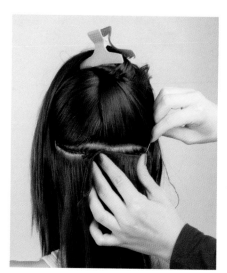

Sewing an extension in

Bonded techniques

The benefits of bonded techniques are that:

- flat styles that require no movement can be achieved
- they are quick and easy to apply
- they are ideal for an immediate fashion look
- they are easy to remove.

The disadvantages of bonded techniques are that:

- they do not last very long, as areas start to loosen and detach from the hair
- oil-based products can't be used
- an allergic reaction to the adhesive might occur.

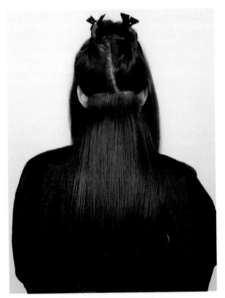
Client prepared for bonded extension

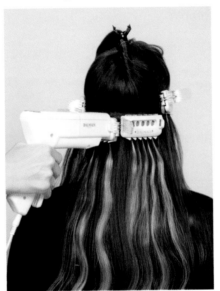
Attaching bonded extensions

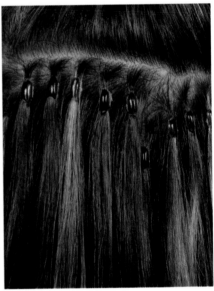
Bonded attachments

Ring techniques

The benefits of ring techniques are that:

- they are longer lasting
- there is no gluing – the hair is just clipped in
- they are easy to remove
- the hair looks natural.

The disadvantages of ring techniques are that:

- the process is time-consuming
- they are more costly to put in.

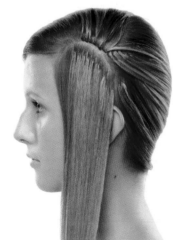
Bond infusing colour

Taped weft techniques

The benefits of taped weft techniques are that:

- the hair wefts are re-usable
- they are easy to remove
- they look natural.

The disadvantages of taped weft techniques are that:

- oil-based products can't be used on the hair
- an allergic reaction to the adhesive tape might occur.

Fusion techniques – including cold bonding (latex)

The benefits of fusion techniques are that:

- there is access to the scalp to aid cleansing or applying products
- they allow for maximum movement
- they look natural.

The disadvantages of fusion techniques are that:

- oil-based products can't be used on the hair
- they can cause hair loss
- the removal process is time-consuming
- an allergic reaction to the adhesive might occur.

Sectioning, tension and securing the hair

The sectioning technique you choose will depend on the technique used to attach the hair. Take the sections you need and ensure that the hair is divided cleanly and evenly to suit the attachment.

You must section hair in a way that will allow the added hair to lie in the direction required. Secure the hair not being extended out of the way, so the hair you are working on is clearly visible.

As you add the hair and secure it, you must ensure that the point of attachment is hidden well. Add the hair in a way that suits the hair's density, texture, direction and fall, which will also avoid any damage to the hair.

As you attach and secure the added hair, you must ensure that you maintain suitable and even tension throughout, to avoid discomfort to your client or damaging their hair follicles, which could lead to hair loss and the first signs of alopecia. If your client shows signs of discomfort, then you must apply less tension. Check periodically that they are still comfortable.

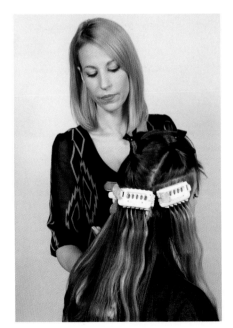

Hair sectioned for bonded attachments

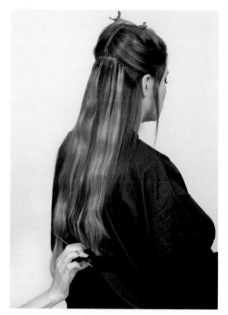

Cutting extension hair

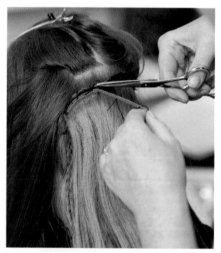

Removing a sewn-in weft

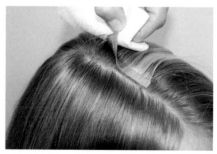

Removing a glued-in weft

Adapting cutting techniques

Once the added hair attachments have been secured in place you will need to blend them with the natural hair. You need to cut and texturise the added hair and sometimes the natural hair too. Bear in mind that hair grows only 1.25cm (½ inch) a month and the style is temporary, so you should not cut too much from the natural hair.

You will need to adapt your cutting technique and take into account certain factors, such as density and texture, to ensure that the hair does not look too thick or bulky. Use freehand cutting techniques to blend the artificial extensions with the natural hair, using either a razor, thinning scissors or texturising cutting techniques. Some hair extensions will be made of artificial hair and razoring the hair may not be a suitable cutting technique for this type of hair.

Removing hair attachments

You should always recommend that clients have their attachments professionally removed in the salon to avoid damage to their hair. However, clip-in hair attachments may be removed by the client and can be re-used to recreate the look themselves.

You must follow the MFIs when removing added hair, using the correct products to remove each type of attachment. Some attachments require a glue removal solution, which will need to be used in a well-ventilated area.

Once the added hair has been effectively removed, you will need to carry out a thorough shampoo and conditioning treatment on the hair. This will ensure that the hair and scalp are free from products, hair attachments and debris.

Removing clip-in and grip-in wefts

These can be easily removed by unclipping the hairpieces and brushing the hair to remove tangles. For grip-in wefts, brush out the backcombing, starting each brush stroke further towards the roots than the previous one.

Removing sewn-in wefts

Carefully cut the stitches, making sure you don't cut the natural hair.

Removing glued in or taped-in wefts

Apply the glue-removing product to soften the glue and remove the tape. Remove the weft.

Removing bonded wefts

Section the hair, use the removal tool to crush the bond, protecting the hair as you apply the removal solution. Once the adhesive breaks down, crush the bond again and pull the extension gently away.

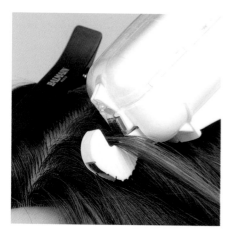

Using a removal tool to crush the bond of an extension

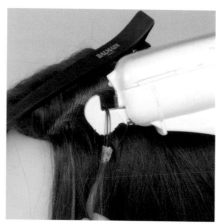

Pulling the extension gently away

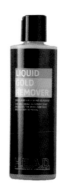

Removal solution

Providing advice and recommendations

Your aftercare advice for this type of service is very important. Not only could your clients lose the desired result quickly if they are not advised on how to maintain it, but they may also cause permanent damage to their hair.

You need to ensure that you provide accurate advice and recommendations on how to maintain the temporary hair extensions and attachments, which products should or shouldn't be used, which styling options are available to the client and how to remove the attachments if relevant.

Removal

If your client has purchased a clip-in attachment, it can be removed easily without damaging the natural hair. You should advise your client on how to remove the clip and store it safely, so that it may be reused. Advise how to remove the band from the ponytail and brush the hair through, starting each stoke further towards the roots. The client can then shampoo and condition their hair as normal.

Advise clients who have had grip-in wefts that it would be more suitable for the salon to remove them because of the backcombing method used. If it is not possible for the client to return to the salon, you must guide them through the removal process. The client should unhook the grip-in wefts and store them safely for future use. Removal is carried out by brushing out the backcombing from the hair, by sectioning the hair and gently brushing the hair through, each stroke starting further towards the roots, until all tangles and backcombing have been removed. You should recommend a treatment to be used on the hair after it has been backcombed, as it can cause the cuticle layer to feel rough and the hair to tangle.

Maintenance

Clients who have longer-lasting extensions should have a lifestyle that supports the time and effort required for home maintenance. Clients should not remove these attachments themselves, as they might damage their hair or scalp. You should advise your clients when to return to the salon, and tell them what signs to look for as a guide to when the extensions are in need of removal. This may include:

- the wefts starting to loosen from the glued areas
- stitching and plaits coming undone
- hair from the attachment starting to come free.

To prolong the longevity of these attachments, you should advise that your clients wear a hairnet in bed. These may not be the most attractive nightwear, but they will prevent the hair from tangling and loosening. The alternative option is to tie the hair back when sleeping or plait it loosely but securely.

You should advise your clients against swimming because the artificial hair might tangle and chlorine could cause hair to become dry and unmanageable. Equally, clients should avoid headwear such as protective helmets, which may loosen the attachments.

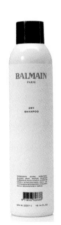

Dry shampoo for hair extensions

Products

Clients may naturally feel that they want to shampoo and apply conditioning treatments to the hair while the attachments are in place. Of course shampoo is required if the attachments are in for more than 24 hours, but only gentle effleurage massage movements should be used. You need to demonstrate this technique to your client and show them what not to do! Rotary massage movements will cause the hair to tangle and loosen. Excessive conditioner and treatments must be avoided, as these might cause the attachments to slip from the hair and the glue to weaken.

You should advise your client to use a moisturising shampoo and a mild conditioner, avoiding the root area. Most temporary hair extensions have their own aftercare products which you can recommend.

The use of hairspray will be advisable, and is one of the most useful products for your clients.

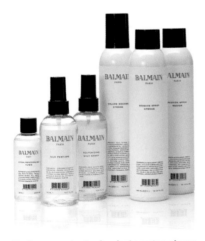

Styling products for hair extensions

Equipment

Some of the attachments will limit flexibility and options for styling the hair. You can't use heated appliances on artificial hair, because it can't withstand the high temperature and will melt. Some styles don't allow a clean parting and therefore the client can't change the way they wear their hair.

To brush and detangle the hair, advise your client to use either the specialist comb recommended with the attachment, or a large wide-toothed comb and a soft bristle brush.

If your client shows signs that they are unsure that the desired result will be achieved, you should give them suitable reassurance. You should explain what you are doing and how this will achieve the expected result. If a client is unhappy with the end result, offer to change the look (if reasonable) either on the same day or as soon as possible.

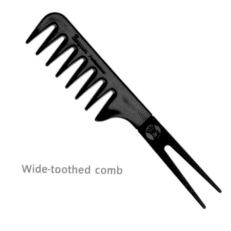

Wide-toothed comb

HANDY HINT

You should be aware of your salon's policy for referring clients to other professionals such as a trichologist or general practitioner and the specialist services they can offer in case your client is in need of their services.

Attach hair to enhance the style – review

Prepare for hair attachment services

When preparing for hair attachment services, you should:

- maintain your responsibilities for health and safety throughout the service
- prepare your client to meet the salon's requirements
- protect your client's clothing throughout the service
- prepare the added hair, when required, to meet the manufacturer's instructions
- prepare your client's hair in a way suitable for the technique to be used.

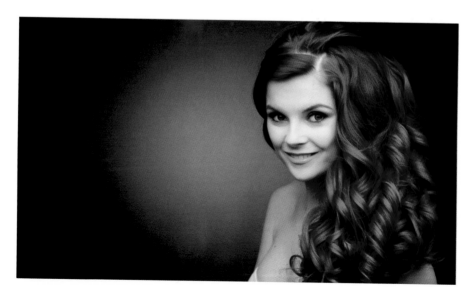

Work safely and hygienically

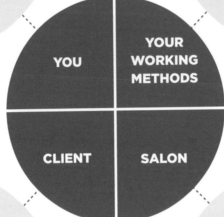

YOU

- Ensure your own posture and position whilst working minimise fatigue and the risk of injury
- Ensure your personal hygiene, protection and appearance meets accepted industry and organisational requirements

YOUR WORKING METHODS

- Minimise the risk of damage to tools
- Minimise the wastage of products and dispose of them correctly
- Minimise the risk of cross-infection
- Make effective use of your working time
- Ensure the use of clean resources
- Minimise the risk of harm or injury to yourself and others
- Promote environmental and sustainable working practices

CLIENT

- Ask your client appropriate questions to establish any known contra-indications to the temporary hair attachment service
- Record your client's responses to questioning
- Identify any factors that may affect the service
- Conduct any relevant tests on your client's hair and skin

SALON

- Keep your work area clean and tidy throughout the service
- Follow workplace and suppliers' or manufacturers' instructions for the safe use of equipment, materials and products

Consult with clients

To consult with clients:

- check the comfort of your client at regular intervals throughout the service
- give reassurance to your client, when necessary
- confirm with your client the look agreed at consultation prior to and during the service.

Select suitable tools, equipment and products

You will need to select and use added hair which is of a suitable:

- texture
- colour
- length
- width.

You will also need to ensure added hair is secure and the point of attachment is hidden.

Carry out plaiting and twisting services

During the service you will need to:

- complete the service within a commercially viable time
- part the sections cleanly and evenly to meet the requirements of the temporary attachment systems to be used
- section the hair in a way that will allow the added hair to lie in the direction required
- secure any hair not being extended to keep each section clearly visible during the service
- ensure added hair is secure and the point of attachment is hidden
- add hair in a way that takes into account the factors influencing the service and avoids potential damage to the client's hair
- maintain a suitable and even tension throughout the process
- adapt your cutting techniques to take account of factors that influence working on added hair
- identify and report any problems occurring during the service to the relevant person
- ensure, on completion, that the added hair is blended with the client's own hair in a way that achieves the style enhancement agreed with the client.

HANDY HINT

Check throughout the service that your client is comfortable and that you are maintaining an even, balanced result.

HANDY HINT

If you encounter or identify any problems you must refer these to the relevant person in your salon.

Remove attachments

You need to make note of the following points when removing attachments:

- use the correct tools, minimising damage to your client's hair
- leave your client's hair free of residue and product build-up

- leave your client's hair clean and prepared ready for the next service
- remove pieces of hair following the manufacturer's instructions
- use the correct products to remove pieces of hair, avoiding damage to your client's hair.

Provide advice and recommendations

Throughout the service and at the end, give your client advice and recommendations on the service provided to ensure that they can:

- maintain their look at home
- know which products would aid home styling and home maintenance
- remove clip-in attachments themselves at home without causing damage to their hair and discomfort to the scalp
- know what future services and products they would benefit from
- know when to return for additional or future services.

Techniques

Clip-on techniques

Clip-on hair attachments are quick and easy to attach. First, the natural hair is styled into position and then a clip-in hair attachment is added securely.

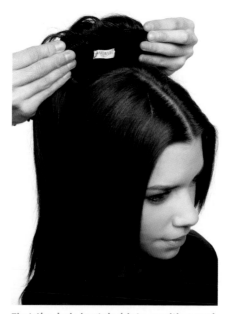

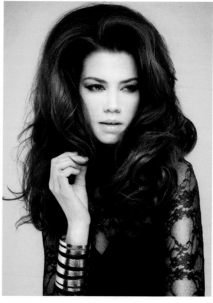

First the hair is styled into position and then a clip-in attachment is added

Clip-in attachments – final look

Grip-in techniques

Grip-in attachments are often in the form of wefts. These are long widths of hair that are cut to size and gripped into backcombed hair. The natural hair is laid over the top to hide the grips and backcombing, if used.

Sewn-in techniques

Hair is plaited into cornrows that form the base, and then the attachments are sewn to the plaits and secured with stitching.

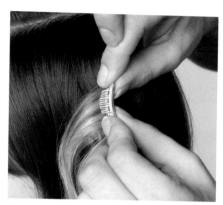

Attaching the grip-in weft

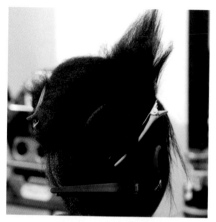

STEP 1 – The same method is used for sectioning as with the clip-in method. Hair is plaited into cornrows that form the base. The number of rows is dependent on client requirements.

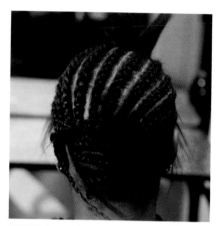

STEP 2 – A fine cornrow is made around each horseshoe section. Use postiche netting, and secure in position at the front, back and each side of the parting.

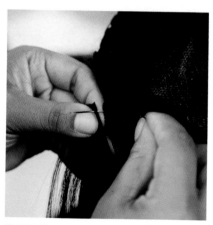

STEP 3 – Using waxed double thread, stich around the hairline, securing the netting to the whole of the head so that it fits snugly, like a skullcap. Blanket stich the wefts to the cornrows.

WHY DON'T YOU...
Look up videos of blanket stitching online.

Bonded techniques

Wefts of hair are cut to size. Glue is either applied to the root area of the natural hair or the hair weft will have a strip of glue already attached. This needs to be removed. The hair wefts are then secured in place by the glue or glue strip.

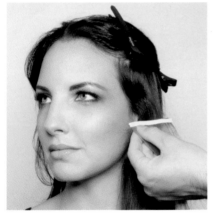

STEP 1 – Section the hair and prepare the weft to be attached according to the client's requirements.

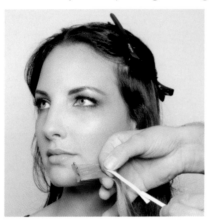

STEP 2 – Remove the sticky back from the strip of glue on the weft.

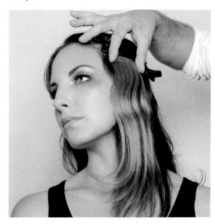

STEP 3 – Attach the glued area of the weft to the hair.

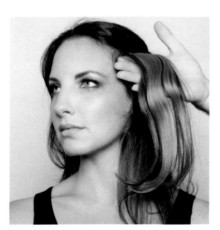

STEP 4 – Continue to add wefts until desired results are achieved.

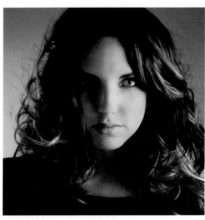

STEP 5 – Final look.

Answers in the back of the book.

1 Why is it important for the stylist to question the client before starting the service?

a   To avoid legal action

b   To avoid contracting diseases

c   To ensure both parties like the results

d   To ensure both parties agree on the details

2 **Statement one**

Clip-in attachments usually take up to 20 minutes to apply.

Statement two

Sewn-in techniques usually take at least 2 hours to apply.

Which **one** of the following is correct for the above statements?

a   True   True

b   True   False

c   False   True

d   False   False

3 Which one of the following is the usual amount of time that a sewn-in attachment should last?

a   Up to 2 weeks

b   Up to 3 weeks

c   Up to 5 weeks

d   Up to 6 weeks

4 Which **one** of the following describes traction alopecia?

a   Small circular bald patches

b   General thinning due to ageing

c   No hair on the head or the body

d   A receding hairline or wide partings

5 Which **one** of the following is a contra-indication to any type of attachment service?

a   Recent colouring service

b   Very dense, curly hair

c   Recent chemotherapy

d   Very curly, long hair

6 Which one of the following is the best cutting technique to blend in added hair?

a   Club cutting

b   Slice cutting

c   Scissor over comb

d   Clipper over comb

7 **Statement one**

When matching the wefts to the natural hair colour, it is best to match it to the mid lengths and ends.

Statement two

Long periods of using added hair that is over 50% of the natural hair length can cause traction alopecia.

Which **one** of the following is correct for the above statements?

a   True   True

b   True   False

c   False   True

d   False   False

8 Which **one** of the following is **not** a client benefit to using clip-in attachments?

a   It is easy to attach

b   It does not last long

c   There is no client commitment

d   It is good for quick transformations

9 **Statement one**

Plaited techniques for adding hair are good for increasing density in fine hair.

Statement two

Plaited techniques rarely look natural.

Which **one** of the following is correct for the above statements?

a   True   True

b   True   False

c   False   True

d   False   False

10 Which **one** of the following is the most common disadvantage of using fusion techniques?

   a Oil-based products cannot be used

   b The removal process is time-consuming

   c An allergic reaction to the glue may occur

   d Areas start to loosen and detach quite quickly

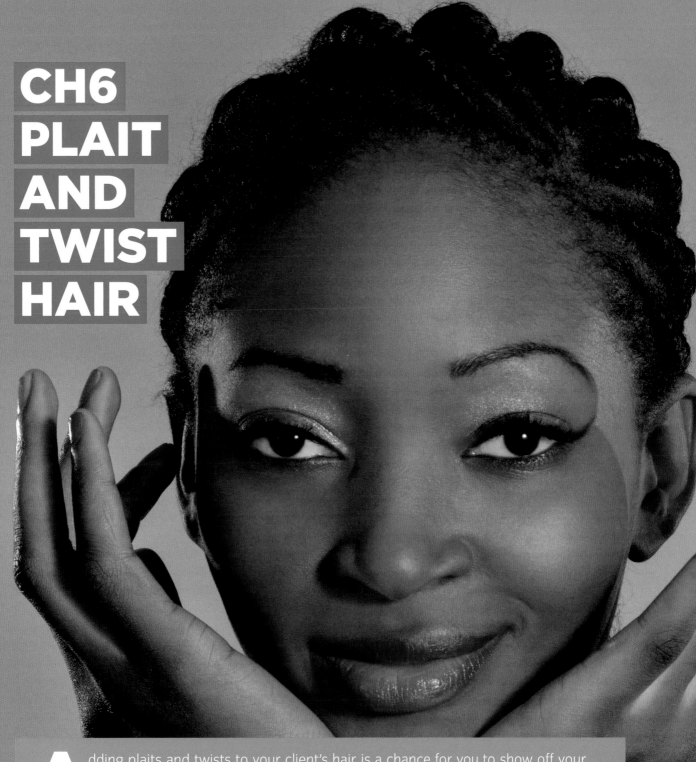

CH6
PLAIT
AND
TWIST
HAIR

Adding plaits and twists to your client's hair is a chance for you to show off your creativity and artistic flair while enhancing your potential to increase your client base. These styles can be functional, as they help to keep the hair away from the face, but are also popular and fashionable. You'll need to demonstrate your dexterity while working with and controlling very small sections of hair, and maintaining even tension throughout. These intricate styles can be seen from the catwalks to the high street, with celebrities bringing these great looks to life and to the forefront of everyday living.

After reading this chapter you will:

- know how health and safety affects plaiting and twisting services
- understand the factors that influence plaiting and twisting services
- know the tools, equipment, products and techniques used to plait and twist hair
- be able to plait and twist hair.

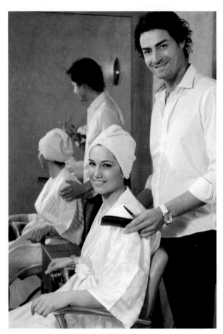

Always protect your client effectively

HEALTH & SAFETY ⚠️

Refer to the health and safety and salon policies chapter to refresh your memory of the main health and safety Acts.

VALUES & BEHAVIOURS

Refer to the values and behaviours chapter for more information on: maintaining effective, hygienic and safe working practices, ensuring personal hygiene and protection meets accepted industry and organisational requirements ('Values'), and maintaining salon standards of behaviour ('Behaviours').

HANDY HINT

Always cover any open wounds and avoid going to work if you have a contagious illness or disease. Maintain a healthy, balanced diet and exercise regularly.

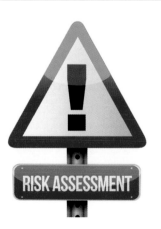

RISK ASSESSMENT

Health and safety

As with all hairdressing services, for plaiting and twisting it is still important that you protect your client with a gown, towel and sometimes a shoulder cape, and to ensure that your client is comfortable and sitting with their back supported by the back of the chair, in an upright position. To guarantee a balanced result, your client should sit evenly with their legs uncrossed and their feet flat. This service involves your client holding their head at various angles to enable you to plait and twist, so you must always check that your client is comfortable.

Own responsibilities under health and safety

As with all services it is important to maintain health and safety to ensure that you, your client and others are not put at risk of harm or injury.

Your responsibilities include:

- following the health and safety legislation – to maintain legal responsibilities and maintain health and safety practices
- gowning your client – to protect their clothes and skin
- maintaining personal hygiene – so as not to cause offence to others and cross-contaminate
- protecting yourself and others from infection and infestation – to avoid cross-contamination and maintain good health
- following salon rules for presentation – to ensure you look professional and represent your salon and the industry's image
- working safely – to avoid risks of injury
- keeping the work area clean and tidy – to prevent cross-contamination and maintain a professional image.

Hazards and risks

In most chapters we have covered the potential hazards and risks that exist in the salon environment. These hazards and risks include slippery services, faulty electrical equipment, use of chemicals or substances, risks of injury and skin conditions.

Activity

On your own, list as many potential salon hazards as you can think of. Now compare this list with a colleague in pairs. Share and discuss your pair's findings with another pair.

Safe working practices

Safe working practices include looking after your clients – protecting them in line with your salon requirements and suitably for the service. Ensure that both you and your client are comfortable, particularly as the plaiting and twisting services can be time-consuming. The client will be sitting and you will be standing for long periods of time. Standing correctly and evenly positioned will help prevent risk of injury and fatigue. Ensuring that your clients sit correctly and comfortably will ensure the desired outcome can be achieved.

Keep your tools and equipment positioned nearby and on your correct side of working for ease of use and to maintain a good posture. Ensure you follow the suppliers' and manufacturers' instructions for the safe use of your equipment and for the materials and products you use. This is not only for health and safety reasons but also to help you to produce the best result for your client.

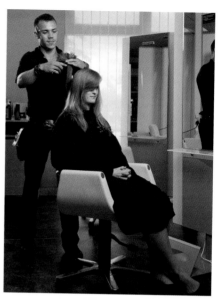

Position your client comfortably for the service

Use safe working methods

Ensure that you work safely, following the Health and Safety at Work Act to minimise the risk of harm to yourself and others. You must use your tools and equipment correctly, and for their intended purpose, to prevent damage and misuse.

Your own standards of personal health and hygiene must be maintained – always shower, wear fresh, clean clothes and use deodorant. This will ensure that you look professional, avoid cross-infection and infestation and that you will not offend your clients.

Follow COSHH

When you are working with products you must follow the Control of Substances Hazardous to Health (COSHH) regulations. Always ensure that you follow the manufacturers' instructions (MFIs), your salon's policy and the local by-laws.

When using your products always follow SHUD:

- **S**tore correctly – keep products out of harm's way. Do not store them too high up, or in high temperatures and always replace the lids after use.

- **H**andle correctly – wear PPE when necessary and follow the MFIs.

- **U**se correctly – use the correct amount and follow the MFIs; do not overload the hair.

- **D**ispose of correctly – place empty containers in the designated salon waste bin and dispose of them following the MFIs and local by-laws to protect the environment.

HANDY HINT

Avoid overstretching and maintain an even balance to prevent backache, injury and fatigue. This service is particularly demanding on the stylist as you may need to bend in different directions to be able to follow the shape of the head as you plait/twist.

HANDY HINT

Always position your work trolley to the right if you are right-handed, and to the left if you are left-handed. This will help you work methodically, avoid strain, save time and maintain a professional image.

HEALTH & SAFETY

Refer to the health and safety and salon policies chapter for more information on environmental and sustainable working practices.

HANDY HINT

You must minimise your wastage of products to prevent overloading the hair, to help preserve the environment and to maintain the salon's profits.

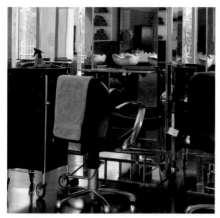

Maintain a clean and tidy work area throughout the service

HANDY HINT

Always speak clearly and use open questions, starting with 'what', 'why', 'how' and 'when' to find out information and closed questions to confirm requirements. Closed questions generally require 'yes' or 'no' or one-word answers.

VALUES & BEHAVIOURS

Refer to the values and behaviours chapter to refresh your knowledge on:

- maintaining client care
- having a flexible working attitude and being a team player
- verbal and non-verbal communication skills
- greeting clients and treating them with respect.

Environmental and sustainable working practices

You should always follow environmental and sustainable working practices such as:

- reduce energy use – switching off lights, electrical items and taps after use
- use organic and hypoallergenic products and those with environmentally friendly packaging
- offer FairTrade tea and coffee to your clients
- reduce waste and use the correct amount of products
- recycle, re-use and dispose of waste safely.

Preventing dermatitis

For your own health and safety, always wear personal protective equipment (PPE), wash and dry your hands after each service and use a hand cream to help prevent contact dermatitis. Contact dermatitis is a condition that affects the skin and the hands in particular in hairdressing. It can be recognised by a red, itchy rash that can blister and weep.

Preventing cross-infection and infestation

Keeping a clean and tidy workstation helps you to prevent cross-infection and infestations. Always ensure that your tools and equipment are cleaned with warm, soapy water and then disinfected or sterilised before being used on any client.

You can use disinfectant sprays, solutions and wipes to clean, a UV light cabinet to keep tools sterile, or an autoclave to sterilise. Disinfecting and sterilising your tools and equipment will ensure you do not cross-contaminate.

Importance of questioning clients

During the consultation process you will find out what your client wants to achieve from their hair. It is important that you question your client effectively to get as much information from them as possible. This may include:

- what they want or like
- what they don't want or like
- any hair or scalp problems
- their lifestyle and time to maintain their look
- products and equipment they have at home to maintain the look.

During the service it is important to continually ask questions to ensure you are meeting the client's requirements and to check they are comfortable during the plaiting and twisting process.

Factors that may influence services

As with all services, your salon will have an expected service time for plaiting and twisting services. These times may vary from one salon to another and also with each service. The client requirements, the length, density and characteristics of the hair can all affect service times.

Activity

Find out your salon service times for the following services:

- multiple cornrows
- French plaits
- fishtail plaits
- flat twists.

In an average working day (7½ hours) how many clients could you fit in for a full head of cornrows? How many French plaits could you do in 7½ hours?

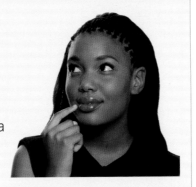

As with all styles, you'll need to consider the hair characteristics and classifications, the shape of the face and head, the scalp condition and the client's lifestyle to be able to confirm that the desired look can be achieved.

Always carry out a thorough consultation with your client to determine how long the style needs to last, what the client's expectations of the finished image are and to ensure you have time to consider all the factors.

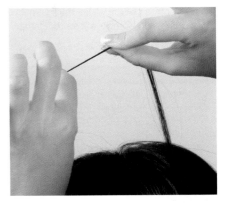

Elasticity test

Hair characteristics

Before you begin French/fishtail plaits or twists you'll need to consider the density, texture, porosity and elasticity of the hair.

Density, texture, porosity and elasticity

Abundant hair may create thick, chunky plaits or twists that may not produce the desired outcome, and fine hair may produce plaits/twists that look too thin and show too much scalp.

Hair that is thinning, porous or weak in elasticity may break or not be able to withstand the tension required for plaiting and twisting.

Normal to average amounts of hair that have good porosity and elasticity will produce the most satisfying end result. Always carry out an elasticity test on the hair to ensure it is strong enough to withstand the tension when plaiting/twisting.

Activity

Compare the hair density and texture among your colleagues and identify who would have the best hair type for this service, and discuss your reasons why.

Hair growth patterns

Some hair growth patterns can affect the plaiting and twisting service. Consider how a widow's peak for instance can affect the finished shape of a plait or twist if it is styled from one side of the head, over the front hairline area and onto the other side. Cornrows can also be affected by a widow's peak, due to the end result shape along the front hairline. Suggest that your client has a small fringe area that is not plaited or cornrowed if they have a widow's peak. Alternatively plait the hair lower onto the face to cover the widow's peak.

Nape whorls can also affect the end shape of plaits and twists by causing the nape and neck area to look a little untidy. Adding the hair into the plait at the nape area can cause client discomfort, so don't apply too much tension on the hair.

Double crowns and cowlicks can be controlled effectively into a plait or twist with tension, clean sections and good stylist dexterity.

Hair classifications

Hair classifications can also affect the services you can offer.

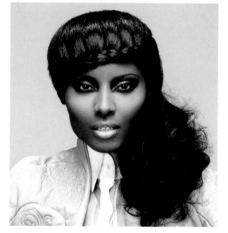

Plait covering a widow's peak

HANDY HINT

A cowlick can also be called a cow's-lick or a calf's-lick. Use the internet to search where the word 'cowlick' came from.

HANDY HINT

Hair that is not suitable in density, texture or elasticity may produce an unsatisfactory style or limit your style choices.

Hair classification	Effect on service
Straight hair 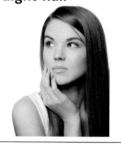	Fine or thin straight hair will potentially create small cornrows and expose a lot of scalp. Twists will also look much thinner. This type of hair tends to be soft and shiny, so is difficult to control and can also look oily quickly too. Medium straight hair has lots of volume and body and can be great hair to work with and create good results. Coarse straight hair can be extremely straight and should be controlled with serum and hair products to achieve the desired results.

Hair classification	Effect on service
Wavy hair 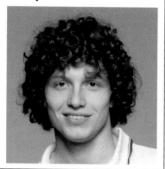	Fine/thin wavy hair can give the same problematic end result as fine/thin straight hair, where too much scalp is visible and twists, cornrows and plaits are too thin. Medium wavy hair can sometimes be frizzy. This can be controlled with styling products, such as serum, oils and creams. Coarse hair can be resistant to styling generally but controllable with plaiting and twisting. The hair can be very frizzy, so again control it with products.
Curly hair 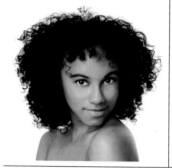	Loose curls are often of combination texture – the hair can be thick with lots of body too. Plaiting and twisting can work well, as long as the frizz is controlled with products, the sections are small and the hair handled with care to avoid discomfort when parting or sectioning the hair. Tight curls will need to be controlled carefully and the hair handled gently. Oil-based products will be required to aid control.
Very curly hair	Soft curly hair tends to be very fragile, so when sectioning the hair you must be very careful. This type of hair will not withstand significant tension and breakage could occur. Wiry curly hair is also very fragile and tightly coiled, so the same precautions are required. Very curly hair is also prone to tangling much more easily, so be careful and ensure your client is comfortable at all times.

Head and face shapes

As you know, every style will suit an oval face and you should aim to create this face shape with your finished result. For plaits and twists, the hair is often pulled back off the face. Therefore, round faces may look rounder, square faces may look squarer and oblong or rectangular faces more so.

You must also consider the shape of the head. Plaits and twists sit closely on the head – you are unable to add height or soften squarer edges. Always feel the shape of the head during the consultation to check that it is suitable for this service and whether it will enhance the client's features rather than draw unwanted attention to them.

HANDY HINT

If the face shape is not suitable for plaiting and twisting, the result may be unflattering. You should soften the face shape by leaving out the fringe area or bringing hair onto the face and not including it in the style.

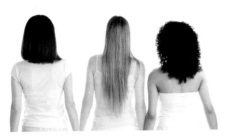

Clients with different types and lengths of hair

Hair length

The length of your client's hair is also important. Is it long enough to plait, twist and cornrow? Although very short hair can still be plaited or twisted, controlling the hair can be harder and you may apply more tension trying to hold the hair – this could cause client discomfort. Very long hair can be plaited and twisted, but the volume of hair should be considered, so that it is not too bulky.

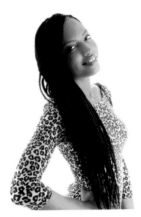

Long hair cornrows

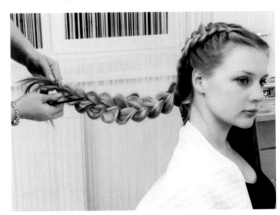

Long hair plait

Scalp condition

You must visually check the condition of the scalp before plaiting or twisting the hair. It will be difficult to clean the hair effectively while the plaits and twists are in place. Excessively oily hair will need regular shampooing with a shampoo designed for oily hair and scalps, but avoid using any massage techniques other than effleurage. If your client has a dry scalp, the flakes of skin will be visible and difficult to remove once the plaits and twists are in place: you should offer a scalp treatment before the service.

Desired look

When considering the client requirements and what your client wants, you have to consider how achievable the look is. If the hair is too fine or thin, too much scalp will be seen. If it's too thick and abundant, the size of the plaits, cornrows or twists may not be suitable. If the hair is too long or too short, you'll need to advise your client accordingly. Equally with hair growth patterns, check that these will suit and work with the style desired. Consider all these factors when advising your client on whether their desired look can be achieved.

Although plaiting and twisting are short-term looks, they require maintenance: if your client has a busy lifestyle they may struggle with the time needed to recreate the style, and those with sporty lifestyles may find that the look does not last as long.

HANDY HINT

The weak temporary hydrogen bonds are softened by water and heat, and hardened by drying and cooling the hair.

THE CITY & GUILDS TEXTBOOK

Physical effects of styling on the hair structure

Hair is held in its natural state by permanent and temporary bonds. The main bonds that are softened when styling the hair are the temporary bonds, which are hydrogen bonds.

Hair in its natural state of curly, wavy or straight is in an alpha keratin state. When hair has been wetted, stretched and dried into a new shape, it is in a beta keratin state.

Consequences of excessive tension

If you apply too much tension to the hair, or plait and twist weak hair that is fine or sparse around the hairline, you risk causing **traction alopecia**.

Traction alopecia can be identified by hair loss or thinning. Further symptoms of traction alopecia are a receding hairline and a sensitive scalp.

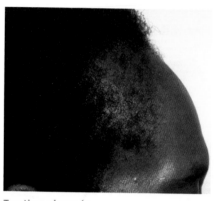

Traction alopecia

Traction alopecia

Hair loss or thinning, due to excessive tension on the follicle.

Tools, equipment and products

Tools and equipment available for use

For the main part of this service you need only a few tools and pieces of equipment. It is always good practice to shampoo and dry the hair prior to the actual plaiting or twisting, so you'll need tools and equipment for styling. However, for the plaiting and twisting itself you will need only the following:

Tools and equipment	Use
Detangling brush	Detangle dry hair prior to sectioning for the plait or twists.

Tools and equipment	Use
Section clips	Hold the sections of hair in place or out of the way.
Detangling comb	Detangle the hair as you section, plait and twist.
Pintail comb	Used to take clean, intricate sections of hair to plait or twist.
Bands Small hairdressing bands Covered bands	Professionally covered elastic bands (or you could use very small hairdressing bands) are used to secure the plaits.
Pins and grips Pins Grips	Used to secure the plaits and twists in place.
Accessories	Hair accessories or hair jewellery can be used to complete and enhance the finished style.

Securing the hair

As you complete each twist or plait, you need to secure it in place effectively. You should use hairgrips, clips or bands to secure each individual plait/twist in place. When you style the hair with French or fishtail plaits you should use a covered band or tiny clear professional elastic bands to hold the plaited hair securely in place, without damaging the hair. You could use ribbons or other hair accessories to complete the look.

Products available for use

The main products that you'll use during plaiting and twisting are serum, gel and hairspray.

Product	Purpose of product	When and how to use the product
Serum	Silicon-based products help smooth the cuticle and prevent tangles when sectioning the hair. Be careful not to overload the hair and make it look oily.	You should use serums prior to plaiting and twisting the hair. Follow the manufacturers' instructions on how to use them.
Gel	Used to help you control and smooth the hair, and tame any stray hairs. Be careful not to overload the hair, otherwise it may look crispy or oily.	Use gel products while plaiting and twisting the hair. Follow the manufacturer's instructions on how to use it.
Spray	Used to ensure longevity of the style. It can also aid you in controlling the hair and taking clean sections during the service. Again, be careful not to overload the hair with product.	Hairspray is used once the plaiting and twisting are complete. Follow the manufacturer's instructions on how to use it.

Activity

Can you identify any other suitable products from your salon's product range that could be used when plaiting and twisting?

Using products cost-effectively

It is important to use products effectively and not waste them. Overloading the hair with products can make plaits and twists look oily, crispy and crunchy. It is also wasteful and costly to the salon.

Activity

To help you smooth the cuticles during a plaiting service you use Wella Velvet Amplifier style primer. This costs the client £10.80 to buy for home use and the product is 50ml. On average you use a 3ml pump of product each time you style their hair.

If you advised the client on how to use this product correctly, how many 'pumps' would your client get before she needed to buy more? How much would each application cost?

If you did not advise your client on how much product to use and they used 5ml instead, they would waste product and their money. Compare your above result with a client using 5ml each time. How many applications would they get for their £10.80? Work out how much each pump would cost the client.

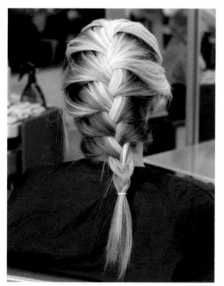

Loose French plait – poor result

HANDY HINT

Remove your rings and bracelets as these may catch on the hair as you section it, ruining your hard work.

Effects of plaits and twists

Whether your client would like multiple cornrows, plaits or twists you will need to control and section the hair, and apply a degree of tension.

Controlling and sectioning the hair

During your consultation you must agree and confirm the result required. You should continue to do this throughout the service, agreeing the section patterns as you go. It is very important that you have control when you section the hair. You will need to demonstrate your dexterity by holding the hair close to the scalp and intricately sectioning the hair. You should secure the hair that is not being plaited out of the way, to ensure the hair being plaited is visible to you.

As you section the hair, work in a methodical manner to ensure you achieve clean partings and an even result. Section and part the hair accurately to suit the direction of the plait or twists.

Tension

As you section the hair to twist or plait, you will need to apply tension and follow the shape of the head to ensure that the section does not become baggy or loose. Ask your client to reposition their head as required to help you maintain the correct tension.

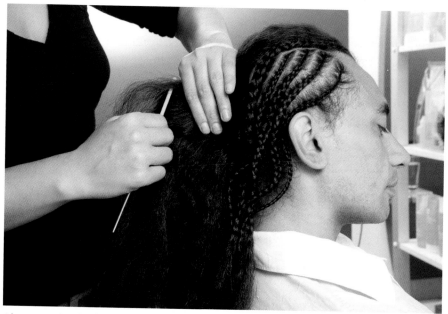

Always maintain the correct tension

How to create different plaits and twist

See the creations in the 'step-by-step' section at the end of the chapter for guidance on how to create cornrows, French plaits, fishtail plaits, two-strand twists and flat twists.

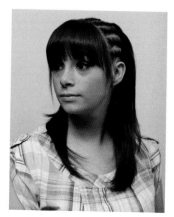

Cornrows

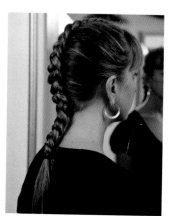

French plait

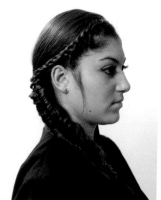

Fishtail plait

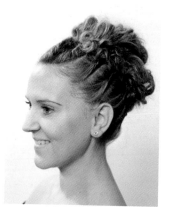

Two-strand twists

Providing advice and recommendations

Throughout the service, and particularly at the end, you should offer your client some aftercare advice for maintaining their style at home, and tell them how to unwind the plaits and twists themselves when the style needs to be removed.

You may need to warn your client to expect to see a small amount of hair loss. This is natural hair loss that would normally be caught in a brush or fall out, but as the hair is secured in a twist it cannot fall away. If your client is worried, remind them that we can each lose up to 100 hairs a day.

How to maintain their look

As you finish the service, make recommendations for products that your client can use to maintain their new style, and give them a tip for keeping any stray hairs less obvious: use the tail of the comb and spray them back into place. You should recommend that your client avoids friction or rubbing of the hair, as this will cause stray hairs to come away from the plaits or twists, and the style will lose its effect.

Removing plaits and twists

It is possible that you will not be the person removing the plaits or twists from the hair: it is more likely that your client will do this at home. You will need to advise your client on how to do this so that they do not cause any damage to the hair or discomfort to themselves.

For cornrows, as you complete part of the service, but before you have secured all the cornrows, demonstrate to your client how to remove one. This visual demonstration will help the client to understand the correct method to use without causing damage to the hair. Advise the client to remove the grips carefully and then untwist the hair from the point to root. Advise brushing through the hair to remove tangles before shampooing and conditioning.

To remove the plaits and twists from the hair, advise your clients to remove all bands and pins first, and then gently unwind the hair from point to root. If they encounter any tangles, remind them to use a detangling brush, not a comb, and work in the direction of the cuticle layer, each time starting the brushing stroke from nearer the root, and working in sections and stages, to avoid damage to the cuticle and cortex layers.

Then advise your client that, after a thorough cleansing shampoo to remove any products, dirt and oils, the hair will benefit from a good conditioning treatment to replace any lost moisture and to smooth the cuticle layer, in particular treating the ends of the hair.

Present and future products and services

Throughout the service you may have discussed other services that the client is interested in. At the end of the service you should revisit this discussion to identify whether your client would like to book for a future service or purchase any recommended products.

HANDY HINT

Using the tail of a pintail comb can help the client to untwist their hair.

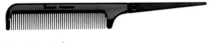

Pintail comb

HANDY HINT

Advise your client on how to remove the band correctly from the hair so as not to cause any damage.

WHY DON'T YOU...

Cornrow your own hair and practise removing the cornrows from the hair, so that you can identify how it will feel for your clients.

HANDY HINT

Always ensure you speak clearly and offer advice and recommendations accurately and constructively. You must use positive body language and check your client's understanding with open and closed questions.

THE CITY & GUILDS TEXTBOOK

Plait and twist hair – review

Prepare for a plaiting and twisting service

Remember that you should always:

- prepare your client to meet your salon's requirements
- protect your client's clothing throughout the service
- position your client to meet the needs of the service without causing them discomfort.

Work safely and hygienically

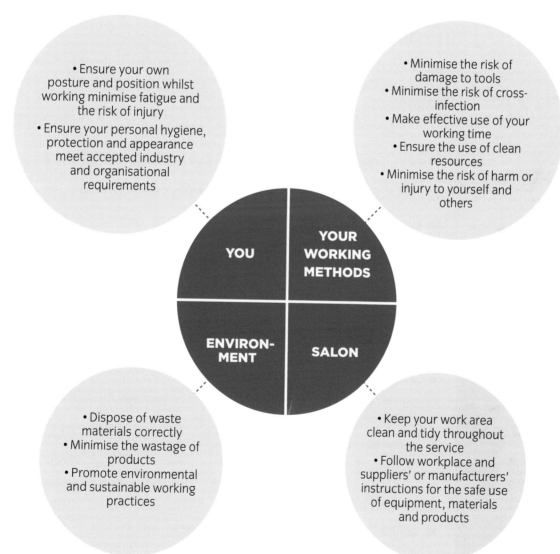

- Ensure your own posture and position whilst working minimise fatigue and the risk of injury
- Ensure your personal hygiene, protection and appearance meet accepted industry and organisational requirements

- Minimise the risk of damage to tools
- Minimise the risk of cross-infection
- Make effective use of your working time
- Ensure the use of clean resources
- Minimise the risk of harm or injury to yourself and others

YOU

YOUR WORKING METHODS

ENVIRON-MENT

SALON

- Dispose of waste materials correctly
- Minimise the wastage of products
- Promote environmental and sustainable working practices

- Keep your work area clean and tidy throughout the service
- Follow workplace and suppliers' or manufacturers' instructions for the safe use of equipment, materials and products

Consult with clients

It is important to consult with your client before and during the service to ensure the desired look is achieved and the client is comfortable:

- confirm with your client the look agreed at consultation prior to and during the service
- consult with your client during the service to ensure the tension is comfortable
- establish the factors likely to influence the service.

Select suitable tools, equipment and products

Before you start the service, set up your trolley with suitable tools. Choose suitable products to use and always follow the manufacturers' instructions.

Carry out plaiting and twisting services

When performing plaiting and twisting services, you should:

- complete the service within a commercially viable time
- control your tools to minimise the risk of damage to the hair and scalp and of client discomfort, and to achieve the desired look
- part the sections cleanly and evenly to achieve the direction of the plait(s) and twists
- secure any hair not being plaited or twisted to keep each section clearly visible
- maintain a suitable and even tension throughout the service
- control and secure your client's hair throughout the plaiting and twisting processes
- apply suitable products, when necessary, to achieve the style requirements
- consult with your client during the service to ensure the tension is comfortable
- adjust the tension of plaits and/or twists, when necessary, avoiding damage to the hair and minimising discomfort to your client
- ensure the direction and balance of the finished plait(s) and/or twists achieve the desired look
- confirm your client's satisfaction with the finished look.

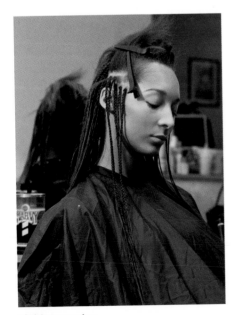

Plaiting service

Provide advice and recommendations

Throughout the service and at the end, give your client advice and recommendations on the service provided to ensure they:

- can maintain their look at home
- know which products would aid home styling and home maintenance
- can remove the plaits or twists themselves at home without causing damage to their hair and discomfort to the scalp
- know what future services and products they would benefit from.

Step by steps

When you begin any plaiting or twisting service, ensure that you double check the client's requirements so that you achieve the correct balance and direction of the plait(s) or twists.

Multiple cornrows

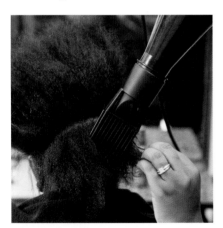

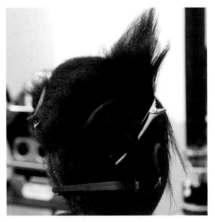

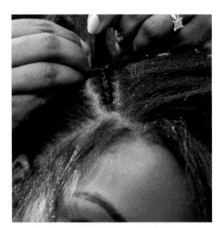

STEP 1 – Apply suitable styling products. Blow dry the hair in preparation for plaiting. Apply a small amount of dressing cream or oils to moisturise the scalp if required.

STEP 2 – Section and separate the hair into manageably sized sections.

STEP 3 – Start plaiting the hair in cornrows away from the front hairline, leaving out some of the hair around the front to soften the hairline.

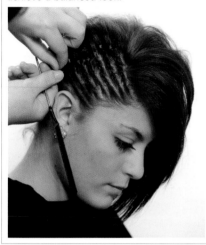

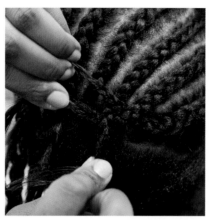

STEP 4 – Plait the ends of the cornrow tails across the back of the hair so the plaits are neat and as flat as possible.

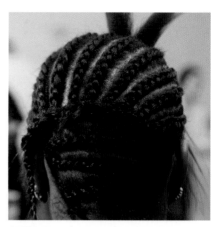

STEP 5 – The completed cornrows. Prepared for hair addition service – see chapter CH7.

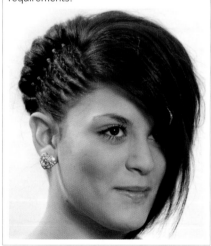

French plait

To complete a French plait, start with a 'V' section. The point of the 'V' is at the front hairline and extending back towards the crown. Divide this 'V' section into three and cross the right stem over the middle stem and then the left stem over the new middle stem.

Add a new section of hair to the right stem, take this new, enlarged right stem over the current middle stem, and add hair to the left stem, taking that enlarged left stem over the current middle stem. Continue this pattern for the whole head of hair.

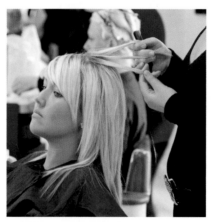

STEP 1 – Section the hair at the middle of the front hairline into three stems ready to start the French plait.

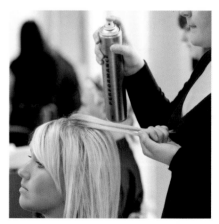

STEP 2 – Apply hairspray to aid control of the hair.

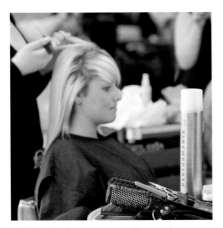

STEP 3 – Have your trolley and equipment to hand.

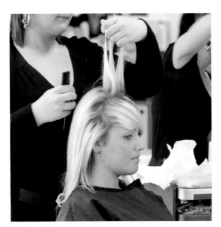

STEP 4 – As you section the hair, ensure your client's head is upright, otherwise the plait may be too loose.

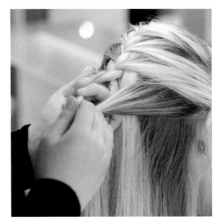

STEP 5 – Add hair to the right stem, then cross the right stem over the middle stem.

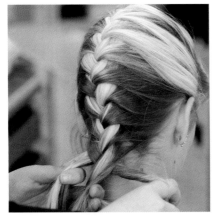

STEP 6 – Continue this process, adding hair to the left stem and crossing it over the middle.

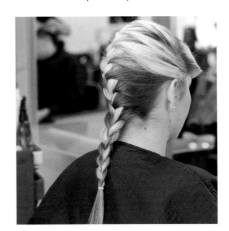

STEP 7 – Secure the completed plait with a professional band.

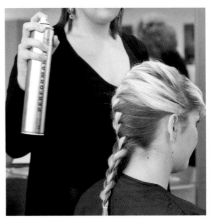

STEP 8 – Apply hairspray to the completed French plait to aid longevity.

HANDY HINT

To add extra interest, try plaiting the top in a side three-strand plait and secure it to the fishtail plait.

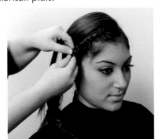

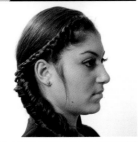

Fishtail plait

STEP 1 – Secure a ponytail with a hairband.

STEP 2 – Divide and section the hair into two equally sized stems.

STEP 3 – Take a small section from the outer edge of stem one and pass it across and over to the inner edge of stem two.

STEP 4 – Now take a small section from the outer edge of stem two and pass it across and over to the inner edge of stem one.

STEP 5 – Continue taking sections from each stem and crossing them over to the opposite side.

STEP 6 – Continue this technique to the ends and secure the hair with a professional band.

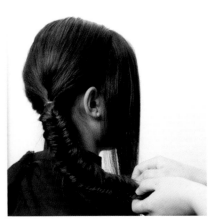

STEP 7 – The finished look.

Two-strand twists

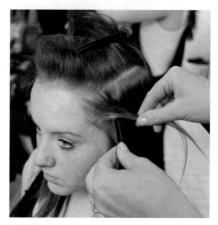

STEP 1 – Section the hair into two equally sized stems.

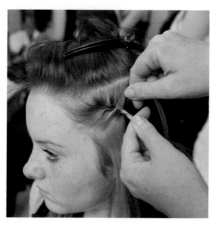

STEP 2 – Twist each stem individually, place the left twisted stem over your right hand, and twist the hair.

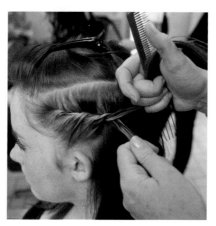

STEP 3 – Take another section from the left and add this to the section in your left hand and twist, then place this over the existing twisted section in your right hand, and twist.

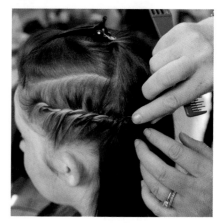

STEP 4 – Continue adding hair from the left side and twisting and swapping over the sections with the right hand until all the hair is twisted. Secure the hair with a professional band.

Flat twists

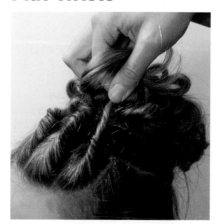

STEP 1 – Take a section of hair and twist it at the root area. Continue this process with more sections.

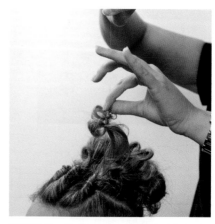

STEP 2 – Secure the untwisted hair at the end with grips and pins into the style.

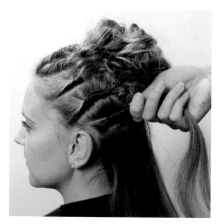

STEP 3 – Continue twisting the sections of hair and secure with a band or grip.

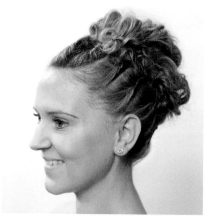

STEP 4 – Check the end result for balance and ensure that your client is happy with the result.

Activity

Practise these styles on your family and friends and ask them to be honest with you about how comfortable they felt and whether you used too much tension.

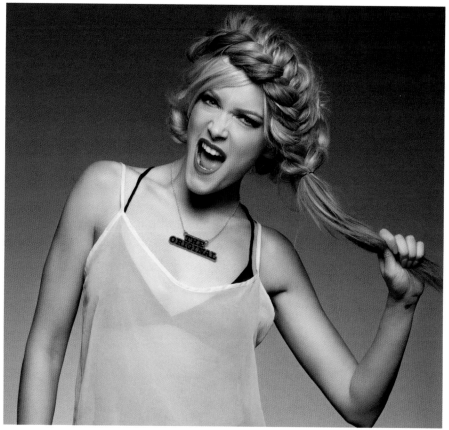

Be creative with colour and plaits

Answers in the back of the book.

1 Which **one** of the following is the best way to protect the client when plaiting and twisting hair?

   a Use a waterproof cape

   b Remove all jewellery

   c Use gown and towel

   d Stand correctly

2 **Statement one**

Reducing energy by switching off electrical items after use will help to save the environment.

Statement two

Salons must use organic and allergy-free products to avoid legal action.

Which **one** of the following is correct for the above statements?

   a True   True

   b True   False

   c False   True

   d False   False

3 Which **one** of the following is the expected service time for fishtail and French plaiting?

   a 50 minutes

   b 40 minutes

   c 30 minutes

   d 20 minutes

4 A client's scalp is showing and the plaits look too thin. Which **one** of the following hair characteristics should have been considered?

   a Texture

   b Density

   c Porosity

   d Elasticity

5 Which **one** of the following is the best advice to give a client who has a widow's peak and wants cornrows?

   a Have a twist in the nape area

   b Have a French plait at the sides

   c Have a small fringe which is left unplaited

   d Have a small amount of added hair at the temples

6 Which **one** of the following is a risk involved with plaiting wiry hair?

   a Client complaints

   b Hair breakage

   c Porous hair

   d Headaches

7 **Statement one**

The temporary hydrogen bonds in the cortex are softened by heat and hardened by water.

Statement two

Hair in its stretched state is called alpha keratin.

Which **one** of the following is correct for the above statements?

   a True   True

   b True   False

   c False   True

   d False   False

8 **Statement one**

Traction alopecia can be identified by hair loss and thinning around the hairline and a sensitive scalp.

Statement two

Traction alopecia can be avoided by using a scalp treatment.

Which **one** of the following is correct for the above statements?

   a True   True

   b True   False

   c False   True

   d False   False

9 Which **one** of the following is the best method of controlling the hair when plaiting?

a Ask the client to hold sections not being worked on

b Use oil-based products and apply heat

c Work methodically and apply tension

d Hold hair close to the scalp

10 What is the best aftercare advice to give to a client following a plaiting service?

a To avoid a sticky result, hairspray should not be used

b To avoid the style loosening, avoid friction

c Remove the plaits at the end of the day

d Untwist the hair from root to point

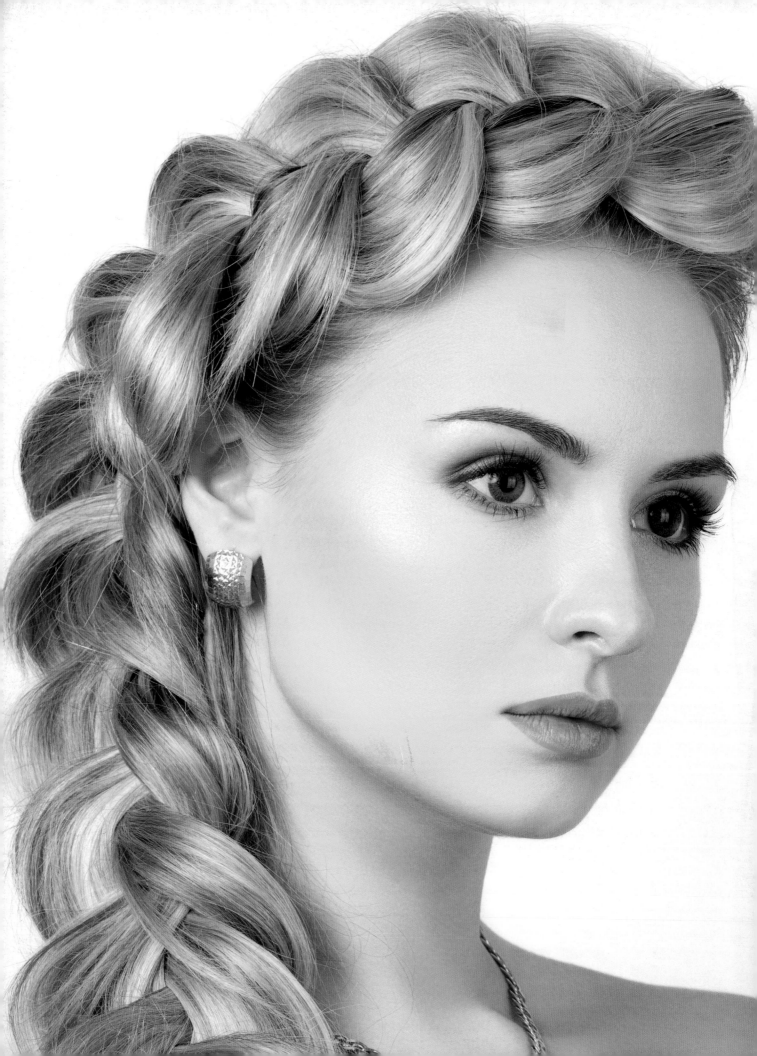

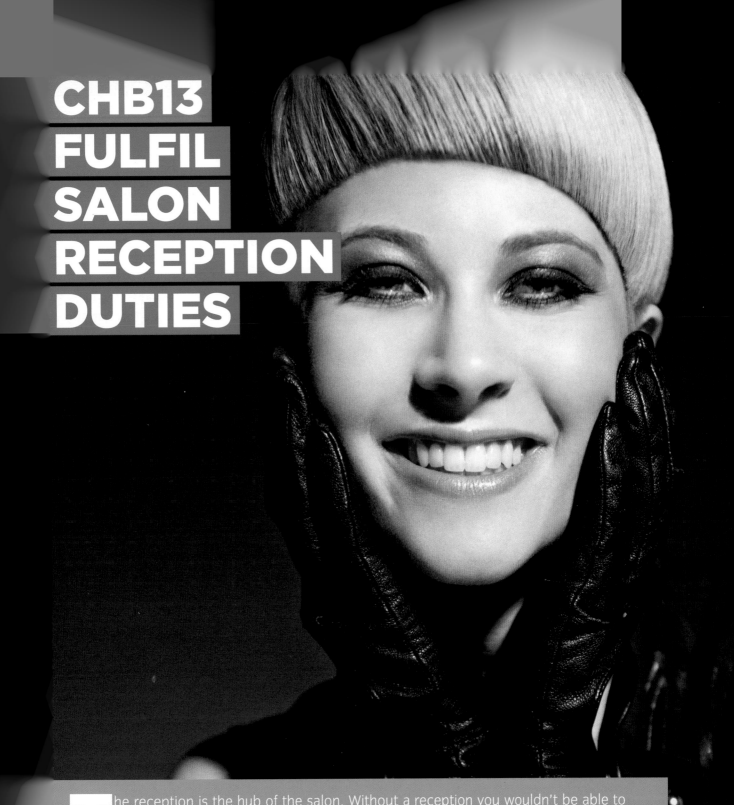

CHB13 FULFIL SALON RECEPTION DUTIES

The reception is the hub of the salon. Without a reception you wouldn't be able to meet and greet your clients, book their appointments or receive payments for your services. It is the first area that your clients see, so first impressions of the salon start here. Clients may drop in for advice on their hair or to buy products, so it is important that the reception area always looks great. The receptionist's role is an important one, and it is essential that the receptionist is effective and efficient when working.

After reading this chapter you will:

■ understand salon and legal requirements for carrying out salon reception duties

■ know the operations of the salon

■ be able to fulfil salon reception duties.

Salon and legal requirements

Salon procedures

Each salon will have its own salon procedures for maintaining the reception area and maintaining client care. This is likely to include keeping the reception area neat and tidy and maintaining stationery levels, retail stock levels and the security of the salon.

Client care and maintaining the reception area

The reception is the 'front of house' and the first area of the salon that your clients see when they pass the salon or walk through the door. Salon reception areas must always look neat and tidy and be well maintained.

At the start of each day, the receptionist must deal with any answerphone messages that have been left overnight and ensure that the reception area is prepared for the day ahead.

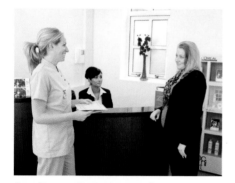
Greeting a client at reception

The daily activities of a receptionist might include:

- maintaining a clean, tidy and well-stocked reception area
- meeting and greeting clients
- maintaining the salon's hospitality and offering refreshments to clients
- dealing with enquiries and bookings
- checking that clients have had any relevant hair and skin tests
- solving problems at reception, such as services running late or clients arriving late
- providing information about salon services and retail products
- answering the telephone
- checking emails and any other electronic methods of communication
- organising the salon's post and distributing it to the relevant people
- taking messages and passing them on to the relevant people
- maintaining communication between clients and stylists
- handling payments and promoting the sale of retail products
- preparing client record cards
- maintaining confidentiality of clients' records
- maintaining salon security at the reception area.

HANDY HINT

When writing messages always write clearly and accurately. When responding to emails, ensure that you use correct English and not 'text speech'. Keep the message professional and check your spellings, punctuation and grammar before you send the message.

Activity

Sort the following 'record cards' into alphabetical order by surname:

Mrs Howards

Mr Jackson

Mr Singh

Mrs Havard

Miss Mackintosh

Mr Harrod

Miss Homeworth

Mrs Harvey

Mr Goshi

Mrs Ohi

Mr Henderson

Miss Hramczuk

Mr O'Shaugnessy

Miss McGrady

VALUES & BEHAVIOURS

When you are working on reception it is very important that you are meeting accepted industry and organisational standards of appearance and hygiene. You must have a willingness to learn, a flexible working attitude and be a team player. Your customer care skills are very important; you need a positive attitude and should have excellent communication skills. Refer to the opening 'Values' section of the values and behaviours chapter to refresh yourself on key areas.

Keep the reception area clean and tidy

As a receptionist you must ensure that the salon is always well presented and portrays a professional image. You must always make sure that the seating area is clean, tidy and welcoming. Neaten any magazines and clear away any used refreshment crockery. You must ensure that the reception area surfaces and floor are free from dust and hair.

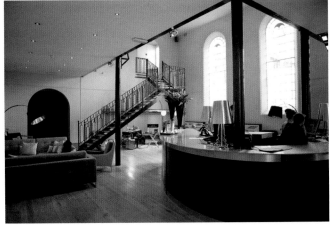

Smart reception

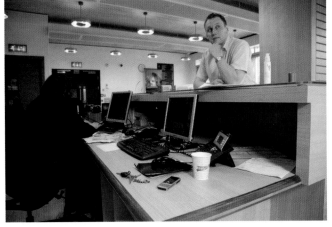

Untidy reception

Maintain retail stock displays

The salon retail stand should look impressive! You must manage your stock levels and display the products in an eye-catching manner, ensuring that product displays have the right level of stock at all times. The retail companies spend thousands of pounds researching what attracts clients to their products, so if the products are displayed effectively, more clients are likely to make purchases. Always make sure you have dusted the shelves and the products. Always check the quality of the goods displayed, ensure that they are not leaking or damaged, that there is no loose packaging and that the goods are in date.

Clearly display the prices so that clients don't have to ask about costs, which they may feel uncomfortable about. If you have any special offers on the salon retail stock, clearly display the information close to the retail stands.

Part of your job role as a receptionist will be to maintain the stock levels and report to the relevant person when stock orders need to be made. Always keep a stock **inventory** of your retail stand.

Inventory

A list of the goods you have in stock.

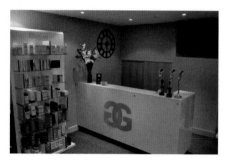

Well-presented retail stand and tidy reception area

HANDY HINT

Your salon is likely to use an electronic till to calculate any retail purchases, but keep a calculator to hand just in case you are asked to work out any retail discounts for your client.

HANDY HINT

Always ensure that you deal with enquiries within the limits of your own authority and refer other enquiries to the relevant person.

Activity

Try to work out the following discounts in your head and then check your results with a calculator.

Your client Mr. Sheriff buys American Crew Fibre at £12.50 and Lock, Stock and Barrel Matte Putty at £11.95. How much will he pay in total:

- at full price?
- with a 10% discount?
- with a 15% discount?
- with a 20% discount?

Maintain the salon's security

Each salon will have a different policy for maintaining the security of the premises, the stock and the safety of staff and clients. Some salons may have a shutter that covers the salon doors and windows when it is closed for the day; others may have a 'buzz' entry or video entry system, which allows entry to authorised clients and salon visitors only. Most salons will have a front door which allows access and entry to all; this is often best kept closed for everybody's personal safety. To prevent breaches in security you must follow your salon's policy for the reception area. This could include:

- storing minimal cash in the till
- keeping the till drawer locked at all times and the key removed when the receptionist leaves the reception area
- rarely leaving the reception area unattended
- keeping staff personal belongings in a locker or secured in the staff-only areas
- ensuring clients keep their personal belongings with them at all times
- displaying retail stands either behind the reception desk, away from the entrance door or in a lockable glass display cabinet.

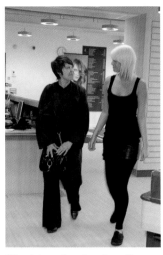

Client keeping her handbag with her

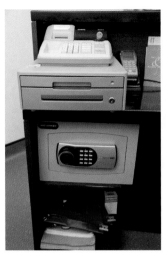

Lockable cabinet

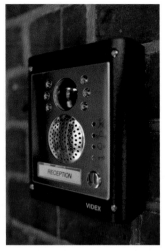

Buzz entry system on salon entrance

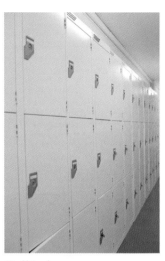

Staff lockers

Activity

If a salon had one retail product stolen from its retail stand every week that was priced on average at £11.95 retail, how much money would have been lost to the salon over a year (52 weeks)?

If this product actually cost the salon £7.45 + 20% VAT to purchase, how much money would the salon have lost?

Maintain stationery stock levels

As the receptionist you are responsible for ensuring that the stationery levels are maintained. This will help the salon to run smoothly and effectively.

You should:

- maintain the appointment systems
- ensure a notepad or message pad is to hand for taking messages
- maintain an appropriate level of appointment cards and price lists, and notify the salon manager when these are running low
- know your salon price structures and display the salon price list for services and retail products
- check stationery supplies, such as pens, pencils, erasers, etc
- keep records of the stylist job sheets – this is particularly important if the salon does not have an electronic computer system and the stylists are on a **commission basis** for the sale of services and products.

HANDY HINT

You must follow your salon's procedures if you suspect fraud and ensure you obtain authorisation for non-cash payments when these are over the salon's limit.

Commission basis

Where stylists receive a percentage of the sale value that they create.

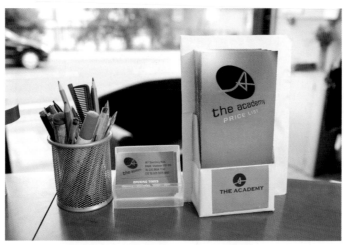

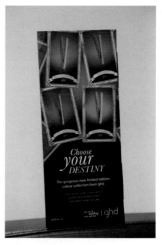

Well-maintained reception desk

Adverts for retail equipment

Your responsibilities

It is important to the salon's business that all staff communicate effectively and know when and how to ask questions. Asking questions is not a sign of weakness or inadequacy, unless you ask the same questions day in and day out. If you come across a new situation and you are not sure how it should be dealt with, then you must seek help from your supervisor.

When working at the reception area it is vital that you work within your own limits of authority and report to your supervisors any problems that you cannot solve.

Make sure you know and follow your limits of authority:

- for what stationery and how much of it should be kept at your reception area
- for how many retail products should be displayed and re-ordered
- when attending to people and enquiries – this may include what discounts and promotions are available
- when making appointments – particularly ensuring that staff are available to cover the clients and that you have allowed for lunch breaks and considered working rotas, etc
- if carrying out skin tests or hair tests – make sure you have had the relevant training before carrying them out and always follow the MFIs
- if you are dealing with payment discrepancies or taking payments
- if a client makes a complaint.

Activity

Find out who you would refer reception problems to in your salon. Who would you refer problems to when this person is on holiday or has a day off?

Taking messages

If the relevant person is not available to deal with a telephone call themselves, it is your responsibility to take a message and clearly record the details of the conversation. When that person is free, make sure you pass on the message promptly, to ensure that the salon runs smoothly.

When taking a message for someone, always record:

- who the message is for
- the date and time the message was left
- a brief but accurate description of the message
- who the message is from
- the contact details of caller/visitor
- the action to be taken, such as to return their call, the best time to call and preferred number
- whether the message is urgent or a general enquiry.

Attending to clients and enquiries

You will need to attend to clients and deal with enquiries, both via the telephone and face to face. In some salons you will also deal with electronic enquiries, which may be via text message or email. Whichever way your enquiries arrive, you must always respond to clients promptly and politely.

The reception area can be very busy at times and you will have to balance people's needs. Clients visiting the salon in person can see how busy you are, but people telephoning the salon cannot, so try not to let the telephone ring more than three times before you answer it.

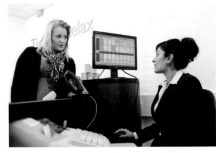

Client being booked in at reception

You'll need to identify who needs your attention first and avoid upsetting those who are still waiting to be seen. When you're rushed off your feet, apologise to clients for keeping them waiting, suggest they take a seat, offer them refreshments, keep them informed about the situation and reassure them that you will not keep them waiting for longer than necessary. If you are really busy, ask for help from the salon team.

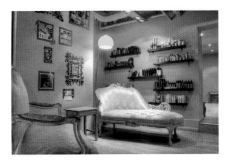

Professional waiting area

You should always greet your clients promptly and warmly. Offer to hang up their coats, show them to the seating area and offer refreshments and magazines to read. Some salons offer TVs, electronic tablets or computer games to entertain clients while they are waiting for their service and during development times. Once you have informed the stylist that their client has arrived, keep the client informed as to how long they may have to wait. You must maintain a friendly yet professional approach at all times.

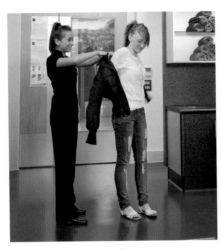

Helping a client with her coat

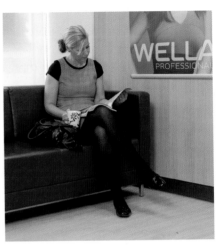

Client sitting comfortably

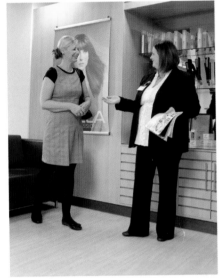

Receptionist taking a client to the stylist

Client arrivals

As clients arrive, always confirm their appointment details to ensure the booking is correct, then promptly inform the relevant stylist of their client's arrival.

Checking that the appointment has been correctly booked in enables you to know in advance if there are likely to be any future problems, such as delays in the service or double bookings, and enables you to adapt to any service changes that the client may request.

Effective salon communication starts with the receptionist who should help to make sure that the salon image is enhanced and business is improved. This will ensure the smooth running of the salon and that the stylists work efficiently.

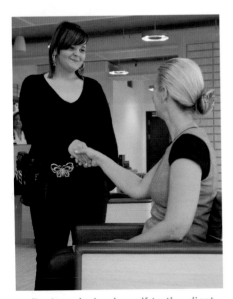

Stylist introducing herself to the client

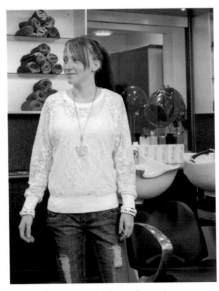

Lost client, wondering where to go

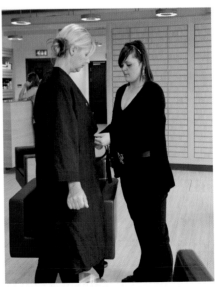

Client being gowned for service by stylist

Salon enquiries

For all salon enquiries it is important that you clearly identify the purpose of the enquiry. As a receptionist, you may deal with the following types of enquiry, either on the telephone, face to face or electronically:

- appointment enquiries
- salon opening and closing times
- costs for services and products
- product representatives selling or promoting their stock
- wholesale deliveries.

It is important that you can answer and deal with these enquiries professionally and **adeptly**, and give accurate information to any visitor of the salon.

Adeptly

Expertly and effectively.

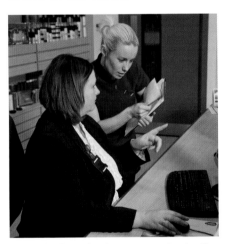

Receptionist referring an enquiry to the manager

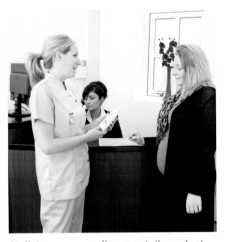

Stylist recommending a retail product

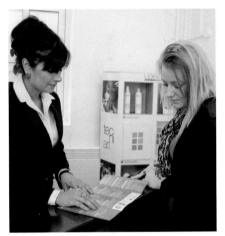

Receptionist showing a client the price list

Speaking clearly and suitably for the situation

As a stylist, and indeed as a receptionist, you will meet a variety of people with different needs and expectations and you will need to speak clearly in a way that suits each situation. You might encounter:

- an unexpected client who has, or at least thinks they have, booked an appointment
- double-booked appointments
- children who need to be treated suitably and may need reassuring
- a client who wishes to change their appointment service
- a client who is unsure of what service to book and when to book it
- a confused client
- an angry client
- a client who wants to complain
- a client with mobility needs.

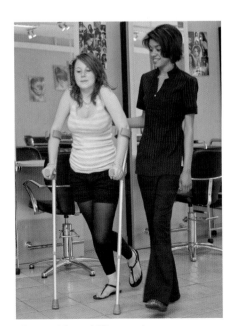

Client with mobility needs

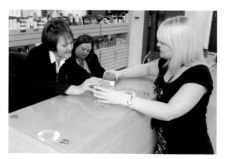

Confused client

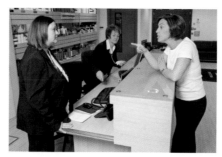

Angry client

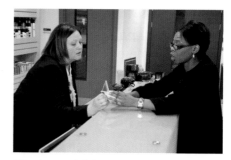

Client complaining

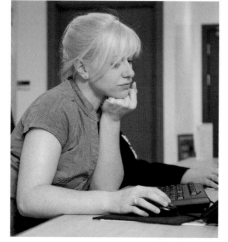

Receptionist with poor posture appearing to show lack of interest

Listening and adapting what to say

When communicating with clients, you must do so politely at all times. Always speak clearly and pronounce your words distinctly. If your client is confused or English is not their first language, you should avoid technical jargon and adapt your language style to suit their needs and the situation. Always show your client that you are listening carefully by maintaining eye contact and nodding, even if your client does not pause for breath, and use positive body language and suitable verbal responses. If you need to encourage a client to move a conversation forward, keep to the subject matter and the purpose of the discussion and summarise any agreed points.

Activity

What would you do and say if a client enquired about the whereabouts of a stylist who had recently left your salon? Discuss.

Adapting your body language

It may also be that you need to adapt your body language as appropriate for different clients and conversations.

VALUES & BEHAVIOURS

When you are communicating with the salon's clients it is very important that you meet the salon's standards of behaviour, and greet the clients respectfully and in a friendly manner. You need to make sure the client feels valued and that you meet their expectations. You'll need to select the most appropriate way to communicate with the client and check they have fully understood what has been agreed. You'll need to be able to recognise the information that a client may find confusing or complicated and check their understanding. Refer to the 'Behaviours' section of the of the values and behaviours chapter for more information.

Activity

In the values and behaviours chapter we explored body language in depth. If you need more information or help with the activity that follows, see the 'Non-verbal communication' section of this chapter.

From the list below, place each point into a category – either 'positive body language' or 'negative body language'.

- Eye contact
- Open body language
- Scratching behind the ear
- Crossed arms
- Smiling
- Open palms
- Rubbing the back of the neck
- Talking behind a hand
- Keeping a little distance
- Poor posture.

Information required to make an appointment

To be able to book your client in for their appointment, you will need to know what services they would like and whether or not additional services are required, such as a cut and finish, after a colour service. If you are booking a client in for a colour service, you'll need to confirm they have had a skin test and check their age, ensuring that they are over 16 years of age. You'll need to know when the client wishes to attend – the date and time and who their preferred stylist is.

Confirming and making appointments correctly

If appointments are booked incorrectly then the salon cannot run smoothly, clients may turn up at the wrong times or dates or stylists may not be available, so it is important that appointment details are checked and confirmed.

Once you have booked an appointment, always repeat back to the client what you have booked, for example, 'Okay Janet, I have booked you in for a half head of woven highlights and a cut and finish with Puru on Tuesday 16 December at 1.30pm. Your skin test has been carried out today. If you have any problems, please contact us and Puru will discuss this with you.' Some salons may request that you inform the client of the duration of the services and the costs too.

A typical conversation between a receptionist and a client (Sarah) may be similar to this:

Receptionist: Hi Sarah, how are you? How can I help you?

Sarah: I'm fine, thank you, Natasha. I'd like to book an appointment for a colour and cut please.

Receptionist: Which stylist do you normally see for your cut and colour?

Sarah: Amraf does my cut and Tina usually does my colour.

Receptionist: When would you like to come in for your appointment?

Sarah: Any chance you can fit me in on Saturday?

Receptionist: Amraf is free and can cut your hair at 2pm, but Tina is on holiday. Would you mind if Julia coloured your hair?

Sarah: No, that's fine, thank you.

Receptionist: Great. Are you having your usual colour or do you fancy a change?

Sarah: No, thank you. I would like my usual highlights, but just the top section this time please.

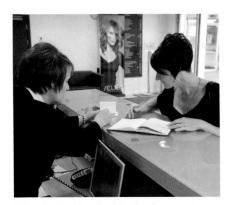

Client being booked in for her next appointment

Receptionist: Okay Sarah. Is 12.15 a suitable time for your colour?

Sarah: Yes, perfect, thank you.

Receptionist: Just to confirm then, Sarah, I have booked you in with Julia at 12.15 for your half head of highlights and then Amraf will cut your hair at 2pm. Is that okay?

Sarah: Perfect, thank you. See you Saturday. Bye.

Receptionist: Goodbye – have a lovely day!

Appointment systems

Common systems available for making appointments include manual appointment systems, where clients are booked in using a pencil and a diary page, or electronic systems, where salon staff can book clients in electronically onto the computerised diary page. Some electronic reception application systems even allow the clients to view the booking system online and they can book their own appointments too.

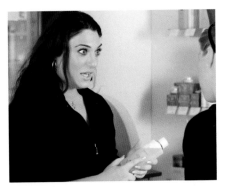

Selling inferior quality products can be illegal

Your legal responsibilities and client confidentiality

When working at reception you are responsible for following the Acts relevant to selling retail products and services, ensuring that you abide by the salon rules and regulations for confidentiality, as well as following the Data Protection Act. You must also check that your client has had any relevant hair and skin tests to ensure that services can go ahead as planned once the client arrives.

The Supply of Goods and Services Act 1982

The Supply of Goods and Services Act 1982 is an Act that requires traders to provide services to a proper standard of workmanship. Furthermore, if a definite completion date or a price has not been fixed then the work must be completed within a reasonable time and for a reasonable charge.

In addition, any material used or goods supplied in providing the service must be of satisfactory quality. The law treats failure to meet these obligations as a breach of contract and consumers would be entitled to seek compensation, if necessary through the civil courts.

Data Protection Act 1998 and confidentiality

As the receptionist, you will need to take client contact details when making appointments or recording messages. Make sure that the contact details are accurately written down and read back the telephone number to the client to double check. Never leave client contact details lying around for unauthorised people to see. Always keep these details confidential and secure.

Part of your role could mean that you access client service records and prepare record cards for the stylists. Salon staff must comply with the Data Protection Act, and if staff or client information is kept on a computer, your salon manager must register the salon with the Data Protection Registrar.

The other rules of the Data Protection Act state that all records must:

- be kept up to date
- hold accurate information
- be kept in a secure location
- be used only for professional purposes which relate to salon services
- not be shared with unauthorised personnel or a third party
- be kept only for as long as the client remains a client
- be disposed of securely, such as by shredding
- be available for clients to see if they wish.

Operations of the salon

It is important you give the right amount of attention to individual clients and balance your time fairly between everyone, especially during busy periods. If you are very busy at the reception area, you should ask if anyone from the salon could assist you, to ensure that the salon runs smoothly.

Services

Salon services, their costs and duration will vary immensely between salons. Some small local salons may charge very little to the weekly clients for a blow dry or set compared with a city salon offering a blow dry for an elegant night out, or a blow-dry bar. A hairstyling service for an elegant night out may be charged at a much higher price, but the quality of service and time spent in the salon may be considerably more too.

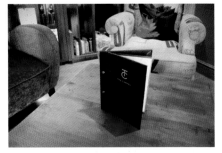

Salon services 'menu'

Activity

Use the internet to search for the nearest blow-dry bar in a local residential area. Compare this with the number of blow-dry bars available in a big city.

Below is a list of services that an average salon may offer, a guide to the cost of the service and its duration.

Salon service, price and duration guide

Salon service	Salon appointment abbreviation	Price guide (depending on salon and stylist experience)	Duration of service
Ladies' cut and finish	CBD	£25–55	From 45 minutes
Ladies' restyle	RESTYLE	£30–65	From 60 minutes
Ladies' wet cut	W/C	£17–45	From 30 minutes
Blow dry	BD	£17–35	From 30 minutes
Hair-up	HAIR-UP or H/up	£19–40	From 30 minutes
Straighten	IRONS	£12–20	From 15 minutes
Shampoo and set	SS	£7.50–20	From 60 minutes
Wrap set	WRAP	£12–25	From 90 minutes
Men's cut and finish	M-CBD	£17–35	From 30 minutes
Men's restyle	M-RES	£20–45	From 30 minutes
Men's wet cut	M-WC	£13–30	From 15 minutes
Beard trim	BEARD	£3–25	From 15 minutes
Wet shave	SHAVE	£15–55	From 30 minutes
Full set of highlights	WHL	£65–95	Up to 2.5 hours including development
½ head of highlights	½ WHL	£40–70	Up to 2 hours including development
Part head of highlights	PART or PHL	£30–45	Up to 1.5 hours including development
Roots and packets (H/L)	ROOTS&PKTS or ROOTS&HL	£65–80	Up to 2.5 hours including development
Full head colour	FHC	£40–60	Up to 2 hours including development
Root colour	ROOTS	£30–50	Up to 1.5 hours including development
Men's shoe shine	S-SHINE	£15–30	Up to 1 hour including development

Men's shoe shine

A colour technique where colour is applied to a foil strip and then applied to the top of the hair as if shining shoes. The colour coats the top layer only and is often cut out with the next haircutting service.

Salon service	Salon appointment abbreviation	Price guide (depending on salon and stylist experience)	Duration of service
Semi/quasi	SEMI or QUAS	£15–30	From 45 minutes including development
Gloss colour	GLOSS	£10–15	Up to 45 minutes including development
Creative colour – ladies	C/COL	On quotation	Can be many hours
Creative colour – men's	M-C/M-COL	£25+	Can be many hours
Colour correction	COL CORR	On quotation	Can be many hours
Hair extensions	H-EX	On quotation	Can be many hours
Protein blow dry	P-BD	From £65	Up to 1.5 hours including development
Wedding hair	WEDD	On quotation	Varies depending on service
Perm services (or permanent wave service)	PW or PERM	On quotation	From 1.5 hours including development
Chemical rearranger	REARRANGE	On quotation	Up to an hour, then add perm service time
Relaxing services	RELAX	On quotation	From 1.5 hours including development

Activity

Compare these services and their prices and duration to those of your salon.

Activity

How does your salon abbreviate the following?

1 Half head foil highlights and cut and blow dry
2 Full head of highlights and blow dry
3 Wedding hair
4 Perm and cut and blow dry
5 Cut, shampoo and set
6 Cut, blow dry and straighten
7 Blow dry and tongs
8 Hair up
9 Two-tone full-head colour and blow dry
10 Regrowth tint with woven highlights.

WHY DON'T YOU...
Find out if these abbreviations differ from your salon's system.

Varied pricing structure

The majority of salons have a pricing structure that varies between stylists depending on their experience. It would not be unusual to see a price list that varies by 50% or more between the owner or a director/artistic designer and a newly qualified stylist.

There may be occasions when you have to calculate a varied bill. For example, a colour service by a stylist and a cut and blow dry by a director. If you are then adding a retail product to the bill, you can see that it can start to get complicated.

Activity

Using the price list below, which includes VAT, calculate costs for these services:

Service	Stylist – Nolan	Director – Sabina
Cut and blow dry	£29.50	£55.00
Woven highlights	£69.00	£77.00
Regrowth colour	£38.00	£45.00
Blow dry	£19.00	£37.00

- Chris had a set of woven highlights with Nolan and a cut and blow dry with Sabina.
- Elaine had a regrowth colour with Sabina and a blow dry with Nolan.
- Jill had a set of woven highlights, and a cut and blow dry with Sabina.
- Jean had a regrowth colour, and cut and blow dry with Nolan.

Products available

The retail products sold in salons vary greatly. Some salons may stock more than one brand, or have different brands for styling products and shampoo ranges, or different ranges for men and women. Add to that any beauty products or equipment and you can see that many items can be displayed and sold at the reception area.

Activity

Find out from your salon whether you use more than one product range and find out the prices of six products.

WHY DON'T YOU...
Research the cost of your salon's retail products and services and compare them with those of a competitor or a salon on the internet.

Activity

Three of your clients (from the previous maths activity) bought retail products. Using the retail price list below, add the retail costs to their service bills. What is now the total price for the hair services and retail?

Product	Cost
Volumising shampoo	£12.99
Smoothing conditioner	£12.49
Colour Stay shampoo	£12.99
Colour Stay conditioner	£12.49
Funk sticks	£9.49
Funk paste	£8.99
Funk gel	£7.99
Naturally Moved mousse	£11.49
Naturally Moved root lift	£9.99
Naturally Moved hairspray	£10.99
Flat Iron heat protector spray	£9.99
Heat protector Moroccan oil	£13.99

- Elaine purchased Funk paste.
- Jill purchased Colour Stay shampoo and conditioner.
- Jean purchased Naturally Moved root lift enhancer, flat iron heat protector spray and Naturally Moved hairspray.

Book and confirm client appointments

When you make appointments for the salon's clients you need to ensure they are booked carefully, to suit the needs of the business, as well as the client. Your role will involve dealing with client requests and accurately identifying their requirements.

How to accurately identify client requirements

For you to be able to identify what your client's requirements are, you'll need to ask a series of open questions. These types of question often start with 'what', 'when', 'where', 'why', 'who' and 'how', and enable you to obtain full answers from your clients.

Some examples of these types of question are:

- What service would you like?
- Could you describe the style you're looking for?
- What is your usual styling routine?

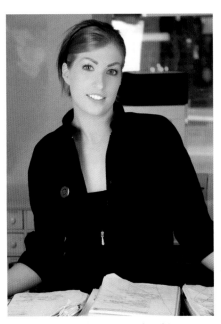

Paper-based appointment booking system

HANDY HINT

Closed questions are good for confirming what has been said and are quick and easy to answer for less articulate people. Open questions provide more in-depth information but can be more difficult to answer, especially for shy or nervous people.

VALUES & BEHAVIOURS

The client will want you to locate the information they need quickly and efficiently. You'll need to provide them with information about salon services and products and explain clearly if for any reason their needs or expectations cannot be meet. Refer to the 'Behaviours' section of the values and behaviours chapter for more information.

HANDY HINT

For clients wanting to book for a colouring service, you must find out when they last had a skin test or colour service. Always check your salon's policy on skin tests.

HANDY HINT

Electronic booking systems vary greatly and you must be trained by your salon manager before using a system. Written appointment systems tend to follow a similar format from salon to salon.

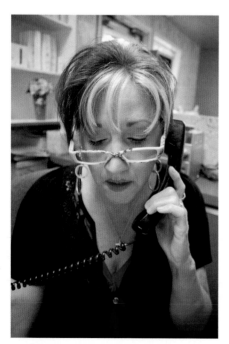

Booking an appointment by phone

- What other times and dates can you make?
- If Suzie is not available on this day, who could look after you?

Activity

Can you think of some more open questions that might be asked at reception?

To clarify the booking of the appointment, you should switch to closed questions, which require 'yes' or 'no' or one-word responses.

Some examples of these types of question could be:

- Is 3pm on Tuesday suitable for you?
- Can you confirm that you would like a cut and finish after your colour service?

Activity

Can you think of some more closed questions that might be asked at reception?

Scheduling the appointments

Once you have confirmed with the client the type of service required, the preferred time and date, and which stylist will service the client's hair, you must record the appointment either in the appointment book or on a computer.

Appointment times

Most salons will have slightly varying appointment times and scheduling procedures. You must always check your salon's policy before booking in any clients. However, most appointment systems have booking spaces for every 15-minute interval, such as 10.00, 10.15, 10.30 and so on.

Many salons will allow about 15 minutes for a consultation for technical services and then the salon assistant will prepare or shampoo the client's hair ready for the service. These times may not be seen in the appointment book. Below is a timing guide for salon bookings (not including development times) for a variety of services.

Service	Time allocated
Wet cut	30 minutes
Cut and blow dry	45 minutes
Blow dry	30 minutes
Regrowth tint	30 minutes
Full head colour	45 minutes

Service	Time allocated
Full head woven highlights	60–90 minutes
Half head highlights	45 minutes
Perm	45 minutes

When booking appointments, not only must you know the abbreviations and the timings, but you must understand how long services take to develop. For example, if you booked Mrs Rossi for a full head of woven highlights followed by a cut and blow dry at 10.00am on Wednesday with Melanie, the appointment might be recorded as follows:

Time	Melanie
10.00	Mrs Rossi
10.15	WHL
10.30	
10.45	
11.00	
11.15	
11.30	Mrs Rossi
11.45	CBD
12.00	
12.15	

From this example, Melanie would be free to take another service at 12.15pm, but what the receptionist has not thought of is the development time of the colour and the colour removal process. As a guide, if we say that Mrs Rossi's woven highlights would take 60 minutes to be developed and removed, Melanie could complete another service (Linda for a long haircut and blow dry and straightening) in this 60-minute gap. The appointment page should look like this:

Time	Melanie
10.00	Mrs Rossi
10.15	WHL
10.30	
10.45	
11.00	
11.15	
11.30	Linda
11.45	L/ hair CBD
12.00	Straighten

Time	Melanie
12.15	
12.30	Mrs Rossi
12.45	CBD
1.00	
1.15	

Melanie would now be free for her next service at 1.15pm, or she may be scheduled for a lunch break.

If, after Melanie's one-hour lunch break, she has Siobhan in for a cut, followed by a long hair perm service and a diffuser dry, the appointment book might now look like this:

Time	Melanie
10.00	Mrs Rossi
10.15	WHL
10.30	
10.45	
11.00	
11.15	
11.30	Linda
11.45	L/ hair CBD
12.00	Straighten
12.15	
12.30	Mrs Rossi
12.45	CBD
1.00	
1.15	
1.30	Melanie
1.45	LUNCH
2.00	
2.15	Siobhan
2.30	C & P/W
2.45	Long hair
3.00	
3.15	
3.30	Aimee
3.45	CBD
4.00	
4.15	Siobhan
4.30	Diff-dry
4.45	

As you can see, this would allow Melanie to complete Aimee's cut and blow dry service while Siobhan's perm was being developed and neutralised, and Melanie would now be available for the next service at 4.45pm. It is extremely important that you book the services accurately, as incorrect timings can mean that:

- services do not run to time
- clients may be irritated by the inconvenience, which may lead to client losses
- the stylist's time is not used effectively, which can lead to a loss of revenue for the salon and the stylist.

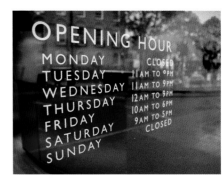

Keep to time in the salon

Activity

Practise booking some appointments. Using the time guides previously, book in the following clients with stylists Luka and Donna.

Luka works 10.00am until 7.00pm and his lunch break is usually 1.30–2.30pm.

His clients for the day are:

- Angela, who would like a half head of highlights and a cut and blow dry at 4.00pm
- Nina, who would like a cut and blow dry at 10.30am
- Chelsea, who would like a regrowth tint and blow dry and straighten in her lunch break, and can be flexible with the times from 12.30–2.30pm
- Kristian, who would like a wet cut in the morning
- Abagebe, who would like a restyle any time after 3.00pm
- Scott, who would like a wet cut after work, from 5.30pm onwards.

Donna works from 8.30am until 5.30pm and her lunch break is around 1pm for an hour.

Her clients for the day are:

- Louise, who would like a cut and blow dry after she has collected the children from school, from 3.30pm onwards
- Gemma, who would like a full head of woven highlights and a cut and blow dry at 11.00am
- Parneet, who would like a cut and blow dry late morning
- Sue, who would like a perm and a trim and blow dry, any time from midday
- Becky, who would like a restyle as early as possible in the morning and must be finished by 11.00am to go to work.

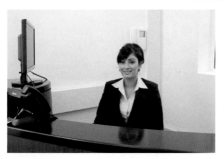
Maintain eye contact when talking to clients

Face-to-face bookings

When you have booked a client appointment, you should ensure that you have entered their name correctly and have taken a contact number. You must then complete an appointment card for the client, clearly stating the date and time. You must always confirm the stylist's name, the service that has been booked and the approximate cost of the service. The appointment card must show the salon name and contact details in case the client needs to change their appointment.

Telephone bookings

For telephone bookings, try to answer the phone promptly, use a pleasant and friendly tone of voice and speak clearly. Smile while you talk on the phone and you will have a happier voice. As you answer, state the salon name, as per your salon policy, and say something along the lines of, 'Good morning/afternoon, Grateful Heads salon, Usman speaking. How may I help you?'

You would book the service in exactly the same way as a face-to-face booking, but as you can't see the client's hair length you may need to ask a few extra questions to ensure you allow sufficient time for the stylist. Some salons send text message reminders to their clients instead of an appointment card, so always ensure their contact details are up to date. You must verbally confirm the booking details with the client prior to completing the call.

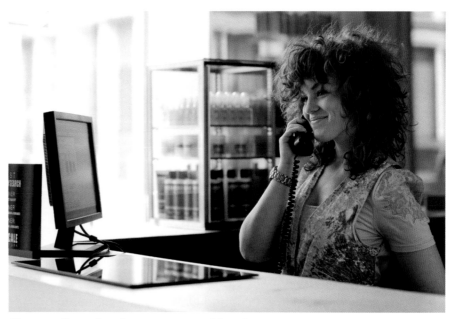
Always smile on the phone – you sound happier

Electronic bookings

Some salons receive booking enquiries via email or text message. You must always send a reply to the client, confirming the details in the same way you would face to face or on the telephone. If the request of the client can't be met, then a further few emails/text messages may be required to offer alternative times and confirm the appointment. You may need to contact them by telephone to clarify any complications.

HANDY HINT

When you send written electronic responses, always ensure your spelling and punctuation are correct and the message reads well, before you press the send button.

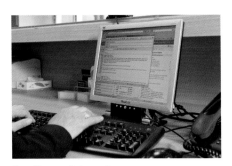

Email appointments

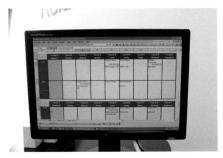

Computer appointment booking system

Identifying discounts and special offers

You should clearly display any special offers and discounts so they are visible to clients in the salon and to people walking past. Check with your salon manager what offers are available, and know which days and stylists they apply to, for example, a new stylist promotion. Some salons advertise discounts and special offers for certain services only. This could be to promote new business or encourage the sale of services that are not as popular as others.

Activity

A walk-in client sees an advert in your window stating 'Buy three products and receive a 25% discount on all three'. If this client buys the following products, what is her bill before and after the discount?

Funk sticks	£6.49
Funk paste	£6.99
Funk gel	£5.99

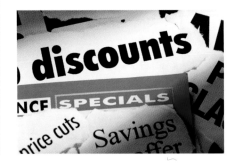

Calculating payments

It is very important that the receptionist is competent at accurately totalling the client's bill at the end of the service. You must be knowledgeable on the pricing structure for the salon services and retail products. Services and retail products are subject to value added tax (VAT) and prices should be displayed inclusive of VAT. If the prices shown exclude VAT, you will need to be able to calculate this with a calculator or electronic till. VAT is charged at 20% in addition to the basic cost. If the government changes the VAT amount, you, as the receptionist, would need to be able to revise the prices to reflect this.

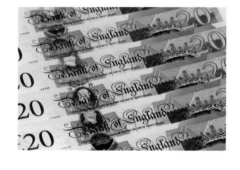

Activity

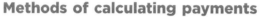

A few years ago the VAT in the UK was calculated at 17.5%. It may change again from 20% in the future. With this in mind, calculate the following bill.

The client's total bill before VAT is £75.00.

1 If VAT returned to 17.5%, what would the total bill be?

2 Calculate the total bill at today's VAT of 20%.

3 If VAT increased to 22%, what would the total bill be?

Methods of calculating payments

Although working through these tasks and calculating the bills with a calculator is good practice, it is likely that your salon will have an automated computer system that works out the cost for you. To calculate a client's bill you could use:

- a calculator
- a pricing scanner
- a till
- an electronic point of sale device
- a pen and paper.

Informing clients of the costs

When you are confirming the total bill to your client, you should do so politely and courteously. Explain the service cost first, then any retail products and then give them the overall cost. This will give your client the opportunity to cancel the retail products if the costs are higher than expected. However, with clearly displayed retail product prices and by previously informing clients of the likely charge for the service, you should be able to avoid any embarrassment or surprises regarding the bill.

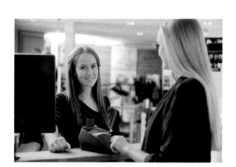
Client buying retail products

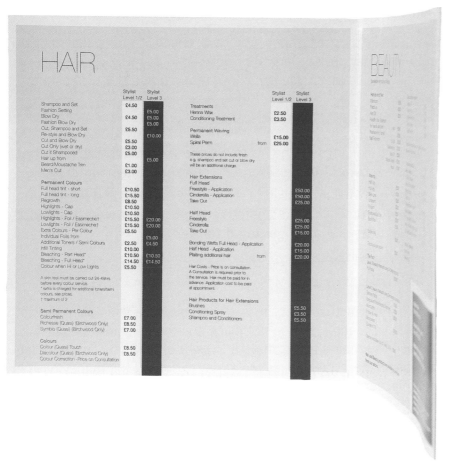

Price list for services

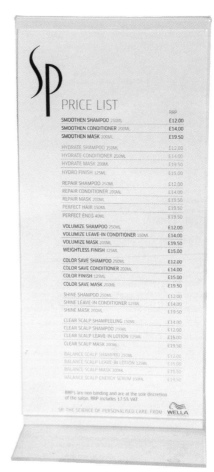

Price list for retail products

Handle payments securely

Maintaining salon security is very important: always keep the till locked and reception manned. If the salon has been very busy, then transferring large amounts of cash to the salon safe may be the securest option, or taking the money to the bank and depositing it.

You must also ensure that client records and/or credit/debit card payment slips are kept securely at the reception area to keep clients' details confidential. If clients pay by card using a chip and PIN machine, you should discreetly look away as they enter their PINs (personal identification numbers).

Types of payment

Once you have calculated the cost of the services and any retail goods to be purchased, you will need to establish your client's preferred method of payment and record the sales correctly, following your salon policy.

HANDY HINT

Never put your own safety at risk (or the safety of others) – do not cash up the till with the doors open or unlocked, or in view of the general public.

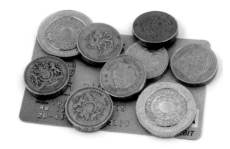

Payment by cash or card?

Payment by cash

If your client chooses to pay with cash, check all notes and coins to verify that they are not forged or defaced in any way. There are several ways in which you can check that the notes and coins are genuine.

- The type of paper – does it feel 'normal'?
- Distinct markings on the notes – is the watermark visible? Is the colour accurate? Is the silver strip present throughout the note?
- Is the note still in circulation? Notes are updated and there is a period of time where old notes can be used, but after this period, these notes are no longer **legal tender**.
- The weight of a coin – is it heavy enough?
- The markings on the coins – are the correct markings present?

If you are happy that the cash is acceptable, take your client's money and count it, but do not place it in the till until your client has received their change: leave it in sight of both you and the client. Cash payment discrepancies are easier to solve if the money has not been placed in the till, and you can confirm exactly how much money the client gave you.

If you think you have been given a forged/counterfeit note, check the note with your salon manager and inform the client. Politely ask them for an alternative method of payment. Always follow your salon's policy and ensure you know what to do if you encounter unacceptable cash or non-legal tender.

Once you have calculated the required change, count this out as you hand it to your client, so that you both agree that accurate change has been given. Ask your client to check the change and then issue a receipt.

WHY DON'T YOU...
Visit http://www.bankofengland.co.uk/banknotes/current for more information about banknotes.

Legal tender
Money that is legal in a given country.

HANDY HINT
Check your salon's policy for accepting £50 notes and confirming that the notes are genuine.

WHY DON'T YOU...
Sadly, in some wallets you'll find a forged coin or note. Check your wallet for forged currency and familiarise yourself with the correct markings.

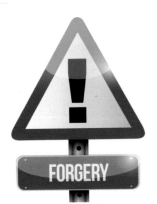

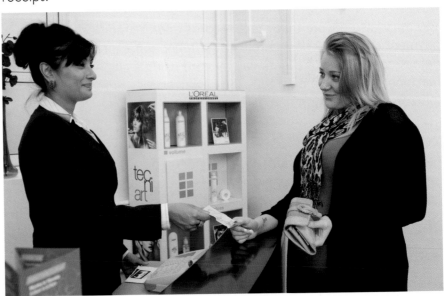

Ensure you give accurate change

THE CITY & GUILDS TEXTBOOK

Payment by cash equivalents

Your client may wish to pay with cash equivalents such as:

- gift vouchers
- discount vouchers
- special offer promotions – 'buy three, pay for two' or 'buy one get one free'
- introductory offers
- loyalty card points
- travellers' cheques.

Cash equivalents are used instead of cash payments but work in the same way. Some salons may give cash or vouchers as change, if the total bill does not match the gift voucher's value, but you must check this against your salon policy. Salons rarely give cash as change when accepting discount offers or loyalty points as payments.

Clients may need to add payment to a voucher to cover the outstanding bill. Be careful to calculate this correctly, making sure that the client is not over- or undercharged, and that the till is balanced at the end of the day.

When taking these types of payment, you must record what the value is, the bill total and check that the voucher is in date and valid. Often, the receptionist signs the vouchers to state they have been used. They should be dated and recorded on the takings sheet, for cashing up purposes and till balancing.

Payment by card

Cards have become very popular and are an easy payment method for clients to use. However, credit cards are costly to the salon and not all salons accept card payments.

If your salon takes card payments and this is your client's chosen payment method, then you need to identify whether your client is using a debit or credit card.

With debit cards the payment is taken immediately from the client's bank account and issued to the salon's bank account when the payment system is processed at the end of the day. Credit card companies request payment from the client on a monthly basis, but pay the salon when the payment system is processed at the end of the day. Therefore banks often charge salons for this service.

Gaining electronic authorisation for payment

Your salon will have a floor/salon limit, which states the amount of money the salon can take in one transaction. To accept payments above this, your salon will require authorisation from the card

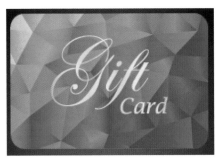

Salon gift card

HANDY HINT

If your salon accepts travellers' cheques, these must be treated differently from all other cash equivalents. Travellers' cheques must be signed in front of you and a passport or photo ID must be produced as identification. Always check that the signature on the identification matches the signature you witness.

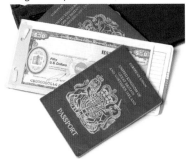

Travellers' cheque with valid ID

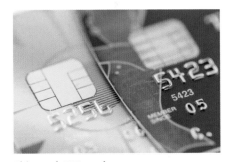

Chip and PIN cards

HANDY HINT

Chip and PIN cards are designed to prevent fraud. Only the cardholder knows the PIN and they are the only person who needs to touch the card, unless there is a query. Remember to look away discreetly when your client enters their PIN.

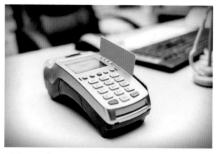
Chip and PIN machine

HANDY HINT

You may need to obtain authorisation from the relevant person when accepting non-cash payments at reception.

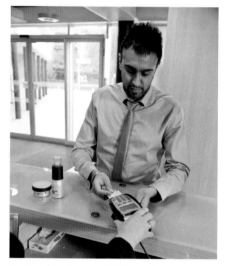
Paying by chip and PIN card

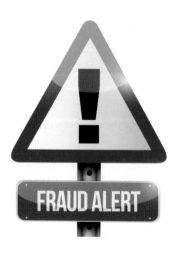
FRAUD ALERT

company. You will need to know what the salon's limits are before you process any credit card payments.

The procedure for paying with a debit or credit card is the same, and you will use a chip and PIN machine called either a 'merchant machine', a 'card reader' or a 'chip and PIN terminal'.

Once you have agreed the cost with the client:

1 Key in the amount and press enter.
2 Hand the merchant terminal to the client to insert their card.
3 Ask the client to check the amount, type in their PIN and press 'enter'.
4 Once the payment has been authorised, ask the client to remove their card.
5 Issue the client with their copy of the receipt and place the salon copy in the till.

Resolving payment discrepancies

As the receptionist, it may be part of your role to identify and resolve payment discrepancies or disputes, and you must ensure that you do so within the limits of your own authority.

Suspected fraud and invalid forms of payment

Suspected fraud does not mean you are accusing your client of fraud: it may simply be that the card is declined by the merchant terminal, the card cannot be authorised or the card company suspects fraudulent spending on the card.

Suspected stolen cheques

If you suspect that a client is providing you with a stolen cheque, ask them for ID to confirm the cheque matches their identification. Alternatively, as cheque payments are not guaranteed, you should ask for an alternative method of payment.

Suspected stolen cards

If you suspect fraud is taking place, excuse yourself from your client, take the card with you and inform your salon manager.

Counterfeit payments

If the merchant terminal informs you that the card is stolen or counterfeit, you must follow the step-by-step instructions on the merchant terminal. This may tell you that you must retain the card, and, in some cases, call the police.

Invalid currency

Invalid currencies could be notes that have expired, those with incorrect markings or even foreign currency. Some salons in the UK accept euros, particularly those in tourist areas. Check your salon policy about receiving payment in euros.

Invalid cards

An invalid card may be unsigned, out of date, look or feel counterfeit, have an unclear hologram, or the cardholder's name may not match the client's name. Alternatively a warning may appear on your card machine when an attempt is made to use it.

Incorrect completion of cheques

Cheques that have been incorrectly completed may have the incorrect amount in figures or words, have an incorrect date or may not be signed by the client.

Payment disputes

Any payment discrepancies or disputes that are outside your authority must be referred to the relevant person. Payment disputes could be disagreements over the total bill, over- or undercharging, insufficient funds, suspect tender or invalid payments.

For all of the above, and if you suspect a client is offering you suspect counterfeit tender, you would need to inform the client tactfully that their payment has been declined or can't be accepted and ask for an alternative payment method. If the client does not have an alternative payment method, then ask your salon manager what you should do.

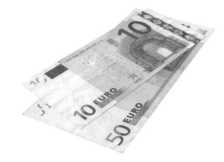

Check your salon policy on accepting euros

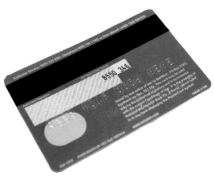

An unsigned card is invalid

HANDY HINT

Always check that payments made are correct and tactfully inform clients if authorisation for payments is not accepted.

HANDY HINT

Always try to solve payment discrepancies or disputes as simply and discreetly as possible to avoid embarrassment to clients and staff, to avoid loss of profit and so that the till balances at the end of the day.

WHY DON'T YOU...
Ask your salon manager how you should deal with the following discrepancies:
- counterfeit payments
- invalid currency
- suspected stolen cheques or cards
- invalid cards
- incorrect completion of cheques
- payment disputes.

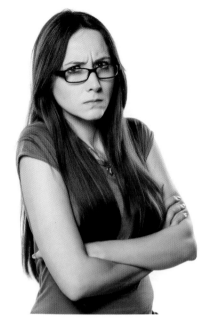

Clients will be unhappy if overcharged

Consequences of failure to handle payments correctly

Failing to handle payments correctly and itemising bills incorrectly can lead to discomfort and embarrassment to you and the client. Clients will be unhappy if they are overcharged and the salon will lose money for any uncharged items.

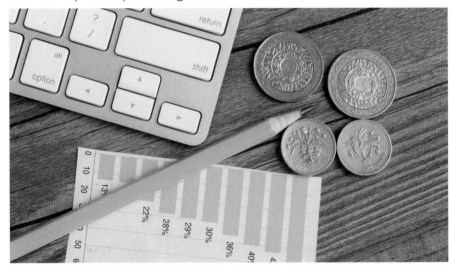

The salon will lose money for uncharged items

Fulfil salon reception duties – review

Maintain reception area

When working at the reception area, you must:

- ensure the reception area is clean and tidy at all times
- maintain the agreed levels of reception stationery
- ensure the product displays have the right level of stock at all times.

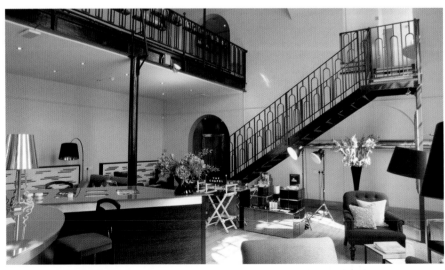

A welcoming reception area

TEST YOUR KNOWLEDGE ANSWERS

Health and safety and salon policies

1 a, 2 b, 3 a, 4 d, 5 a,
6 b, 7 b, 8 c, 9 b, 10 c

Values and behaviours

1 a, 2 d, 3 a, 4 b, 5 b,
6 c, 7 d, 8 a, 9 b, 10 b

CHB12 Develop and maintain your effectiveness at work

1 b, 2 b, 3 a, 4 c, 5 a,
6 b, 7 a, 8 b, 9 d, 10 c

CHB9 Advise and consult with clients

1 b, 2 c, 3 a, 4 d, 5 c,
6 b, 7 c, 8 b, 9 b, 10 d

CHB11 Shampoo, condition and treat the hair and scalp

1 a, 2 d, 3 a, 4 d, 5 b,
6 a, 7 a, 8 b, 9 a, 10 b

CH1 Style and finish hair

1 a, 2 c, 3 b, 4 b, 5 a,
6 a, 7 a, 8 c, 9 a, 10 d

CH2 Set and dress hair

1 a, 2 a, 3 d, 4 c, 5 d,
6 b, 7 a, 8 d, 9 b, 10 c

CH3 Cut hair using basic techniques

1 c, 2 a, 3 b, 4 b, 5 d,
6 c, 7 d, 8 d, 9 c, 10 a

CB2 Cut hair using basic barbering techniques

1 a, 2 c, 3 d, 4 a, 5 c,
6 b, 7 d, 8 d, 9 b, 10 c

CB3 Cut facial hair to shape using basic techniques

1 a, 2 c, 3 c, 4 a, 5 b,
6 c, 7 a, 8 d, 9 d, 10 d

CH4 Colour and lighten hair

1 d, 2 b, 3 d, 4 b, 5 a,
6 c, 7 c, 8 b, 9 a, 10 b

CH5 Perm and neutralise hair

1 b, 2 a, 3 d, 4 a, 5 a,
6 c, 7 a, 8 c, 9 b, 10 b

AH2 Relax hair

1 b,	2 d,	3 d,	4 c,	5 b,
6 d,	7 c,	8 c,	9 a,	10 d

CH7 Plaiting and twisting

1 c,	2 b,	3 c,	4 b,	5 c,
6 b,	7 d,	8 b,	9 c,	10 b

CH6 Temporarily attach hair to enhance a style

1 d,	2 a,	3 d,	4 d,	5 c,
6 b,	7 a,	8 b,	9 b,	10 c

CHB13 Fulfil salon reception duties

1 d,	2 c,	3 b,	4 a,	5 d,
6 c,	7 b,	8 c,	9 b,	10 d